Fundamentals of Anaesthesia and Acute Medicine

Neuroanaesthetic Practice

Dedicated to Gretchen, the continual source of my
energy and inspiration.

Fundamentals of Anaesthesia and Acute Medicine

Neuroanaesthetic Practice

Edited by
H Van Aken
Professor and Chairman, Department of Anesthesiology and Intensive Care Medicine, University Hospitals, Westfälische Wilhelms-Universität Münster, Germany

Series editors
Ronald M Jones, MD, RCA
Professor of Anaesthetics, St Mary's Hospital Medical School, London

Alan Aitkenhead
Professor of Anaesthesia, University of Nottingham

and

Pierre Foëx
Nuffield Professor of Anaesthetics, University of Oxford

BMJ
Publishing
Group

First published in 1995
by the BMJ Publishing Group, BMA House, Tavistock Square,
London WC1H 9JR

British Library Cataloguing in Publication Data
A catalogue record for this book is available
from the British Library

ISBN 0-7279-0909-6

Typeset in Great Britain by
Apek Typesetters Ltd, Nailsea, Avon
Printed and bound in Great Britain by Latimer Trend & Co., Plymouth

Contents

Contributors

AL Baert
Director
Department of Radiology, University Hospitals K.U. Leuven, Belgium

I Bone, FRCP
Department of Neurology, University of Glasgow, Southern General
Hospital, Glasgow, UK

N Mark Dearden
Department of Anaesthesia, Middlemore Hospital, Otahuhu, Auckland,
New Zealand

W Fitch, MB ChB, PhD, FRCA, FRCP(G)
Professor of Anaesthesia
University Department of Anaesthesia, Glasgow Royal Infirmary, UK

Adrian W Gelb, MB ChB, FRCP(C)
Professor and Chairman
Department of Anaesthesia, University Hospital, London, Ontario,
Canada

DI Graham, PhD, FRCPathol
Professor
Department of Neuropathology, University of Glasgow, Southern General
Hospital, Glasgow, UK

A Inglis, MB ChB, FRCA
Research Registrar
University Departments of Neurosurgery and Anaesthesia, Institute of
Neurological Sciences, Southern General Hospital, Glasgow, UK

Eberhard Kochs, MD
Professor of Anesthesiology and Chairman
Institute of Anesthesiology, Technical University of Munich, Germany

J Adam Law, MD, FRCP(C)
Clinical Neuroanaesthesia Fellow
Department of Anaesthesia, University Hospital, London, Ontario,
Canada

JAR Nicoll, MD, MRCPathol
Department of Neuropathology, University of Glasgow, Southern General
Hospital, Glasgow, UK

Glenda J Oldroyd
Department of Anaesthesia, Middlemore Hospital, Otahuhu, Auckland,
New Zealand

C Plets
Director
Department of Neurosurgery, University Hospitals K.U. Leuven, Belgium

P Ravussin, MD
Consultant Anaesthesiologist
Department of Anaesthesiology, University Hospital Centre, Lausanne,
Switzerland

Michael M Todd, MD
Professor of Anesthesiology
University of Iowa, USA

Concezione Tommasino, MD
Assistant Professor of Anesthesiology
University of Milan, Italy

H Van Aken
Professor and Chairman
Department of Anesthesiology and Operative Intensive Care Medicine,
University Hospitals, Westfälischen Wilhelms-Universität Münster,
Germany

Jan Van Hemelrijck, MD, PhD
Associate Professor
Department of Anesthesiology, University Hospitals, Catholic University
of Leuven, Belgium

Marleen Verhaegen, MD
Staff Member
Department of Anesthesiology, University Hospitals, Catholic University
of Leuven, Belgium

David S Warner, MD
Professor
Departments of Anesthesiology, Neurobiology, and Surgery,
Duke University Medical Center, Durham, North Carolina, USA

Christian Werner, MD
Associate Professor of Anesthesiology
Institute of Anesthesiology, Technical University of Munich, Germany

OHG Wilder-Smith, MB ChB, MD
Staff Anaesthesiologist
Department of Anaesthesiology, Geneva University Hospital, Switzerland

G Wilms
Professor of Radiology
Department of Radiology, University Hospitals K.U. Leuven, Belgium

Foreword

The pace of change within the biological sciences continues to increase and nowhere is this more apparent than in the specialties of anaesthesia, acute medicine, and intensive care. Although many practitioners continue to rely on comprehensive but bulky texts for reference, the accelerating rate of biomedical advances makes this source of information increasingly likely to be dated, even if the latest edition is used. The series *Fundamentals of anaesthesia and acute medicine* aims to bring to the reader up to date and authoritative reviews of the principal clinical topics which make up the specialties. Each volume will cover the fundamentals of the topic in a comprehensive manner but will also emphasise recent developments of controversial issues.

International differences in the practice of anaesthesia and intensive care are now much less than in the past, and the editors of each volume have commissioned chapters from acknowledged authorities throughout the world to assemble contributions of the highest possible calibre. Three volumes will appear annually and, as the pace and extent of clinically significant advances varies among the individual topics, new editions will be commissioned to ensure that practitioners will be in a position to keep abreast of the important developments within the specialties.

Not only does the pace of advance in biomedical science serve to justify the appearance of an international series of this nature but the current awareness of the need for more formal continuing education also underlines the timeliness of its appearance. The editors would welcome feedback from readers about the series, which is aimed at both established practitioners and trainees preparing for degrees and diplomas in anaesthesia and intensive care.

RONALD M JONES
ALAN R AITKENHEAD
PIERRE FOËX
July 1995

Preface

The field of anaesthetics has, during the past decade, been significantly enhanced by advances in technology, the manufacture and clinical validation of new equipment, and the development of new drugs. In combination with advances in electrophysiological monitoring, these tools have expanded the research upon which neuroanaesthetics is now built. This enriched foundation has, in turn, resulted in a greater understanding of neurophysiology, neurobiochemistry, neuropharmacology, and neuropathology.

Advances in neuroanaesthetics have also enabled neurosurgeons to expand their own field while anaesthetists can provide more appropriate perioperative management, superior postoperative care, and improved management of acute and chronic pain. Indeed, as our expanding abilities become applicable to a larger and more diversified patient population, neuroanaesthetists are now faced with new challenges in providing assistance to colleagues in radiology, neonatology, critical care, and other specialties.

Subspecialties emerge as a result of an expansion of knowledge. The *Oxford English Dictionary* defines a "specialist" as an "authority who particularly or exclusively studies a single branch of his profession or subject." The authors of the different chapters of this book have certainly devoted their lives to becoming authorities in the subspecialty of neuroanaesthetics.

I would like to thank these colleagues for accepting the onerous task of writing yet "another review" and hope that others who are involved in this area of anaesthesia will find it of value and interest.

Outcome is the most important attribute of any anaesthetic intervention of critical care experience. Brain damage can cause severe emotional and financial consequences—consequences that we can most fully appreciate when the damage affects someone close to us—a colleague, a friend, or, in particular, a member of our own family.

I hope that this book will be an indispensable source of up to date knowledge and practical clinical advice for all anaesthetists who strive to provide neurosurgical patients with the most appropriate care and the best possible outcome.

H VAN AKEN
July 1995

1: Physiology and metabolism of the central nervous system: anaesthetic implications

A INGLIS, W FITCH

Introduction

The central nervous system (CNS) comprises the brain and spinal cord. Its specialisation is based on "excitable cells"—neurons that allow the transmission of impulses by alterations in membrane permeability. Implications for anaesthesia range from the difficulty in assessing patients with gross CNS impairment to the process of free radical generation in ischaemia.

In addition to neurons, which are specialised conducting cells, the CNS contains around 10–50 times as many connective tissue cells or neuroglia. These are of three types:

1 Astrocytes, which have supportive functions including transmitter uptake
2 Oligodendrocytes, which are involved in the formation of myelin sheaths
3 Microglia, which are scavenger cells from the immune system.

There are around 10^{12} neurons in the CNS. Although morphology is very varied the classic model of a spinal motor neuron is useful (fig 1.1): a receptive field of dendrites feeds a cell body and an extended axonal process terminates in branches with synaptic knobs.

Neurons, similar to other cells, contain a higher concentration of potassium ions ($[K^+]$) than the surrounding interstitial fluid (about 150 mmol/l compared with 4·5 mmol/l) and a lower sodium ion concentration ($[Na^+]$) (about 15 mmol/l compared with 140 mmol/l). This imbalance is maintained actively by the membrane pump, Na^+/K^+ ATPase, which extrudes $3Na^+$ from the cell and takes in $2K^+$ for each mole of ATP. It is estimated that this membrane pump uses 33% of all cell energy. In neurons the resting membrane permeability to K^+ is much greater than that to Na^+. Thus K^+ will tend to diffuse out of the cell until a balance is reached between the concentration effect (outward diffusion) and the electrical charge (inward

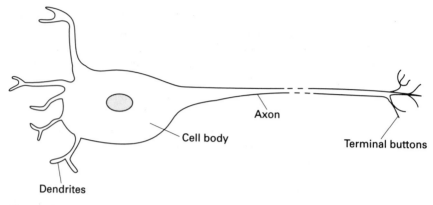

Fig 1.1 Spinal motor neuron: classic model (not to scale)

attraction). This point can be predicted from the Goldman constant field equation;[1] the greater resting permeability to K^+ means this predominates and gives a resting membrane potential of -70 mV (inside negative). When the membrane is exposed to an adequate stimulus, changes in the membrane permeability occur. Initial depolarisation to -55 mV causes an increase in Na^+ permeability and the membrane potential reaches $+35$ mV.

Repolarisation is produced by an increase in K^+ permeability (fig 1.2). This change in membrane charge produces an action potential which self propagates along the axon.

Impulse conduction between neurons is via synapses. Presynaptic and

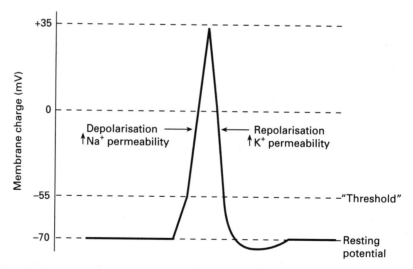

Fig 1.2 Generation of an action potential

postsynaptic cells are separated by a cleft 30–50 nm wide. An action potential, reaching the presynaptic knob from the axon, causes transitory opening of calcium ion channels, which allow calcium ions to enter the synaptic knob; vesicles of neurotransmitter are released into the synapse. Neurotransmitter diffuses across the synaptic cleft and reaches specific receptors on the postsynaptic cell (on dendrites in the classic model). The binding of transmitter to receptor triggers changes in the postsynaptic membrane (for example, opening cation entry channels) which produce postsynaptic potentials that may be summated, temporally or spatially, to reach the depolarisation threshold and generate an action potential. The synapse mechanism allows one way conduction of impulses thereby regulating communication.

It is estimated that each neuron forms an average of 1000 synaptic junctions, giving around 10^{15} synapses in the CNS. Each spinal motor neuron averages 10 000 synapses and in the human forebrain a neuron may receive up to 40 000 synapses.

Synaptic conduction may vary from the simple axon–dendrite excitatory junction. A synapse may be inhibitory, that is, the net result is to make the postsynaptic neuron less likely to fire. Inhibition may be produced directly (postsynaptic) with an inhibitory neuron acting on a postsynaptic neuron. Alternatively, inhibition may be indirect (presynaptic) where the inhibitory neuron synapses onto the synaptic knob of a presynaptic neuron; this reduces the amount of neurotransmitter released and effectively inhibits the postsynaptic neuron.

Neurotransmitters

There are a variety of substances which serve as neurotransmitters; over 40 have been identified including amines, amino acids, purines, and polypeptides. Some neurotransmitters have more than one receptor type and may serve different functions in different areas of the CNS. In some neuronal pathways the neurotransmitters are well characterised. The diversity of neurotransmitters gives potential for both pharmacological and pathological manipulation (for example, anaesthesia or parkinsonism). Additional research may provide further therapeutic options in this area.

Glutamate

Glutamate, an amino acid, is known to be the neurotransmitter in 75% of excitatory brain transmission; it is also the transmitter in spinal cord monosynaptic stretch reflexes. Three types of glutamate receptor have been identified: NMDA (*N*-methyl-D-aspartate), kainate, and quisqualate. The NMDA receptor is a complex cation channel; it is normally blocked by

3

magnesium ions and unblocked by depolarisation. Glycine facilitates NMDA receptor function. Ketamine and phencyclidine bind to a site in this receptor, these drugs causing sensations of dissociation and amnesia. Release of glutamate in ischaemia and its actions at NMDA receptors feature in the "excitotoxic" theory[2] allowing calcium ions to enter into neurons, and ultimately precipitating cell death. Studies continue into the use of NMDA antagonists with potential clinical uses including strokes, head injuries, and perinatal hypoxia. Evidence supports the effectiveness of NMDA antagonists in reducing infarct size in cases of focal ischaemia.[3 4]

The kainate receptor is a cation channel allowing, when open, Na^+ influx and K^+ efflux. Two subtypes of quisqualate receptor have been demonstrated, one of which, the AMPA receptor (α-amino-3-hydroxyl-5-methyl-4-isoxazole-propionic acid), is a cation channel. There are suggestions that AMPA antagonists may be more effective than NMDA antagonists in cases of global ischaemia (for example, cardiac arrest).

γ-Aminobutyrate

γ-Aminobutyrate (GABA) is an amino acid; it is the neurotransmitter that mediates indirect inhibition (presynaptic). GABA produces an increase in membrane permeability to chloride ions, which stabilises the membrane potential, rendering the membrane less liable to depolarisation. GABA is found throughout the CNS and may be present at up to one third of all synapses.

GABA is formed by the decarboxylation of glutamate. The reaction is catalysed by the enzyme glutamate decarboxylase, which requires pyridoxal phosphate as a cofactor—a derivative of pyridoxine, vitamin B_6. Thus vitamin B_6 deficiency is associated with GABA depletion, signs of hyperexcitability, and convulsions.

Benzodiazepine drugs facilitate GABA actions at synapses and have a marked anxiolytic, sedative effect. Barbiturates, phenytoin, and alcohol also act in part by facilitating chloride ion (Cl^-) conductance at the same Cl^- channel. Drugs that increase GABA concentrations in the CNS are used in the management of epilepsy, for example, sodium valproate inhibits the breakdown of GABA. In acute liver failure there is an increase in the number of GABA, glycine, and benzodiazepine receptors which may be important in the development of hepatic encephalopathy.

Glycine

Glycine is an amino acid neurotransmitter which mediates direct inhibition at synapses in the spinal cord. As with GABA, glycine acts by increasing Cl^- conductance and thus stabilising membranes. Glycine also facilitates the action of glutamate at NMDA receptors in the brain. Glycine is antagonised

4

by tetanus toxin and strychnine which produce muscle spasm and convulsions.

Serotonin

Serotonin (5-hydroxytryptamine, 5HT) acts as a neurotransmitter in the hypothalamus, limbic system, cerebellum, brain stem, and spinal cord. Seven types of serotonin receptor have been described. In some animal models serotonin has been shown to mediate indirect (presynaptic) inhibition by prolonging the effect of an action potential. In the forebrain serotonin is involved in regulation of the sleep–wake cycle, temperature control, and aggression. In the spinal cord serotonin is thought to mediate a descending control pathway which modulates sensitivity to pain. Much of the serotonin released at synapses undergoes active reuptake into the neuron and is inactivated by the enzyme monoamine oxidase (MAO). The potential exists to modify the actions of serotonin with MAO inhibitors and tricyclic antidepressant drugs as in psychiatry.

Acetylcholine

Acetylcholine acts via two principal types of receptor. Nicotinic receptors are found in many parts of the CNS; they act by increasing Na^+ conductance. Of the four types of muscarinic acetylcholine receptor, type M1 are widespread in the CNS and act by increasing calcium influx. Acetylcholine is found in spinal cord motor neurons and cranial nerve motor nuclei. It also acts as a modulator in the basal ganglia, hippocampus, and brain stem. Patients with affective disorders have increased cholinergic receptor density whereas this is reduced in patients with Alzheimer's disease. Tricyclic antidepressant drugs block cholinergic receptors and manic symptoms may be treated with physostigmine which, as an anticholinesterase, decreases the breakdown of acetylcholine.

Dopamine

Dopamine acts as a neurotransmitter in the basal ganglia and limbic system. Degeneration of the nigrostriatal dopaminergic pathway (from the pars compacta of the substantia nigra to the putamen of the striatum) leads to the development of parkinsonism. Symptoms can be reduced by altering the relative balance of dopamine and acetylcholine, using dopamine agonists or anticholinergic drugs. In the limbic system dopamine pathways are implicated in the development of schizophrenia. Many antipsychotic drugs have antidopaminergic effects. Dopamine is also involved via the chemoreceptor trigger zone, in nausea and vomiting, and via the hypothalamus, in

5

suppression of prolactin secretion. Antidopaminergic drugs such as meto-clopramide are often used clinically in these disorders.

Noradrenaline and adrenaline

Noradrenaline (norepinephrine) acts as a neurotransmitter in parts of the hypothalamus, brain stem, cortex, cerebellum, and spinal cord. Neurons actively reuptake noradrenaline; this is reduced by tricyclic antidepressant drugs. Adrenaline (epinephrine) functions as a neurotransmitter in the hypothalamus, thalamus, periaqueductal grey matter, and the spinal cord.

Endogenous opioids

Endogenous opioid neurotransmitters are found in the hypothalamus, pituitary, brain stem, and spinal cord and were first identified in 1975. There are several types of receptor (μ, σ, κ, etc) with distribution of the μ receptor matching that of enkephalins which are thought to act as inhibitory transmitters in pain pathways.[5]

Spinal pathways

Sensory pathways

Nerve fibres for painful stimuli enter the spinal cord in the dorsal root (fig 1.3a). Two fibre types are involved: myelinated Aδ fibres and slower conducting unmyelinated C fibres.[6] The dorsal horn of the spinal cord grey matter is divided into nine laminae.[7] Aδ fibres terminate in laminae I and V, and C fibres end in laminae I and II. From here further neurons run in the spinothalamic tract. Substance P is a polypeptide neurotransmitter which is believed to act as the mediator in pain pathways. The gate control theory of pain[8] proposes that large diameter Aα fibres from the dorsal column send collateral branches which inhibit pain transmission (hence "gating"). This is thought to occur in the substantia gelatinosa, laminae II and III of the dorsal horn, with enkephalin acting as the presynaptic inhibitory transmitter. Clinically, this theory may help explain the pain relief produced by transcutaneous (TENS) or dorsal column stimulation. It is thought that postherpetic neuralgia results from loss of Aα collateral fibres and that polyneuropathy results from increases in Aδ fibres.

From the dorsal horn second order neurons mediating pain and tempera-ture cross the midline of the spinal cord anterior to the central canal and run cephalad in the lateral spinothalamic tract (fig 1.3b). Some second order neurons mediating touch sensation cross the midline and run as the anterior spinothalamic tract (fig 1.3a). The functional distinction between the two components of this anterolateral system is not absolute. The tracts are joined

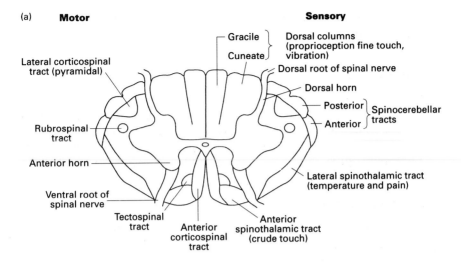

(a) **Motor**   **Sensory**

Gracile ⎤
Cuneate ⎦ Dorsal columns (proprioception fine touch, vibration)

Lateral corticospinal tract (pyramidal)

Dorsal root of spinal nerve

Dorsal horn

Posterior ⎤ Spinocerebellar
Anterior ⎦ tracts

Rubrospinal tract

Anterior horn

Lateral spinothalamic tract (temperature and pain)

Ventral root of spinal nerve

Tectospinal tract

Anterior corticospinal tract

Anterior spinothalamic tract (crude touch)

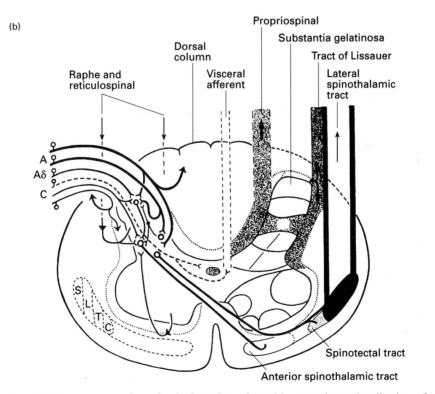

(b)

Propriospinal

Substantia gelatinosa

Dorsal column

Tract of Lissauer

Raphe and reticulospinal

Visceral afferent

Lateral spinothalamic tract

A
Aδ
C

S
L
T
C

Spinotectal tract

Anterior spinothalamic tract

Fig 1.3 Transverse section of spinal cord to show (a) approximate localisation of tracts, and (b) pain pathways

7

by fibres from higher spinal levels and sacral fibres then lie outermost. Spinoreticular fibres run to the reticular formation of the brain stem. In the pons the lateral and anterior spinothalamic tracts join the medial lemniscus and run on to thalamic relay nuclei. Third order fibres run from the thalamus to the postcentral gyrus (sensory cortex). The spinothalamic tract is affected in syringomyelia where enlargement of the central canal of the spinal cord damages decussating fibres. This produces "dissociated anaesthesia"—loss of pain and temperature sensation with preservation of vibration and proprioception.

Fibres mediating proprioception and fine touch ascend in the dorsal columns of the spinal cord. In this tract sacral fibres lie nearest the midline; collateral branches of dorsal column fibres are thought to produce "gating" of pain signals. On reaching the medulla the fibres synapse in the gracile (medial) and cuneate (lateral) nuclei. Second order fibres then cross the midline to form the medial lemniscus and run on to thalamic nuclei. The dorsal columns are damaged in vitamin B_{12} deficiency (pernicious anaemia). The most severe forms may also involve corticospinal motor tracts and cause subacute combined degeneration of the spinal cord.

Motor pathways

The corticospinal and corticobulbar tracts are formed of fibres from the precentral gyrus (Brodmann's area 4 and motor cortex, 40% of fibres), the premotor cortex, anterior to the above (area 6, 30% of fibres), and parts of the parietal lobe (30% of fibres). The fibres pass through the internal capsule, the crus cerebri, and pons into the medulla. Fibres of the lateral corticospinal tracts form the pyramids of the medulla, and fibres of this and associated tracts are often referred to as the pyramidal tracts. Lateral corticospinal tract fibres (80% of corticospinal fibres) cross the midline in the medulla. Ventral corticospinal fibres (20% of corticospinal fibres) continue and do not cross the midline until close to their level of termination in the spinal cord. Ventral corticospinal tract fibres control trunk and proximal limb musculature. Fibres of the phylogenetically younger, lateral, corticospinal tract control muscles in the more distal parts of the limbs.

Damage to the lateral corticospinal tract produces Babinski's sign of dorsiflexion in the great toe, an "upgoing plantar," when the sole of the foot is stroked. Isolated damage to the corticospinal tracts produces flaccidity rather than the classically increased tone in upper motor neuron lesions. This is caused by the involvement of other motor tracts which regulate control of posture and coordination.

The cerebellum

The spinocerebellum receives proprioceptive input from the body and integrates this with motor plans. The more medial area, the vermis, deals with the trunk and proximal parts of the limbs; parts of the cerebellar hemispheres deal with distal limb movements. Lateral parts of the cerebellar hemispheres form the neocerebellum which, in conjunction with the cerebral motor cortex, plans movements. Cerebellar outputs travel via deep cerebellar nuclei to the thalamus, red nucleus, and brain stem. Fibres from the red nucleus form the rubrospinal and rubrobulbar tracts. Cerebellar lesions are characterised by incoordination, ataxia, dysdiadochokinesia, and dysarthria.

The basal ganglia

The basal ganglia are a collection of deep nuclear masses in the forebrain (the substantia nigra is in the midbrain). They are separated from the thalamus by the internal capsule. Inputs are received from the cerebral cortex in corticostriate fibres and from the thalamus. The basal ganglia are involved in the planning and coordination of movements. Outputs from the basal ganglia run to the thalamus and brain stem. The basal ganglia have a particularly high oxygen consumption. Conditions affecting the basal ganglia produce abnormalities of movement and coordination. In parkinsonism, degeneration of the nigrostriatal dopaminergic pathway leads to hypokinesia, rigidity, and tremor. Degeneration of the caudate nucleus produces chorea with rapid jerky movements, and lesions of the lenticular nucleus produce athetosis with slow writhing movements.

Two further tracts that influence posture and movement are the vestibulospinal and the tectospinal tracts (fig 1.3a). These integrate input from the ears and eyes respectively into motor output.

Together these "extrapyramidal" tracts have a net inhibitory effect on muscle tone, so lesions of these tracts are characterised by increases in muscle tone.

Autonomic nervous system

The autonomic nervous system (ANS) integrates visceral function via its two networks. Each consists of central preganglionic cells in the interomediolateral grey column of the spinal cord (or equivalent brain stem motor nuclei) and ganglia outside the CNS. The sympathetic outflow arises from the first thoracic (T1) to the third lumbar (L3) segmental levels and has a chain of paraspinal ganglia. It mediates the "fight or flight" response, the "catabolic nervous system" with noradrenaline as its final transmitter. The parasympathetic outflow is from cranial nerves III, VII, IX, and X, and first to fourth sacral nerves (S2–S4). The ganglia are usually close to the target organs. This mediates the "vegetative," "anabolic" functions with acetylcholine as the transmitter.

Autonomic functions are integrated in the CNS in a hierarchical fashion, some by spinal cord reflexes, respiratory, cardiac, and swallowing reflexes in

9

the brain stem, and pupillary reflexes in the midbrain. More complex functions involve the hypothalamus, Sherrington's "head ganglion of the ANS," through multiple nuclei and with connections to the pituitary, cortex, and limbic system.

Many drugs used in anaesthesia have actions via the ANS. Adrenergic agonists, for example, catecholamines and antagonists such as β-adrenoceptor blockers, act via the sympathetic nervous system. Anticholinesterase drugs which reduce the breakdown of acetylcholine have parasympathomimetic actions, for example, neostigmine used in the antagonism of neuromuscular blockade. Parasympathetic antagonists, such as atropine, may be used in anaesthesia to treat bradycardia or as antisialogogues. Hyoscine (scopolamine) has greater CNS penetration and may produce a "central anticholinergic crisis" with confusion and ataxia, particularly in elderly patients. A number of autonomic reflexes are important in anaesthesia, especially the bradycardia produced by parasympathetic actions as, for example, in the oculocardiac reflex or with traction on the spermatic cord.

Spinal cord

The spinal cord in the adult runs from the foramen magnum of the skull to the level of the intervertebral disc between the first and second lumbar vertebrae. In children the cord reaches lower levels. It serves to mediate reflex arcs and to organise neural impulses into tracts communicating with other spinal levels and the brain. There are 31 pairs of spinal nerves, eight cervical, 12 thoracic, five lumbar, five sacral, and the coccygeal. Sensory or afferent fibres enter via the dorsal root with cell bodies in the dorsal root ganglion. Motor or efferent fibres leave via the anterior root, the cell bodies being in the anterior horn of the spinal grey matter. This arrangement of dorsal sensory and ventral motor fibres constitutes the Bell–Magendie law.

The effects of localised cord damage can be predicted by considering the tracts involved (fig 1.3).[9] For example, a hemisection of the cord will produce the Brown–Séquard syndrome with ipsilateral loss of dorsal column sensation, but with loss of contralateral spinothalamic sensation. Trauma, particularly from road traffic accidents (around 55% of acute cord injuries), may produce reflex depression ("spinal shock") with bradycardia and hypotension. Anaesthetic intervention may be required to maintain ventilation. The principal nerve supply to the diaphragm is the phrenic nerve which arises from cervical roots III, IV, and V. Particular care is required with airway manoeuvres in patients with suspected cervical trauma because further cord damage may be produced. The circulatory system may also require support in the acute stage and care must be taken not to overlook occult traumatic injuries.

Reflexes subsequently return and become relatively hyperactive as a result of the removal of descending inhibition. In chronic cord lesions, irradiation of afferent impulses may produce a "mass" reflex with complex withdrawal and autonomic effects. This may be used in bladder or bowel control but is a potential hazard in anaesthesia.

Brain stem

The brain stem consists of the midbrain, pons, and medulla. It is of such great importance in integrating neural function that its "permanent cessation of function" as defined by brain death criteria is recognised as a declaration of death.[10] The brain stem contains integrating centres for respiratory and cardiovascular functions. The reticular formation at the core of the brain stem generates the capacity for consciousness whereas the cerebral cortex generates the content of consciousness. It has complex links to ascending pathways, the cerebellum, limbic system, and cerebral cortex.

The nuclei of cranial nerves III–XII lie in the brain stem. The midbrain integrates auditory and visual inputs, and contains the red nucleus. Demonstration of patterns of cranial nerve injury may enable localisation of the lesions. Cranial motor nerves IX, X, and XII, arising from the medulla, mediate the swallowing and gag reflexes. Impairment of these reflexes (for example, in pseudobulbar palsy, a bilateral upper motor neuron lesion usually in the internal capsule in cerebrovascular disease or multiple sclerosis) produces risks of aspiration pneumonia.

Forebrain

The forebrain comprises the cerebral cortex, thalamus, and hypothalamus. The cortex is concerned with functions of memory, language, and conscious thought, and the thalamus and hypothalamus with integrating many neural activities; they are closely linked to the endocrine system. Cortical areas are described by Brodmann's numbers. There is some functional localisation within the cortex. The sensory postcentral gyrus and motor precentral gyrus have already been considered. In addition, the primary visual cortex (area 17) lies on the sides of the calcarine fissure towards the occipital pole and the primary auditory cortex (area 41) lies in the superior part of the temporal lobe. The greater development of the human brain is reflected in the increased size of three "association areas" when compared with other animal species: the frontal, the temporoparietal–occipital, and the temporal areas.

Language function is largely localised to one cerebral hemisphere, the dominant or categorical one. In 96% of right handed people (with 91% of people being right handed) the left hemisphere is dominant. In 15% of left handers the right hemisphere is dominant, in 15% the hemispheres are co-dominant, and in 70%, as for most right handers, the left hemisphere is dominant. This has implications in cerebrovascular disease when damage to

11

the internal capsule causes contralateral motor loss and, if on the dominant side, may cause dysphasia. Lesions of the non-dominant "representational" hemisphere may cause loss of visual memory or unilateral neglect and loss of insight (parietal lesions).

Within the categorical hemisphere there are two areas that are further specialised for language function. Wernicke's area, at the posterior end of the superior temporal gyrus, is responsible for comprehension of auditory and visual information. Lesions here will cause a failure of understanding—a receptive dysphasia. Broca's area lies in the frontal lobes anterior to the inferior part of the motor cortex; it is responsible for producing coordination of speech. Lesions here will produce a non-fluent expressive dysphasia.

Damage to these areas may result from trauma (for example, head injury) or ischaemia, either focal (for example, embolic) or global (for example, cardiac arrest). Areas at the watershed zones, the boundaries between areas supplied by different cerebral arteries, are particularly vulnerable during hypotension.

CNS blood supply

The blood supply to the brain is via the two internal carotid arteries (two thirds) and the two vertebral arteries (one third). The vertebral arteries join to form the basilar artery which with the internal carotid arteries enters the circle of Willis. From here the anterior, middle, and posterior cerebral arteries supply the cortex.

The blood supply to the spinal cord is less predictable. An anterior spinal artery supplies the anterior two thirds of the cord; damage to this produces anterior cord syndrome with loss of the corticospinal and spinothalamic tracts. Two posterior spinal arteries supply the posterior one third of the cord. Superiorly, the spinal arteries receive blood from the vertebral arteries, but throughout the rest of the spinal cord they rely on radicular arteries from branches of surrounding vessels. The arteria radicularis magna (the artery of Adamkiewicz)[11] usually arises from a left lower intercostal or lumbar artery; it is the principal supply to the lower two thirds of the cord. The spinal cord is vulnerable to watershed damage in the same way as the brain, and the lower thoracic cord is especially at risk. Spinal blood supply may be compromised by abdominal vascular surgery.

Blood–brain barrier

Circulation in the CNS differs from other areas in that specialised tight junctions of the capillary endothelium and choroid plexus endothelium form the blood–brain barrier.[12] In ordinary capillary beds the endothelial junctions between cells are about 7 nm; at cerebral tight junctions this is reduced to

1 nm. The cerebral capillary endothelium is surrounded by a basement membrane and outside this lie astrocyte foot processes (fig 1.4). This greatly reduces the rate at which large polar molecules can enter the CNS. Thus, an intact blood–brain barrier is relatively impermeable to catecholamines and bile salts. It is, however, readily permeable to lipid soluble anaesthetic agents. The permeability to other drugs varies; for example, it is permeable to sulphadiazine and relatively impermeable to penicillins and aminoglycosides. Thus, when selecting drugs for actions in the CNS the penetration of the blood–brain barrier must be considered. Permeability is increased in disruption of the barrier as in inflammation, trauma, or acute hypertension. Four areas, the circumventricular organs, lie outside the blood–brain barrier. These include the posterior pituitary (neurohypophysis) and areas that act as chemoreceptor zones.

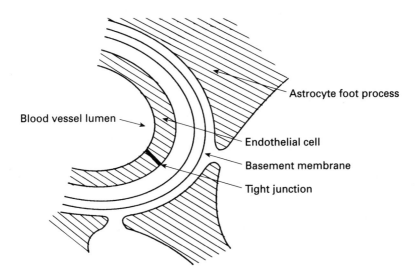

Fig 1.4 Blood–brain barrier

Metabolism

Within the CNS blood flow varies widely;[13] flow in grey matter averages five times that in white matter (grey matter: 110 ml/100 g per min; white matter: 22 ml/100 g per min; overall average: 52 ml/100 g per min). Although the brain is only 2–3% of the body mass (about 1400 g), it receives around 15% of the resting cardiac output (about 750 ml/min) and consumes 20% of basal oxygen requirements (that is, 170 μmol/100 g per min or 3·5 ml/100 g per min or about 50 ml/min) and 25% of basal glucose used

13

(31 μmol/100 g per min). This reflects the brain's high metabolic rate. In normal circumstances 90% of cerebral energy requirements are met by glucose. With starvation the brain can utilise ketone bodies, providing a basal glucose supply is available to regenerate intermediates of the citric acid cycle. The brain is unable to store significant amounts of glucose and reserves are exhausted in under three minutes. Hypoglycaemia produces behavioural changes, often aggression, unconsciousness, and ultimately neuronal damage.

Energy used by the brain is expressed as the cerebral metabolic rate (CMR; for oxygen: CMR_{O_2}). This can be divided into two components: that used to maintain electrophysiological function (60%) and that required to maintain the structural integrity of the cell (40%) (fig 1.5). The functional component (60%) can be progressively reduced by increasing the dose of anaesthetic agents (for example, thiopentone (thiopental), isoflurane, or etomidate) until the basal level is reached. This corresponds to EEG silence. Further increase in anaesthetic dose beyond that required for EEG silence produces no further reduction in CMR_{O_2}.

Temperature also affects CMR_{O_2} but by a different mechanism. Temperature affects the rate of chemical reactions by altering the activation energy required. This can be expressed as a coefficient (Q_{10}), giving the ratio of reaction rates where the temperature differs by 10°C; for most reactions this is about 2. Thus with a fall in temperature from 38°C to 28°C, the CMR_{O_2} is reduced by 55%. Overall, CMR_{O_2} changes by about 7% per °C, hence the importance of avoiding pyrexia in cases where cerebral ischaemia is likely. Unlike anaesthetic agents, hypothermia reduces both components of CMR_{O_2} (that is, below the CMR_{O_2} at EEG silence) and at 18°C CMR_{O_2} is only about 10% of the normothermic value.[14]

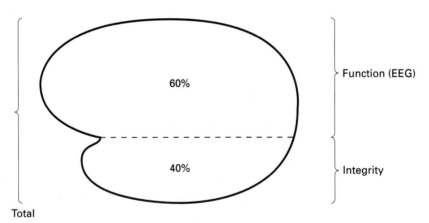

Fig 1.5 Cerebral metabolism: oxygen requirements of normal brain. $CMR_{O_2} = $ 5·5 ml/100 g per min; function = 3·3 ml/100 g per min; integrity = 2·2 ml/100 g per min

Flow–metabolic coupling

Cerebral blood flow (CBF) is normally closely matched to CMR_{O_2}. This flow–metabolic coupling was proposed as early as 1890; Roy and Sherrington stated that "the brain possesses an intrinsic mechanism by which vascular supply can be varied locally or globally in correspondence with local variations in functional activity."[15] The mediator of this coupling is the subject of continuing research; many potential candidates have been suggested (H^+, K^+, adenosine, etc) but the lack of temporal delay in adjusting blood flow is difficult to explain (there is no time for a metabolic intermediate to accumulate before increases in flow). At present, nitric oxide (NO or endothelium derived relaxing factor—EDRF) is being investigated as a possible mediator. In head injuries, although CMR_{O_2} is reduced, the coupling with CBF may be damaged giving rise to a potential for ischaemia.

Autoregulation

Autoregulation is the maintenance of CBF over a range of cerebral perfusion pressures (CPP, calculated as the mean arterial pressure minus the intracranial pressure, that is, MAP – ICP).[16] The normal range of autoregulation is 60–130 mm Hg (fig 1.6). Above a CPP of 130 mm Hg, CBF will increase proportionally with CPP; below a CPP of 60 mm Hg, CBF will decrease. The stability of CBF is accomplished by varying cerebral vascular

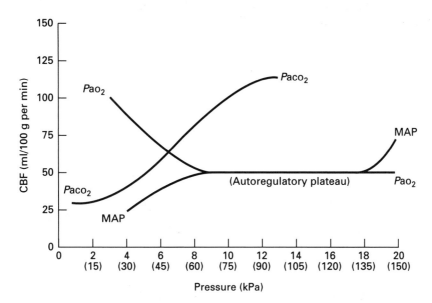

Fig 1.6 Effects on CBF. Values of pressure in brackets are mm Hg

15

resistance (CVR) through alteration of the vessel radius. The Hagen–Poiseuille equation shows that flow is proportional to the reciprocal of resistance and that resistance is proportional to the reciprocal of radius.[16] The mediator of this change is not fully understood. Head injury or other disruption of the blood–brain barrier may render the CBF wholly CPP dependent. The range of pressures covered by the autoregulatory plateau may differ for individuals; thus a patient with chronic untreated hypertension may maintain CBF over a range of CPP of 110–180 mm Hg and CBF will decrease at a CPP of less than 110 mm Hg.

Carbon dioxide

CBF is also influenced by arterial carbon dioxide levels (Pa_{CO_2}). Carbon dioxide diffuses rapidly across the blood–brain barrier and alters the $[H^+]$ (hydrogen ion concentration) of the cerebral extracellular fluid (ECF). At normotension there is a linear relationship between CBF and Pa_{CO_2} over the range 3–10 kPa (fig 1.6). CBF changes by 25% for each kilopascal change in Pa_{CO_2} (or 3% per mm Hg change in Pa_{CO_2}). The effect of a change in Pa_{CO_2} on CBF falls with a half life of six hours, because the cerebral ECF is buffered by bicarbonate ion exchange. As a consequence, prolonged hyperventilation will achieve progressively less reduction in CBF, and a return to normocapnia after a period of hyperventilation risks a rebound increase in CBF.[17] Similar considerations are required if a patient with a chronically raised Pa_{CO_2} as a result of pulmonary disease is ventilated to normocapnia. Another potential disadvantage of hypocapnia is the production of a leftward shift in the oxyhaemoglobin dissociation curve, thus making oxygen less readily released in the tissues. Hypercapnia reduces the range of autoregulation whereas hypocapnia widens this. Pa_{CO_2} reactivity of cerebral vessels is reduced in hypotension, head injury, subarachnoid haemorrhage, and cerebrovascular disease.

Jugular bulb oxygen saturation

There is concern that induced hyperventilation may, by decreasing Pa_{CO_2}, so reduce CBF as to induce ischaemia. Internal jugular venous bulb oxygen saturation (Sj_{O_2}) monitoring is increasingly used in these circumstances.[18] Basically as the CBF is progressively reduced, there will first be a period of increased oxygen extraction, with reducing Sj_{O_2}, until ischaemia is produced. Problems include the variability of venous drainage of the brain. It is not simply a left side to left internal jugular pattern. In general venous outflow from cortical structures drains to the superior sagittal sinus; this drains into the right transverse sinus and to the right internal jugular bulb. Deeper structures drain to the straight sinus, which usually drains into the left transverse sinus and on to the left internal jugular bulb. There is considerable

16

variability in this pattern. Several methods have been proposed to judge which jugular bulb saturation is the most appropriate to monitor in an individual case, such as compressing each jugular in turn, to see which produces the greater rise in intracranial pressure, or assessing the size of the jugular foramina on a computed tomographic (CT) scan. Inaccurate positioning of the catheter tip may lead to contamination with extracerebral blood and a lateral cervical spine radiograph is obtained to show the position of the catheter tip. Bilateral jugular bulb saturations showed a mean difference of 5% in a series of head injured patients.[19] Given these points and the wide normal range quoted, usually 54–75%, Sjo_2 is best interpreted in terms of trends rather than absolute values. The principal use is in indicating patients who are not likely to tolerate hyperventilation and a reduction in CBF. In those with an already low Sjo_2 a further reduction in CBF may precipitate ischaemia.

Hypoxia

Hypoxia is also a potent stimulus for increasing CBF. If Pao_2 decreases to below 6 kPa, CBF begins to increase and doubles as a Pao_2 of 3 kPa is reached (fig 1.6). High Pao_2 values have a small effect on CBF with a 12% reduction at a Pao_2 of 1 atmosphere (101 kPa). Hypoxia impairs autoregulation and this effect may persist in the postischaemic brain rendering CBF pressure dependent.

Intracranial pressure

CBF is one of the principal factors involved in determining ICP. Fundamental to this is the concept of the skull as a box of fixed volume; any changes to the contents of this "box" may vary the pressure within it. Normal intracranial contents are the brain, about 1400 g, CSF, about 75 ml, and the cerebral blood volume, about 140 ml, that is normally around 83%, 6%, and 11% respectively. An increase in volume of one component will cause compression of the others and an increase in pressure.

CSF is produced at the choroid plexus in the cerebral ventricles at a rate of 0·3–0·5 ml/min. The total volume of about 150 ml is normally divided evenly between cerebral and spinal spaces, the total volume being replaced two to three times daily. CSF circulates via the subarachnoid spaces and is reabsorbed at arachnoid granulations into the venous system, a process that is pressure dependent. The primary function of CSF is cushioning the CNS from sudden movements. Anaesthetic agents may alter both production and reabsorption. Enflurane is thought to increase CSF production and reduce absorption, a potentially deleterious combination; by contrast isoflurane has no effect on CSF production and increases reabsorption.[20]

With an expanding intracranial lesion such as a tumour, compensatory

17

mechanisms, such as displacement of CSF to the spinal subarachnoid space, initially forestall any increase in ICP. The ability to compensate is influenced by the time scale involved, with slow growing lesions better tolerated than acute insults. When compensatory mechanisms are no longer sufficient the compliance (change in volume per unit change in pressure, dV/dP) of the intracranial cavity is greatly reduced and ICP rises (fig 1.7). Normal ICP is 7–10 mm Hg; a sustained increase in ICP to more than 15 mm Hg is termed "intracranial hypertension." At an ICP of more than 20 mm Hg areas of focal ischaemia appear, and at values of ICP more than 50 mm Hg global ischaemia supervenes.

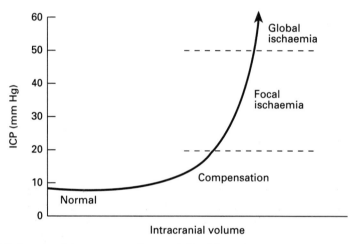

Fig 1.7 Intracranial pressure–volume relationship

The effective perfusion pressure of the brain is the difference between the mean arterial pressure (MAP) and the ICP—cerebral perfusion pressure (CPP). Clinically it is important to ensure that the two constituent readings are zeroed to the same level to give an accurate CPP, for example, both ICP and arterial pressure should be zeroed at the level of the external auditory meatus. There is an additional component to the calculation, further subtracting jugular bulb pressure from the MAP, but this is usually omitted as being insignificant clinically. Although autoregulation of CBF normally occurs over a range of CPP of 60–130 mm Hg, this feature is lost when ICP is over 30 mm Hg. In addition, Sjo_2 has been shown to decrease with values of CPP of less than 70 mm Hg. Attempts to improve CPP by increasing MAP to supranormal levels may reduce ischaemia, but risk increasing disruption of the blood–brain barrier and production of further oedema. A vicious cycle may be established, triggered by an initial insult such as a head injury (fig 1.8).

18

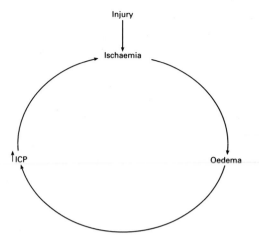

Fig 1.8 Vicious cycle of cerebral ischaemia

Cerebral oedema may arise from one of three mechanisms. In cytotoxic oedema, cell membrane failure leads to the entry of sodium and water into the cell, causing it to swell; this may result from focal or global ischaemia. Vasogenic oedema is caused by disruption of the blood–brain barrier, with a resultant increase in ECF; this may result from trauma, infection, or hypertension. Interstitial oedema is caused by a shift of CSF into the ECF resulting from obstruction of CSF outflow such as in hydrocephalus.

As compensatory mechanisms fail and ICP increases, a continuous monitor of ICP may show Lundberg's waves, first described in 1910.[21] "A" waves last 5–20 minutes and reach pressures of up to 80 mm Hg; they may be triggered by an increase in Pa_{CO_2} causing an increase in CBF. "B" waves have a frequency of 1/min and are associated with brain stem disorders. "C" waves occur at 6/min; they are related to cyclical changes in arterial pressure in the presence of cerebral disorders.

An increase in ICP may cause displacement of intracranial contents. Pressure in the supratentorial compartment can cause herniation of the temporal uncus and a reduction of conscious level. This causes pressure on the third cranial nerve (III, the occulomotor nerve) producing an ipsilateral fixed, dilated pupil.[22] The sixth intracranial nerve (VI, the abducent nerve) is also particularly vulnerable to raised ICP as a result of its long intracranial course. Paralysis of cranial nerve VI causes a lateral rectus palsy. Pressure on the brain stem can cause decerebrate rigidity with extensor posturing in all limbs, and "Cushing's reflex" with hypertension and bradycardia. Increased ICP may cause swelling of the optic nerve head, seen as papilloedema at ophthalmoscopy. Further increases in ICP may impact the cerebellar tonsils in the foramen magnum leading to apnoea and brain death.

CNS monitoring

The EEG records spontaneous cerebral electrical activity.[23] As ICP rises CPP is reduced, CBF decreases, and cerebral electrical activity is reduced (see above about EEG silence when CMR is reduced by 60%). The EEG will slow at CPP of less than 50 mm Hg and is silenced at CPP of less than 30 mm Hg. A scalp EEG records activity in the superficial cortical dendrites. The following rhythm patterns may be identified: α rhythm at 8–15 Hz predominates in conscious adults with the eyes closed and mind wandering; it is best recorded in the parieto-occipital region. The β rhythm at 18–30 Hz is best recorded over the frontal region. The δ rhythm at less than 4 Hz predominates in deep sleep (stages three and four sleep). The θ rhythm at 4–7 Hz is found in normal children. When the eyes are opened α block or desynchronisation occurs. Sleep produces δ rhythm with interspersed α activity. Periods of rapid eye movement (REM) sleep are associated with dreaming and produce irregular low voltage EEG activity.

Increasing anaesthetic depth reduces EEG activity to a burst suppression and then to isoelectricity. The EEG provides a large amount of data but as a monitor of anaesthetic depth it is difficult to interpret and vulnerable to electrical interference.[24] A cerebral function monitor (CFM) processes EEG data into a single value calculated to reflect EEG power; however, it loses much of the EEG data and its product is a hybrid trace which makes interpretation difficult. The cerebral function analysing monitor (CFAM) develops this idea further and records a percentage of α, β, θ, and δ bands. Such processed EEG techniques are occasionally used in anaesthesia for carotid artery surgery. Power spectrum analysis uses a Fourier analysis of sampled EEG data to produce a graph of power versus frequency. It has proved useful in predicting outcome after severe coma.

Evoked potentials measure the "evoked" cortical response to a specific peripheral stimulus. Electrodes over the relevant receiving area can be used in either clinical investigation or, increasingly, during intraoperative monitoring. Visual evoked potentials are used in the investigation of multiple sclerosis. Auditory evoked potentials can be used intraoperatively in dissection of an acoustic neuroma.[25]

Anaesthesia

Central to general anaesthesia is the deliberate depression of conscious level by anaesthetic agents. Clearly the resultant state reflects a reversible neurophysiological change but debate continues as to the exact mechanism. As early as 1901 the Meyer–Overton lipid solubility theory highlighted the correlation between anaesthetic potency (as measured by minimum alveolar concentration or MAC) and the oil/gas partition coefficient (MAC × Oil/Gas coefficient = 2·1);[26] this theory proposes a hydrophobic site of action for anaesthesia. The multisite expansion theory of Halsey in 1979[27] suggests that this site is within the cell membrane. Anaesthetic agents are thought to produce conformational changes and close ion channels. Other theories have suggested a synaptic site of action either by reducing neurotransmitter release, decreased receptor response, or by inducing chronic membrane depolarisation.[28] Increasing evidence of the effects of specific agents at synapses and an improved understanding of neurochemistry will shed light on this fundamental basis of anaesthesia.

1 Ganong WF. *Review of medical physiology*, 15th edn. Norwalk: Appleton Lange, 1991.
2 Choi DW. Excitotoxicity. In: Meldrum BS (Ed), *Excitatory amino acid antagonists*. Oxford: Blackwell, 1991: 216–36.
3 Siesjo BK, Memezawa H, Smith ML. Neurocytotoxicity: pharmacological implications. *Fundament Clin Pharmacol* 1991; 5: 755–67.
4 McCulloch J, Bullock R, Teasdale GM. Excitatory amino acids: opportunities for the treatment of ischaemic brain damage in man. In: Meldrum BS (Ed), *excitatory amino acid antagonists*. Oxford: Blackwell, 1991: 287–326.
5 Pleuvry BJ. Opioid receptors and their ligands: natural and unnatural. *Br J Anaesth* 1991; **66**: 370–80.
6 Erlanger J, Gasser HS. Classification of peripheral nerve fibres. *Am J Physiol* 1929; **88**: 581–7.
7 Melzack R, Wall PD. Pain mechanisms: a new theory. *Science* 1965; **1150**: 971–9.
8 Rexed B. Some aspects of cytoarchitectonics and synaptology in the spinal cord. In: Eccles JC, Schade JP (Eds), *Progress in brain research: organisation of the spinal cord*, vol 11. Amsterdam: Elsevier, 1964: 58–92.
9 Grundy D, Swain A. *ABC of spinal cord injury*, 2nd edn. London: BMJ, 1993.
10 Pallis C. *ABC of brain stem death*. London: BMJ, 1983.
11 Moore KL. *Clinically oriented anatomy*. Baltimore: Williams & Wilkins, 1980.
12 Bradbury M. *The concept of a blood–brain barrier*. Chichester: Wiley, 1979.
13 Fitch W. Brain metabolism. In: Cotterell JE, Smith DS (Eds), *Anesthesia and neurosurgery*. St Louis: Mosby, 1994: 1–16.
14 Michenfelder JD. *Anesthesia and the brain: clinical, functional, metabolic and vascular correlates*. Churchill Livingstone: New York, 1988.
15 Roy CS, Sherrington CS. On the regulation of the blood-supply of the brain. *J Physiol (Lond)* 1890; **11**: 85–109.
16 Young WL, Ornstein E. Cerebral and spinal cord blood flow. In: Cotterell JE, Smith DS (Eds), *Anesthesia and neurosurgery*. St Louis: Mosby, 1994, 17–48.
17 Raichle ME, Posner JB, Plum F. Cerebral blood flow during and after hyperventilation. *Arch Neurol* 1970; **23**: 394–9.
18 Dearden NM. Jugular venous bulb oxygen saturation in the management of severe head injury. *Curr Opin Anaesthesiol* 1991; **4**: 279–86.
19 Stocchetti N, Paparella A, Bridelli F, Bacchi M, Piazza P, Zuccoli P. Cerebral venous oxygen saturation studied with bilateral samples in the internal jugular veins. *Neurosurgery* 1994; **34**: 38–44.
20 Simpson JA, Fitch W. Cerebrospinal fluid: formation, composition and pressures. In: Simpson JA, Fitch W (Eds), *Applied neurophysiology*. London: Wright, 1988: 316–30.
21 Shapiro HM, Drummond JC. Neurosurgical anaesthesia and intracranial hypertension. In: Miller MD (Ed), *Anesthesia*, 3rd edn. New York: Churchill Livingstone, 1990: 51–84.
22 Bullock R, Teasdale G. Head injuries. In: Skinner D, Driscoll P, Earlam R (Eds), *ABC of major trauma*. London: BMJ, 1991: 25–32.
23 Simpson JA, Fitch W. The electroencephalogram. In: Simpson JA, Fitch W (Eds), *Applied neurophysiology*. London: Wright, 1988: 147–53.
24 Levy WJ, Shapiro HM, Maruchak G, Meathe E. Automated EEG processing for intraoperative monitoring. *Anesthesiology* 1980; **53**: 223–31.
25 Grundy BL. Intraoperative monitoring of sensory-evoked potentials. *Anesthesiology* 1983; **58**: 72–81.

26 Miller KW. The nature of the site of general anaesthesia. *Int Rev Neurobiol* 1985; **27**: 1–14.
27 Wardley-Smith B, Halsey MJ. Recent molecular theories of anaesthesia. *Br J Anaesth* 1979; **51**: 619–25.
28 Koblin DD. Mechanisms of action. In: Miller MD (Ed), *Anesthesia*, 3rd edn. New York: Churchill Livingstone, 1990: 51–84.

2: Survey of neurological diseases encountered in an intensive care unit

I BONE, JAR NICOLL, DI GRAHAM

The purposes of this chapter are to acquaint the anaesthetist with the clinical manifestations of disorders commonly encountered in a neurointensive care unit, as well as outlining common pathological features. Allocation and appropriate use of intensive care require well defined admission criteria and, in the context of limited resources, the development of priority categories for specific groups of neurologically ill patients. Several categories can be defined: first, those who are critically ill and deteriorating as a consequence of acute neurological damage; second, patients who are not critically impaired at the time of admission but who are taken into the unit for the purposes of intensive neurological monitoring and anticipated deterioration; and finally critically ill patients already residing in intensive care who develop neurological complications as a consequence of their "critical illness" status.

If one addresses the types of neurological condition in which intensive therapy might positively influence outcome these can be divided into certain groups.

1 Those with acute respiratory depression, that is, either the consequence of central nervous system (CNS) disorders such as a brain stem syndrome or status epilepticus, or as a result of peripheral nervous system disease affecting the nerves themselves, the neuromuscular junction, or muscle.
2 Patients with progressive intracranial mass lesions who probably represent most patients under neurological intensive care. Such lesions may be the consequence of haemorrhage, traumatic contusion, tumour, infarction, or other space occupying mass.
3 A proportion of intensive care patients have acute central nervous system infections such as encephalitis, meningoencephalitis, and brain abscess.

In this section each of these disorders is dealt with briefly in terms of prevalence, clinical manifestations, and pathology. It is important to emphasise at the outset that the diversity of neurological disease results in protean clinical manifestations and that the pragmatic approach to diagnosis, and often to management, is the localisation of pathology to the supratentorial, infratentorial, and spinal compartments, or to the peripheral nervous system. The presentation of hemisphere, brain stem, craniocervical, and spinal lesions is addressed and also that of peripheral nerve, neuromuscular junction, and muscle disorders. A brief outline is also given of specific pathological processes, particularly in relation to tumour classification and ischaemic brain damage. Table 2.1 outlines neurological conditions in which intensive care may be anticipated and effective.

Table 2.1   Conditions resulting in neuro-intensive care admission

1	*Presenting with respiratory depression*
	Peripheral
	Disorder of nerve,
	neuromuscular junction, or muscle
	Central
	Brain stem
	Craniocervical junction
	Status epilepticus
2	*Progressive intracranial mass lesions*
	Infarction
	Haemorrhage
	Trauma
	Tumours
	Hydrocephalus
3	*Acute CNS infections*
	Encephalitis
	Meningoencephalitis
	Meningitis
	Abscess

Peripheral nervous system and muscular disorders

Respiratory failure may develop during the course of many neurological conditions affecting the peripheral nervous system (table 2.2). Conditions

Table 2.2   Peripheral nervous system causes of respiratory failure

Guillain–Barré syndrome
Polymyositis
Myasthenia gravis
Poliomyelitis
Metabolic myopathy (acid maltase deficiency)
Muscular dystrophy
  Duchenne
  Myotonic dystrophy
Motor neuron disease
Poliomyelitis

24

that are commonly encountered in intensive care practice are the Guillain–Barré syndrome, myasthenia gravis, and polymyositis. Respiratory failure is also encountered in other rarer forms of muscle disease such as the dystrophies, and metabolic and congenital myopathy. Rarely, respiratory insufficiency presents in the end stage of motor neuron disease. Recognition of neurological patients with impending respiratory failure is important so that assisted ventilation can be instigated electively rather than waiting for "respiratory arrest." There are major ethical considerations when offering ventilatory support to patients with progressive incurable neuromuscular disorders and full discussion with patients, family, and carers is essential in such circumstances.

Guillain–Barré syndrome

Guillain–Barré syndrome is the most common peripheral nervous system disorder requiring ventilatory support. It has a worldwide incidence of between 1 and 1·5 cases per 100 000 and is characterised usually by a prodromal self limiting infection (viral or bacterial). In most cases the diagnosis is confirmed by the clinical picture of symmetrical muscle weakness affecting proximal limb muscles associated with areflexia and distal paresthesiae. In about 25% of patients cranial nerve involvement is present, usually in the form of a lower motor neuron facial weakness; some 25% of patients admitted to an acute receiving service with Guillain–Barré syndrome will develop respiratory failure as a consequence of diaphragmatic weakness, and this is often associated with cardiovascular instability as a result of autonomic nervous system involvement.[1] Such patients will require admission to a neurological intensive therapy unit for respiratory function monitoring and, if indicated, ventilatory support. Haemodynamic and cardiovascular disturbances are also observed and require that appropriate action be taken.

Guillain–Barré syndrome is assumed to be an immunological disorder, possibly involving both antibody mediated and cell mediated reactions to peripheral nerve. Indeed, antibodies to peripheral myelin and activated "T" cells have frequently been found. The clinical picture is diagnostic, being supported by electrophysiological investigations—nerve conduction and electromyography—as well as lumbar puncture, with an elevated cerebrospinal fluid (CSF) protein and a normal cell count. Antecedent infective triggers, such as Epstein–Barr virus, cytomegalovirus, varicella-zoster virus, and human immunodeficiency virus, are frequently identified. The condition has also been described with infection with *Campylobacter jejuni*, *Mycoplasma pneumoniae*, and many other infections as well as after surgery, trauma, and in association with malignancy. The treatment is not only supportive but also the appropriate intervention with specific immunotherapy. Plasmapheresis (plasma exchange) is an effective treatment in patients showing significant motor deterioration, trials having clearly demonstrated that such patients, when offered plasmapharesis, have a better functional outcome recovery. More recently intravenous immunoglobulin has been offered as an alternative with infusion of 0·4 g/kg body weight daily over a five day period. This treatment appears to be as effective as plasmapharesis but simpler to administer, and is currently the subject of a multicentre randomised trial. In Guillain–Barré syndrome, the outcome is generally good, the mortality rate having declined to between 3% and 5% of survivors; only 15–20% have residual disability and may be unable, on discharge from hospital, to achieve complete functional independence.

Polymyositis

Polymyositis (inflammatory myopathy) accounts for a small number of patients requiring ventilatory support. This condition also has an incidence of one case per 100 000 and in its most severe form can be fulminating and life threatening. Polymyositis appears to be a disorder of cell mediated immunity and very typically presents with weakness affecting proximal muscles in both upper and lower limbs; it usually evolves over weeks and months and is associated with some degree of muscle pain. Muscle wasting does not occur and, unlike the Guillain–Barré syndrome, reflexes are not affected. In severe cases pharyngeal and respiratory muscles can be involved with difficulty in swallowing and in breathing. As many as 40% of patients with this disorder may also have involvement of cardiac muscle and at least 50% have pulmonary involvement resulting in respiratory muscle weakness, a tendency to respiratory infection, and, commonly, respiratory failure. Polymyositis is often associated with other autoimmune disorders such as Sjögren's syndrome, systemic lupus erythematosus, and mixed connective tissue disease.

The diagnosis is established by measuring the level of the muscle enzyme, creatinine kinase (CK), in blood, as well as by carrying out electromygraphy (EMG), which shows low voltage muscle action potentials with abnormal spontaneous activity. The most important diagnostic investigation is, however, that of muscle biopsy, which confirms the presence of inflammatory cells, necrosis, and regeneration of muscle fibres with an increase in connective tissue. The management of polymyositis is essentially one of respiratory support when indicated, as well as specific immunotherapy, initially using prednisolone in high dosage and often combining this in the long term with less toxic immunosuppressive therapy such as azathioprine and occasionally methotrexate or cyclosporin (cyclosporine).[2] Refractory cases may be treated by high dose intravenous immunoglobulin. Patients with polymyositis may require intensive therapy, particularly when the disease appears to have taken a fulminant course with evidence of respiratory involvement. Occasionally patients with a more chronic form of disease also develop respiratory failure, often precipitated by intercurrent infection, and require assisted ventilation.

A host of other muscle disorders can result in respiratory failure; these are often rare, such as acid maltase deficiency, and precipitated by intercurrent infection. A more vexing question is whether to offer respiratory support to patients with incurable progressive peripheral nervous system disorders such as motor neuron disease. This condition has a worldwide incidence rate of about one per 100 000. It is unusual for respiratory failure to be a presenting feature, as this normally occurs in the context of profound limb or bulbar weakness. Patients in whom the phrenic nerves are, however, affected early occasionally develop respiratory muscle weakness that is disproportionate to the rest of the clinical presentation.

Typically, motor neuron disease presents painlessly with wasting and weakness affecting limb and muscles often associated with visible muscle fasciculation. The disorder tends to start in a single limb and then involves all four slowly over months or years. Alternatively, the presentation may initially be cranial with involvement of bulbar muscles, producing difficulty in swallowing and speech in the first instance. Assisted ventilation may be considered in motor neuron disease in patients who present with early respiratory involvement, but should not be considered in those who already have severe limb weakness to the point that they are wholly incapacitated. To prolong life in such circumstances, using assisted ventilation, would hardly seem desirable. Decisions on the management of impending respiratory failure should be discussed at length with patient, relatives, and carers.[3]

Poliomyelitis

In earlier years this was the most common peripheral nervous system disorder requiring ventilation.[4] With the introduction of active immunisation in the late 1960s there was a dramatic decrease in incidence. Today in developed countries only 1·4 per million people present with this condition, although it remains a problem in the developing world. About 10% of patients with poliomyelitis experience life threatening complications such as respiratory failure.

Three strains of polio enterovirus are recognised, spread being by the orofaecal route. Anterior horn cells in both the spinal cord and brain stem are affected selectively. A brief period of gastrointestinal or upper respiratory symptomatology is followed by headache, meningism, and muscle pain. At this stage fasciculation becomes evident in involved limbs and paralysis ensues. The paralytic phase progresses over less than one week, diaphragm, intercostal, and other auxiliary respiratory muscles being frequently affected. Treatment is essentially supportive. When intercostal or diaphragmatic muscle weakness results in respiratory failure then ventilation is introduced.

27

Functional recovery is usually the case but occasionally patients are left in respiratory failure requiring indefinite ventilatory support.

Myasthenia gravis

Myasthenia gravis is an autoimmune disease in which antibodies against N-acetylcholine receptors result in impaired neuromuscular transmission. The condition has an incidence of 2–4 per 100 000 and frequently requires intensive care management either in the context of a myasthenic or cholinergic crisis or in patients who undergo thymectomy. The disorder is caused by an antibody and complement mediated reduction in postsynaptic acetylcholine receptors.[5] Patients typically present with weakness that characteristically shows fatiguability.

Occasionally, the eyes may be affected in isolation in which case acetylcholine receptor antibodies are often not detected in serum. Generally the patient notices fatiguing of ocular movement, limb weakness, difficulty in swallowing, weakness of speech, and breathlessness. These features gradually worsen until the diagnosis is established on the basis of antibody detection, repetitive nerve stimulation, and single fibrillary EMG studies. One important diagnostic test is giving intravenous edrophonium chloride to patients and observing improvement in fatiguable eye movement, speech, or limb weakness. Myasthenia gravis can sometimes be precipitated or present for the first time after a patient has been exposed to certain drugs, for example, antibiotics, anticonvulsants, antiarrhythmics, hypnotics, and tranquillisers. When the diagnosis has been established imaging of the anterior mediastinum should be carried out to exclude the presence of thymic tumour and, if the patient is severely symptomatic, consideration should in any case be given to thymectomy. Assisted ventilation is frequently required in both myasthenic and cholinergic crises, which are often being precipitated by intercurrent infection or by the injudicious use of anticholinesterase drugs.

Lambert–Eaton myasthenic syndrome

This is also an autoimmune disorder of the neuromuscular junction in which antibodies appear to be raised against presynaptic calcium channels. The incidence is less than one per 10^6. Patients are generally older and there is often an association with underlying malignancy; respiratory failure is uncommon. The diagnosis is established by repetitive nerve stimulation tests as well as by the detection of calcium channel antibodies. Drug treatment involves the use of anticholinesterase drugs and 3,4-diaminopyridine, a drug that increases acetylcholine release. As with myasthenia gravis assessment of respiratory function should be carried out in case there is a necessity, albeit rare, for assisted ventilation.

Central nervous system disorders

The brain stem plays a fundamental role in central respiratory control. Various specific centres have been identified:

- The pneumotaxic centre responsible for respiratory switch off
- The centre for the apneustic phenomenon of prolonged respiratory state
- The medullary centre comprising the dorsal and ventral respiratory group which are anatomically related to the nucleus of the tractus solitarius and the nucleus ambiguus respectively, and project through these to the spinal cord to innervate both intercostal and phrenic nerve neurons.

It is not surprising, in view of the location of these respiratory centres, that diseases affecting the brain stem may result in respiratory failure. An acute brain stem disorder presenting in this way is central pontine myelinolysis; this rare condition is associated with hyponatraemia and appears to be the consequence of rapid correction resulting in acute brain stem demyelination. This is generally a disorder from which recovery can be made but, in the acute phase, central respiratory failure frequently occurs and may require ventilatory support. The other more common demyelinating disorder of the brain stem which might result in respiratory failure is multiple sclerosis, a condition that has a prevalence in the United Kingdom of 110 per 100 000. Although brain stem involvement is common, respiratory failure is rare and transient, and should be managed by ventilatory support and steroids given in the form of intravenous methylprednisolone 500 mg daily over a 4–5 day period.

Medullary compression can produce respiratory failure. It may occur in the course of tonsillar herniation resulting from raised intracranial pressure or from compressive lesions at the foramen magnum such as Arnold–Chiari malformation, meningioma, or neurofibroma. Medullary compression as a cause of respiratory failure without raised intracranial pressure is rare.

The most common disease process to affect the brain stem is cerebrovascular disease. The average incidence rate of "stroke" varies considerably throughout the world, the Oxford Community Stroke Study suggesting a total incidence of 690 per 100 000: between 15% and 20% of these are haemorrhagic "stroke," most being ischaemic, of which only 20% are confined to the posterior circulation.

Brain stem infarction can be divided into certain specific syndromes. First, there may be major vessel occlusion, such as basilar artery thrombosis, and second, the long circumflex branches of the basilar artery (superior cerebellar, anteroinferior cerebellar, and posteroinferior cerebellar arteries) may be affected. Finally, vascular disease may be the consequence of occlusion of a small perforating paramedian branch. The clinical syndromes of brain stem ischaemia are complex; respiratory failure, however, is encountered when basilar artery or paramedian vessel occlusion occurs.[6] Such patients usually have demonstrable vascular risk factors such as hypertension, ischaemic heart disease, diabetes, and hypercholesterolaemia. The clinical picture is usually that of acute brain stem dysfunction with symptoms, such as double vision, vertigo, and paralysis, often affecting all four limbs in varying degrees. If pontine infarction occurs, a syndrome referred to as "the locked-in syndrome" results. The features of this condition are quadriplegia, aphonia (lack of speech), and impairment of ocular movement. As the reticular formation is spared the patient remains conscious but initially requires ventilatory support. Patients with this catastrophic type of cerebral infarction usually regain respiratory function in time and are often left profoundly disabled with paralysis of all motor function. Brain stem haemorrhage may produce a similar clinical picture (fig 2.1).

"Status epilepticus" is a term referring to continuous seizure activity without evidence of recovery in between events, persisting seizure activity of longer than 30 minutes being diagnostic. Status epilepticus is one of the most common neurological emergencies; a recent community based study suggested that one per 1000 of the population was affected annually.[7] On the basis of this figure it has been suggested that there are five million cases of status epilepticus annually world wide with mortality rates ranging from 2% to 25%. The most common causes of status epilepticus are drug withdrawal, including alcohol or anticonvulsants, drug injection with recreational drugs, such as cocaine, ischaemic brain damage following cardiac or respiratory arrest, and viral encephalitic illnesses. The neuropathological consequences of this condition are thought to be the result of excitotoxicity, high levels of

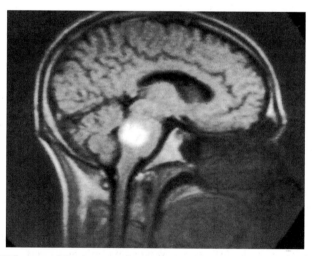

Fig 2.1 MRI scan of brain stem haematoma: 29 year old man presenting with headache, diplopia, and ataxia. Scan shows a pontine haematoma; angiography and coagulation screen normal

intracellular calcium being produced by excessive neuronal activity which, if sustained, might result in irreversible brain damage. During status epilepticus metabolic requirements of the brain increase by 200–300% and this is associated with an increase in cerebral blood flow and systemic hypertension; intracranial pressure is also significantly elevated. Patients in status epilepticus have, as a result of increased muscle activity, excessive levels of carbon dioxide, and ventilatory impairment causes a respiratory acidosis and hypoxaemia. The diagnosis is clinically evident, the patient experiencing continuous clonic, tonic, or tonic–clonic convulsions, and the EEG showing continuous seizure activity.

Management is that of airway support and aggressive anticonvulsant treatment. All drugs employed in attempting control of seizures are respiratory depressants. Initially benzodiazepines are used followed by phenytoin, phenobarbitone (phenobarbital), and paraldehyde in turn. More recently, drugs such as midazolam have been shown to be extremely effective but necessitate intubation and respiratory support, this also being necessary if drugs such as thiopentone (thiopental) are used. When cerebral oedema is suspected control of intracranial pressure with either mannitol or steroids might be justified. Status epilepticus is a life theatening condition requiring proactive management; poor outcome often reflects a conservative approach to an anticonvulsant regimen and a failure to intubate and ventilate electively at the correct stage. In all those presenting with status epilepticus in whom recovery has taken place, an attempt should be made to identify the provoking factor so that recurrence is prevented.

Progressive intracranial mass lesions

Haemorrhagic, traumatic, and other space occupying lesions such as tumours have different modes of clinical presentation, and yet all can result in raised intracranial pressure (ICP), with resultant impairment of consciousness and clinical manifestations of brain shift. The skull is a rigid structure with its contents of blood, brain, and cerebrospinal fluid (CSF) being almost incompressible (the Monro–Kelly doctrine which states that an increase in one constituent or an expanding mass within the skull would result in an increased intracranial pressure).

The craniospinal cavity is divided into four distinct compartments: the falx divides the right from the left hemisphere; the tentorium divides the forebrain from cerebellar structures; and the foramen magnum divides intracranial from intraspinal structures. Of the cranial cavity about 85% of the volume is taken up by the brain, 10% by CSF, and 5–10% by blood. Under normal circumstances ICP is equal throughout all compartments apart from minor hydrostatic differences. When a pathological condition develops, such as a mass lesion or obstruction of CSF pathways, or a general increase in brain volume, pressure gradients develop with consequent movement of

31

brain tissue; this produces certain specific syndromes as a result of the brain shift. An important aspect of neurological intensive care is the monitoring of ICP.

Frontal lobe tumours often present with alteration in personality and mood, temporal lobe tumours sometimes present with seizures in the context of no other neurological abnormality, parietal tumours present with neglect syndromes, sensory inattention, and visual field impairment, and occipital lobe tumours similarly result in visual symptomatology. Seizures occur in about 35% of patients with intracerebral tumour and the development of seizures in adult life should always raise suspicion of such a tumour, necessitating cranial imaging. Intraventricular tumours present with headache disorders and personality change, tumours in the pineal region present with ocular movement disorders, and those in the sellar or parasellar region present with visual field impairment and abnormalities of ocular movement. Tumours of the posterior fossa present with disorders of stance, gait, and posture often associated with limb incoordination. Tumours in the cerebellopontine angle present with impairment of hearing and equilibrium, facial sensation, and weakness of expression and mastication. Skull base tumours present with a constellation of lower cranial nerve signs and symptoms.

If these disorders go undiagnosed and the tumour increases in size, then the development of symptoms and signs of raised ICP are inevitable. The headache of raised ICP has certain characteristics such as early morning onset, wakening from sleep, and short periodicity occurring for 30 or 40 minutes and settling in waves throughout the day. Primary intracranial tumours are relatively rare occurring with an annual incidence of 3–4 per 100 000. Intracranial haemorrhage is more common with an incidence of 25–30 per 100 000.

Finally, diffuse intracranial disorders may also cause raised ICP, in particular, viral or toxic encephalitis, and Reye's syndrome—a worldwide disorder associated with influenza A, B, varicella-zoster infection, and the use of aspirin. Reye's syndrome seems to represent a synergism between viral infection and salicylate which leads to mitochondrial dysfunction. This, in turn, results in cerebral oedema associated with liver abnormality and causes an elevation of blood ammonia and free fatty acids, and hypoglycaemia. The disorder has become relatively less frequent with the avoidance of widespread aspirin use in young children. The condition requires ICP monitoring and, in the context of respiratory failure, ventilatory support in an intensive care unit. The mortality rate of this condition has fallen to about 30%, although children who survive are often left with significant psychomotor retardation and visual abnormalities.

Whatever the pathological process that results in raised ICP, the end result represents a final common clinical pathway with specific brain shift syndromes.

The subfalcine shift occurs early in unilateral space occupying lesions affecting the hemisphere: the medial surface of the frontal lobe slips under the falx occasionally compressing the ipsilateral anterior cerebral artery and resulting in arterial occlusion. Symptomatically this form of shift might result in contralateral lower limb paralysis. Tentorial herniation can occur laterally; a unilateral expanding mass lesion causes uncal herniation as the medial edge of the temporal lobe slips through the tentorial hiatus. This results in compression of the third nerve with pupillary dilatation (mydriasis) and the eye adopting a down and out position. Pressure from the edge of the tentorium may also compress the contralateral cerebral peduncle (Kernohan's notch) and produce limb weakness ipsilateral to the mass lesion. Finally, the posterior cerebral artery may be compressed on the tentorium resulting in a contralateral homonymous hemianopia. These symptoms and signs normally develop gradually, although the rate of development does not depend on the nature of the lesion, but rather on the speed at which it increases in size; intracranial haemorrhage develops rapidly and intracranial tumour more gradually.

A central form of tentorial herniation is also recognised. Here the diencephalon and other midbrain structures are pushed downwards and are thus buckled and distorted; this results in a stretching of the paramedian perforating branches of the basilar artery. The consequence here is one of deterioration of the consciousness level, the pupils initially becoming small, then moderately dilated, and eventually fixed. Pressure on the dorsal aspect of the brain stem at the level of the superior colliculus results in impairment of vertical gaze movement. Finally, downward traction on the pituitary stalk and hypothalamus may result in diabetes insipidus.

The final form of herniation is tonsillar herniation. Here, tonsillar impaction in the foramen magnum produces symptomatic neck stiffness and a head tilt, which is associated with depression of the consciousness level and with respiratory irregularities, as a consequence of compression of medullary respiratory centres and with eventual respiratory arrest. These syndromes are often irreversible, especially tonsillar herniation. The management of raised ICP is that of trying to reduce it rapidly. Various treatment modalities are available such as mannitol infusion, controlled hyperventilation, ventricular CSF withdrawal, barbiturate therapy, and steroids;[8] naturally the cause of the herniation (for example, tumour, haematoma) should also be treated as soon as possible.

Acute central nervous system infections

The most common infective conditions necessitating admission to neurological intensive care are encephalitis, meningoencephalitis, and cerebral abscess. These conditions have taken on a new significance with the increasing recognition of acquired immune deficiency syndrome (AIDS) and the awareness of the unusual opportunistic infections that can result. The use of widespread immunosuppressive treatment in patients undergoing kidney, heart, or lung transplantation, as well as the effects on immunocompetence of malignant disease and its treatment, have significantly increased the numbers of patients with unusual CNS infections requiring intensive care management.

Herpes simplex encephalitis

Herpes simplex encephalitis has an incidence of one per 250 000 per annum, with the mortality rate without treatment being 70%. About 30% of cases represent primary infection, which is usually the case in young people; the rest represent activation of existing infection. Herpes simplex encephalitis is not usually associated with immunosuppression. Access to the subfrontal and temporal lobes is gained along the olfactory nerve by transneural transport.

Pathologically, the temporal lobes, insular and cingulate gyrus, and the frontal basal cortex are affected; the changes are those of inflammation with haemorrhagic congestion, perivascular cuffing, gliosis, and intranuclear inclusions.[9] The clinical history is suggestive with a short prodromal illness of headache and fever, and, thereafter, depression in the consciousness level, personality alteration, memory changes, confusion, hallucinations, and seizures; later hemiparesis develops. A diagnosis is suggested by an influenza like illness followed by convulsions and impaired consciousness. The diagnosis is supported by abnormalities within the temporal lobe on computed tomography (fig 2.2) and magnetic reasonance imaging (MRI), EEG findings of spike and slow wave activity associated with periodic complexes, the detection of virus specific antibodies in CSF and blood, and the detection of herpes simplex virus DNA by the polymerase chain reaction (PCR). Treatment is with antiviral drugs; acyclovir has a low toxicity, inhibits DNA synthases, and results in a substantial reduction in mortality rate (20%). Patients with herpes simplex encephalitis are often critically ill with impaired consciousness, raised ICP, and seizures that are difficult to control; respiratory insufficiency is not uncommon.

Bacterial meningitis

The incidence of bacterial meningitis is 5–10 cases per 100 000 per annum. The diagnosis is based on the presence of symptoms and signs of meningism—headache, stiff neck, vomiting, impaired consciousness level, and the detection of micro-organisms in the CSF. The laboratory diagnosis requires support by CSF microscopy, demonstrating the presence of white blood cells—predominantly polymorphs, as well as Gram stain smears and culture for bacterial pathogens. Bacterial antigen can also be detected using latex agglutination methods. It has recently been shown that components of bacterial cell walls initiate the production of cytokines including tumour necrosis factor and interleukin-1β within the CSF, all of which have

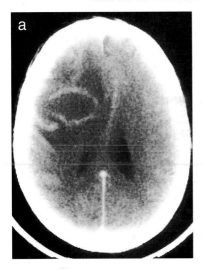
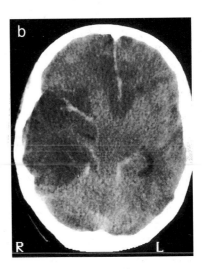

Fig 2.2 CT scan of biopsy proven herpes simplex encephalitis: heterogeneous changes in temporal lobes on MRI indicative of herpes simplex encephalitis: (a) 37 year old woman with history of confusion and seizures. CT scan suggests early swelling of right temporal lobe; (b) 72 hours later, CT scan shows marked changes in right temporal and both cingulate gyri

neurotoxic properties. Cerebral oedema may also result from these changes, as well as obstruction to CSF pathways; this, in turn, results in raised ICP. The common organisms encountered in clinical practice are *Haemophilus influenzae* and *Streptococcus pneumoniae*, *Neisseria meningitidis*, and *Listeria monocytogenes*. Management necessitates an adequate and appropriate antibiotic regimen, dependent on the organism isolated, and intensive care support in patients with a significantly impaired consciousness level. In spite of improvements in antibacterial therapy the mortality rate from bacterial meningitis is still significant, being as high as 20% in adults. The complications of meningitis are also significant, sensorineural deafness occurring in between 10% and 20% of surviving children.[10]

Chronic meningitis

Chronic meningitis produces a meningoencephalitic syndrome which develops over many months or weeks; in the CSF there is generally a lymphocytosis. Patients present with fatigue, headache, a low grade temperature, cranial nerve palsies, focal neurological deficit, seizures, and dementia. Left untreated, complications such as brain oedema, hydrocephalus, and secondary vasculitis develop. The most common cause of chronic meningitis is tuberculosis, usually as a reactivation of previous infection; other organisms such as mycoplasmas, legionellas, *Brucella* sp., and fungi such as aspergilli and cryptococci can present in this manner. The diagnosis is

35

suggested by an increase in white cells in the CSF (lymphocytes), depression of CSF glucose, and elevation of CSF protein. In fungal infection a chest radiograph may show concomitant lung disease; in tuberculous meningitis it may show evidence of previous pulmonary tuberculosis. An MRI scan, with gadolinium enhancement, will demonstrate accentuation of basal meninges. The investigation of these patients is complex and should follow a rigid protocol to ensure that no rare form of chronic meningitis is overlooked. The necessity for exhaustive investigation is supported by the fact that each infection carries its own specific treatment and, if untreated, death is inevitable. Also the longer the delay until diagnosis the higher the probability that recovery will be incomplete.[11]

Human immunodeficiency virus

Neurological involvement is a major feature of infection with human immunodeficiency virus (HIV), more than 50% of patients developing a neurological complication during the course of the illness, often as the initial manifestation. A study at Johns Hopkins Hospital (Baltimore) found that 3% of all critically ill patients were infected with human immunodeficiency virus. Neurological manifestations usually occur in full blown AIDS, although some subtle symptomatology can occur earlier at seroconversion. The most common problems encountered are those of opportunistic infection, toxoplasmosis being the most frequent. Other infections, such as those from *Mycobacterium tuberculosis*, *Cryptococcus*, and *Listeria* spp., however, can develop, as can CNS lymphoma. HIV is not only a lymphotrophic virus, it is also neurotrophic; it can therefore give rise directly to neurological syndromes, the most common of which is AIDS related dementia.

Toxoplasmosis

Toxoplasmosis occurs in between 10% and 20% of AIDS patients; it results from reactivation of dormant infection in individuals who have previously had toxoplasmosis. The condition develops subacutely over a matter of days, the clinical picture depending on lesion site. Usually there is a combination of focal neurological disturbance associated with diffuse encephalitic symptoms. Cranial imaging is highly suggestive, showing multiple areas of ring enhancement (fig 2.3). Lymphoma often cannot, however, be excluded with certainty and serological tests are often unhelpful. As a consequence, when CNS toxoplasmosis is suspected, treatment is started and imaging repeated after 2–4 weeks. If there is no clinical improvement then stereotactic brain biopsy should be performed on an accessible lesion to discriminate from lymphoma or other infection.

Tumours

Introduction

There are significant differences between primary tumours of the nervous

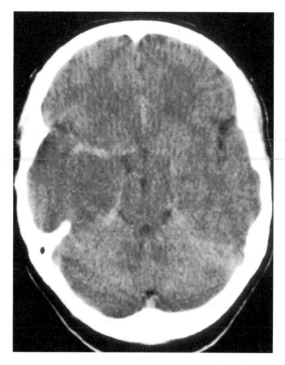

Fig 2.3 CT scan with contrast: biopsy proven toxoplasmosis: 55 year old HIV positive man with encephalopathy, hemiplegia, and seizures. There is a ring enhancing lesion

system and tumours encountered in other organs. Most systemic tumours are divisible into those with benign or malignant behaviour, but this division is not so readily applied to primary brain tumours. In part this is because benign tumours in other organs tend to be well demarcated from the surrounding tissue and are often encapsulated, whereas even those primary brain tumours with a low growth rate tend to have ill defined margins with diffuse infiltration of surrounding tissue by individual tumour cells. As a direct consequence of this it is rarely possible to excise even such slowly growing tumours by surgery, and they often recur. At the other end of the spectrum those primary brain tumours with a high growth rate are rarely truly "malignant" because systemic metastases are exceptionally rare, although such tumours can spread to distant sites in the central nervous system by seeding through CSF pathways (medulloblastoma, ependymoma, and germ cell tumour are particularly prone to do this). As a consequence of these differences primary brain tumours in general are best regarded as occurring in a spectrum ranging from "low grade" to "high grade."

Nervous system tumours are classified largely on the basis of their appearance through the light microscope and the current classification is that drawn up on behalf of the World Health Organization and published in 1993.[12] In this classification tumours with different degrees of malignancy are referred to by name or by a number with I denoting very low grade behaviour and IV denoting high grade behaviour (WHO grades I–IV). Particular care is needed to avoid confusion when a number is used to describe the grade of a tumour, because historically many classification systems have been used for tumours of the nervous system, some of which use only three grades rather than four.

In general the name of the tumour relates to the similarity of the appearance of the tumour cells under the light microscope to that of a normal mature cell or developing cell type.[13–17] The most common tumours are those that resemble glial cells and as a group are known as "glial tumours" or "gliomas;" according to their resemblance to normal glial cell types, they are divided into astrocytoma, oligodendroglioma, and ependymoma.

The presence on neuroimaging of multiple tumour deposits in the central nervous system usually indicates metastatic disease. Primary brain tumours, particularly gliomas and lymphomas, can, however, occasionally appear multifocal as a result of either CSF metastasis with reinvasion of brain or multiple foci of solid tumour within an extensive area of diffusely infiltrated brain. As a further consideration, multiple primary tumours can occur in those patients with a genetic predisposition to neoplasia, for example, neurofibromatosis or von Hippel–Lindau syndrome.

Pathogenesis

In general little is known about the pathogenesis of primary tumours of the nervous system, and this is particularly true of the more common tumours, including gliomas and meningiomas. Oncogene abnormalities, for example, of the p53 gene, certainly occur in some gliomas, although the role of such abnormalities in the pathogenesis of these tumours is not yet clear. It is known, however, that an inherited abnormality of the p53 oncogene can result in the familial occurrence of gliomas in association with tumours outside the nervous system (Li–Fraumeni syndrome). Inherited genetic predisposition to tumours of the nervous system is also seen in the context of neurofibromatosis (particularly peripheral nerve sheath tumours and gliomas) and von Hippel–Lindau syndrome (haemangioblastomas).

The potential roles of oncogenic viruses and other environmental influences in the pathogenesis of tumours of the nervous system are poorly understood. Epstein–Barr virus genome has, however, been identified in lymphomas and is suggested to play a causal role in the genesis of these tumours. Immunological factors also appear to play a role because lymphomas are particularly common in immunosuppressed individuals, including those with AIDS. X-irradiation is a further environmental influence which seems to be of importance because meningiomas occasionally occur at the margins of radiotherapy fields several years after treatment for a different tumour.

Incidence

Primary tumours of the nervous system are relatively rare, accounting for about 1% of all tumours occurring in adults. It is probable that metastatic tumours in the brain are more common than primary tumours, although patients with metastases may not be referred to a neurosurgical centre. It is of particular note that medulloblastoma is the most common solid tumour of childhood, accounting for 3–4% of deaths in this age group.

Effects of nervous system tumours

The pathophysiological effects of such tumours are largely the consequence of a number of special features relating to the nervous system:

1 As a result of the localisation of function to defined anatomical regions within the central nervous system, pathological lesions frequently produce focal neurological deficits.
2 As a consequence of the electrical excitability of adjacent neurons tumours can result in seizures.
3 The brain is enclosed in a bony box of fixed volume and therefore an intracranial space occupying lesion is associated with an increase in ICP. As a result there is a decrease in cerebral blood flow and internal herniations may occur, generating brain stem compression and interference with vital cardiorespiratory functions.
4 Finally, tumours, particularly those located near the ventricular system such as ependymomas, disturb the flow of CSF and may cause hydrocephalus.

Tumour biopsy

When a focal lesion has been identified on a CT or MRI scan a clinical decision is made whether or not it is appropriate to obtain a biopsy for a tissue diagnosis. Different neuroscience centres vary widely in their approach to this question, with some taking the view that all such lesions warrant a tissue diagnosis, whereas others are more conservative. Once the decision to obtain tissue has been made there are a number of alternative surgical approaches. A small tissue sample may be obtained by passing a needle freehand through a burr hole in the skull. Increasingly, needle biopsies are performed using stereotactic coordinates obtained from a CT or MRI scan. Particularly if the patient is experiencing problems with raised ICP, it may be appropriate to perform a craniotomy with a combination of open biopsy and debulking of the space occupying lesion. Spinal extradural tumours may be sampled with a needle whereas intradural tumours usually require a laminectomy and direct visualisation.

Intraoperative diagnosis

In dealing with nervous system tumours it is frequently of benefit to obtain a tissue diagnosis during the course of the surgical procedure. Intraoperative diagnosis allows possible modification of the course of the operation. For example, not infrequently intraoperative examination of tissue biopsies reveals normal or reactive brain or simply necrotic debris, and further sampling of the lesion by the neurosurgeon is recommended. In addition, further laboratory investigation of the tissue may be planned. For example, it may be suspected that electron microscopy will be diagnostically helpful and tissue should be fixed in glutaraldehyde—the optimal fixative for electron microscopy. If DNA analysis is likely to be helpful then fresh, unfixed tissue should be stored frozen. In the small proportion of cases in which a specific diagnosis cannot be made intraoperatively, it is often possible to be able to say that the tumour is of low or high grade, that it is likely to be primary or secondary, or simply that tumour tissue has been obtained which will allow a diagnosis to be made on subsequent histological examination of paraffin sections.

Non-neoplastic pathology may also be identified by intraoperative examination and recognition of this often influences the appropriate handling of the material. For example, if inflammatory tissue is identified it is recommended that fresh tissue be supplied to the microbiology department. Non-tumour pathology, which may be recognised or suspected on intraoperative examination of specimens, includes bacterial, fungal, and tuberculous abscesses, viral encephalitis, multiple sclerosis plaques, infarcts, and, on occasion, progressive multifocal encephalopathy or toxoplasmosis—these last two being of particular importance in AIDS.

To obtain the maximum possible information from a neurosurgical biopsy and to lessen the risk of a non-diagnostic biopsy, good communications between the neurosurgical operating room and the pathology laboratory are essential. Ideally the laboratory is informed in advance when an intraoperative diagnosis is likely to be required. Information that is of help to the pathologist when assessing the microscopic appearances of the specimen include the age and sex of the patient, the clinical history, a previous history of neoplastic disease, including tumours outside the nervous system, a family history of neoplasia, the site of the lesion, and the scan and macroscopic appearances of the tumour.

Histological examination on paraffin section

Most of the tissue remaining after preparation of a smear or frozen section will be fixed in formalin and processed for subsequent histological examination by embedding in paraffin wax. Sections of the paraffin wax embedded tissue are available to be examined 24–48 hours after the operation. The sections are stained with a variety of methods to highlight different structural features in the tissue, the most commonly used stain being haematoxylin and eosin. As the classification of tumours of the nervous system depends largely on recognition of morphological features of tumour cells under the light microscope, such preparations are the backbone of the diagnostic process. The following methods provide additional information.

Immunohistochemistry

The recognition of specific antigens possessed by tumour cells is often of great help in determining the type of tumour. This is particularly so when the tumour biopsy is small, as is often the case, or when the tumour is poorly differentiated. These antigens are recognised by applying specific antibodies to the paraffin embedded tissue sections, followed by the application of a detection system to identify whether or not, and to which cells in the tissue section, the antibody has bound. Antibodies that are of particular use include those to glial fibrillary acidic protein (GFAP—present in most glial tumours) and cytokeratin (usually present in metastatic carcinoma). Specific antibodies also aid in the recognition of neuronal tumours, melanomas, and lymphomas. Antibodies are available to the protein products of oncogenes (for example, p53), although these have not yet been shown to yield information of prognostic value. Specific antibodies are also available to proteins present only in proliferating cells and these may aid in assessing the growth rate of tumours.

Nucleic acid analysis

It seems likely that the demonstration of oncogene abnormalities in tumours will be useful as an indication of prognosis and future classifications of tumours may even be based on such analyses. PCR enables the relevant information to be obtained by generating multiple copies of specific DNA fragments of interest, such as part of an oncogene. Detection of mRNA allows analysis of tumour cell gene expression and this can also be performed by PCR or *in situ* hybridisation.

Electron microscopy

Although largely superseded by immunohistochemistry, electron microscopy still plays a role in the analysis of nervous system tumours. It can, for example, be of use in identifying neuronal differentiation in a tumour.

Classification of nervous system tumours

As mentioned above, tumours are classified largely according to the resemblance of the tumour cells to normal cell types. The cells comprising the central nervous system are principally glial cells (astrocytes, oligodendrocytes, and ependymal cells) and neurons, and consequently many nervous system tumours fall into the categories of astrocytic, oligodendroglial, ependymal, and neuronal tumours. Although some tumours may occur at almost any site within the central nervous system (for example, astrocytoma), others are restricted in their distribution (for example, central neurocytoma). The types of tumour that occur most frequently at specific anatomical locations are shown in table 2.3.

Astrocytic tumours

"Ordinary" astrocytic tumours

The term "ordinary" astrocytic tumours may be used to encompass a group comprising astrocytoma, anaplastic astrocytoma, and glioblastoma. This group contains the most common primary brain tumours. The tumour cells possess cytoplasmic processes containing GFAP. They are diffusely infiltrating tumours which exist in a continuous spectrum of malignancy. Histological grading imposes artificial divisions in this continuous spectrum and, although grading poses a number of problems in practical terms, it provides a useful guide to prognosis and the selection of appropriate therapy. The problems with grading such tumours are as follows:

1 Numerous different grading systems have been applied to astrocytic tumours in the past and confusion can exist between the various systems.
2 A tumour biopsy often provides only a small proportion of the whole tumour for analysis, and this act of sampling raises problems as a result of the non-uniformity of astrocytic tumours.
3 Astrocytic tumours frequently do not remain static in terms of grade but tend to increase in malignancy with time.

It can be seen therefore that it is important to use all the information available in the analysis of an astrocytic tumour. For example, contrast enhancement of a tumour on computed tomography or MRI suggests that the tumour is likely to be of high grade even if the features of a high grade tumour are not present in a small tumour biopsy.

The current WHO grading system is based essentially on the presence or absence of four histological variables: nuclear atypia (that is, variation in the size and staining intensity of tumour cell nuclei), mitoses, proliferation of vascular endothelial cells, and tumour necrosis.

Astrocytoma

Astrocytoma is defined histologically by the presence of nuclear atypia alone or of the four features mentioned above. The most common variant of astrocytoma is the fibrillary astrocytoma which occurs typically in the cerebral hemispheres of young adults and tends to be centred on the white matter. CT and MRI scans usually show an ill defined, low density lesion without contrast enhancement. Macroscopically these tumours may be difficult to distinguish from surrounding brain. They have a homogeneous

Table 2.3   Types of tumours that occur most frequently at specific anatomical locations

Anatomical region	Adults	Children/adolescents
Cerebrum	Astrocytoma Anaplastic astrocytoma Glioblastoma Oligodendroglioma Ependymoma Lymphoma Metastatic tumour Meningioma	Astrocytoma Anaplastic astrocytoma Ependymoma Neuroblastoma (PNET) Neuronal tumour Oligodendroglioma
Lateral ventricle	Central neurocytoma Ependymoma Choroid plexus tumour Subependymoma Meningioma	Ependymoma Choroid plexus tumour Central neurocytoma
Third ventricle	Colloid cyst Ependymoma	
Around the third ventricle	Astrocytoma Anaplastic astrocytoma Glioblastoma Oligodendroglioma Ependymoma	Pilocytic astrocytoma
Pineal region	Pineal parenchymal tumour Germ cell tumour Glial tumour	Pineal parenchymal tumour Germ cell tumour Glial tumour
Pituitary fossa and suprasellar region	Pituitary adenoma Craniopharyngioma Meningioma Germ cell tumour	Craniopharyngioma Germ cell tumour
Brain stem	Astrocytoma Anaplastic astrocytoma Glioblastoma	Pilocytic astrocytoma
Cerebellum	Metastatic tumour Medulloblastoma (PNET) Haemangioblastoma Astrocytoma	Medulloblastoma (PNET) Pilocytic astrocytoma
Fourth ventricle	Ependymoma Subependymoma Choroid plexus tumour	Ependymoma Choroid plexus tumour
Cerebellopontine angle tumour	Acoustic schwannoma Meningioma Epidermoid cyst	
Spinal tumours Extradural	Metastatic tumour Myeloma Nerve sheath tumour	Metastatic tumour
Intradural extramedullary	Meningioma Nerve sheath tumour	Developmental cysts
Intradural intramedullary	Ependymoma Astrocytoma Myxopapillary ependymoma	Astrocytoma

PNET, primitive neuroectodermal tumour.

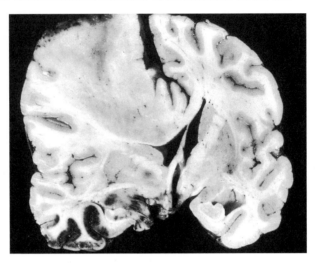

Fig 2.4 A fibrillary astrocytoma involving the superior parietal region in the left cerebral hemisphere. The tumour has an ill defined margin and is diffusely infiltrating cortex and white matter. It has a homogeneous appearance without haemorrhage or necrosis. There is a marked space occupying effect with shift of the midline to the right

appearance, may contain cysts, are abnormally firm in texture, and show a tendency to diffuse infiltration of pre-existing anatomical structures (fig 2.4). In a small biopsy, astrocytoma may be difficult to distinguish histologically from a reactive proliferation of astrocytes. Therapy may involve surgery, although excision is almost certain to be incomplete because of diffuse infiltration by tumour cells of surrounding structures that are still functioning. It is not clear whether radiotherapy is of benefit.

Even these low grade "ordinary" astrocytomas are not regarded as "benign" because all recur postoperatively and most, if not all, eventually undergo transformation to anaplastic astrocytoma or glioblastoma. The mean survival of patients with an astrocytoma is in the region of eight years.

Other variants include the protoplasmic astrocytoma which is usually centred on grey matter. A further variant is the gemistocytic astrocytoma which more readily undergoes anaplastic change than either fibrillary or protoplasmic astrocytomas.

Anaplastic astrocytoma

Anaplastic astrocytoma is defined by the presence of nuclear atypia and mitoses, but without endothelial cell proliferation or necrosis. The peak incidence of such tumours is in the fifth decade of life. Anaplastic astrocytomas do not show contrast enhancement on CT or MRI scan. The histological differential diagnosis is that of a "missed" glioblastoma, referring to absence in a small biopsy of the additional features required to make that diagnosis. The mean survival for patients with an anaplastic astrocytoma is in the region of 2–3 years.

Glioblastoma

Glioblastoma is defined by the presence of all four histological features: nuclear atypia, mitoses, endothelial cell proliferation, and tumour necrosis. Glioblastoma is by far the most common glial tumour and may be derived from malignant transformation of a pre-existing astrocytoma or may arise *de novo* as a high grade tumour. Glioblastomas occur most commonly in patients over the age of 50 years.

CT and MRI scans typically show a central low density area with "ring" enhancement and surrounding oedema. The radiological contrast enhancement may correspond to the presence of endothelial cell proliferation. The differential diagnosis from the clinical and radiological point of view may be that of an abscess and of a metastasis. Macroscopically glioblastomas are firm in texture, and white or yellow in colour, with areas of haemorrhage and necrosis (fig 2.5). Although macroscopically the tumour may appear well circumscribed, on microscopic examination there is nearly always diffuse infiltration of tumour cells beyond the macroscopic margin. CSF dissemination of the tumour may occur, but metastasis outside the central nervous system is very rare. Treatment usually involves radiotherapy, sometimes combined with debulking of the tumour to reduce its space occupying effect. The mean survival for patients with glioblastoma is one year or less.

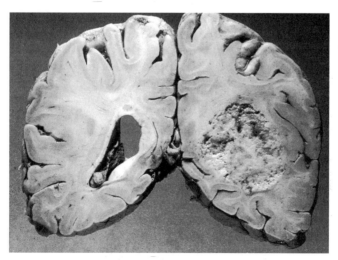

Fig 2.5 A glioblastoma obliterating the lateral ventricle in the right cerebral hemisphere. The tumour contains areas of haemorrhage and necrosis. In this case there is little evidence of space occupying effect, the patient having died from an unrelated cause

Variants include gliosarcoma which is a mixed tumour with both malignant glial and sarcomatous components. This tumour is usually superficially located, well circumscribed, and tough in texture. The clinical outcome is similar to that for glioblastoma.

Other astrocytic tumours

Pilocytic astrocytomas occur in childhood and adolescence and are typically located in the cerebellum, pons, around the third ventricle, or in the optic nerves and chiasma. They are defined histologically by the presence of "hair like" cells with bipolar processes and Rosenthal fibres. Such tumours are of very low grade; they do not tend to recur postoperatively and do not undergo anaplastic change.

Pleomorphic xanthoastrocytoma and subependymal giant cell astrocytoma are both variants which in spite of their bizarre cytology behave as low grade neoplasms. Pleomorphic xanthoastrocytoma typically occurs in a superficial location in the cerebral hemispheres whereas subependymal giant cell astrocytoma is an intraventricular tumour which often occurs in the context of tuberous sclerosis.

Oligodendroglial tumours

Oligodendroglial tumours often appear macroscopically well circumscribed and microcalcification within the tumour or at the tumour margin is common. There is no widely agreed formal grading system for these tumours; however, low cell density and the presence of microcysts have been identified as favourable histological features. The WHO classification allows division into oligodendroglioma and anaplastic (malignant) oligodendroglioma. There is a poor correlation between the histological features of oligodendrogliomas and their biological behaviour. Prolonged survival, sometimes for decades, may occur.

Ependymal tumours

Ependymoma

Ependymomas are composed of cells which are reminiscent of the ependymal cells that line the ventricles. They are frequently located adjacent to the ventricular system and may protrude into the cavity of the ventricle. The fourth ventricle is a common site for such tumours, particularly in childhood, and they may also occur in the spinal cord. Ependymal tumours are divided on histological grounds into ependymoma and anaplastic (malignant) ependymoma, the second being prone to dissemination via the CSF.

Myxopapillary ependymoma

This variant occurs at the lower end of the spinal cord and involves the

46

cauda equina. The characteristic histological features are a papillary architecture and the presence of mucin. These neoplasms are of very low grade and are essentially benign.

Subependymoma

This firm lobulated benign tumour protrudes into a ventricular cavity and, although most are asymptomatic, they may present by causing disturbance of CSF flow.

Gliomatosis cerebri

This uncommon glial neoplasm is characterised by very widespread involvement of different parts of the central nervous system without foci of solid tumour. Clinical diagnosis is difficult and a diagnosis is not usually made on biopsy. As a consequence this entity is usually only recognised on postmortem examination of the brain.

Neuronal and mixed neuronal/glial tumours

This group of tumours contains a number of different variants most of which behave as low grade or very low grade neoplasms. Of particular note is the central neurocytoma, a well circumscribed tumour which occurs in the lateral ventricle. In the past this tumour has been mistaken for an oligodendroglioma as a result of an almost identical light macroscopic appearance; however, it is now identified with certainty by demonstration of neuronal differentiation by immunohistochemistry or electron microscopy.

Primitive neuroectodermal tumours

The category of primitive neuroectodermal tumours (PNET) includes tumours that occur in the cerebellum (medulloblastoma), cerebral hemispheres (neuroblastoma), and the pineal gland (pineoblastoma). Although grouping these tumours together under this heading is contentious they have a number of features in common, including occurrence early in life, the potential for both glial and neuronal differentiation, and highly malignant behaviour with a particular tendency to metastasise via the CSF. By far the most common of these tumours is the medulloblastoma, usually arising in the midline of the cerebellum. Although the biological behaviour of this tumour indicates a high degree of malignancy, therapeutic regimens, including surgery, radiotherapy, and chemotherapy, have been relatively successful.

Choroid plexus tumours

The choroid plexus lies within the ventricular system and secretes the CSF. Choroid plexus tumours therefore have an intraventricular location and may be benign (papilloma) or malignant (carcinoma).

47

Tumours of cranial and spinal nerves

Schwannoma

This benign encapsulated tumour is composed of cells resembling the normal Schwann cells which provide the myelin sheath for peripheral nerve axons. Schwannomas may arise from any cranial or spinal nerve, and the nerve of origin may be seen stretched over the surface of the tumour. They arise most commonly from cranial nerve VIII (the acoustic nerve). Most schwannomas occur sporadically in patients with no apparent genetic predisposition, although individuals with neurofibromatosis often have schwannomas, which may be multiple.

Neurofibroma

In a neurofibroma, in contrast to a schwannoma, the peripheral nerve fibres are diffusely distributed throughout the tumour which is composed of perineural cells and fibroblasts in addition to Schwann cells. This neoplasm is virtually pathognomonic of neurofibromatosis.

Malignant peripheral nerve sheath tumours

These tumours are assumed to arise *de novo* or by transformation of a neurofibroma. Malignant change in a schwannoma is exceptionally rare. Malignant peripheral nerve sheath tumours recur locally and may metastasise.

Meningioma

Meningiomas arise from arachnoidal cells which are situated in the meninges overlying the brain and spinal cord. These tumours are usually entirely benign and well circumscribed and indent the adjacent brain or spinal cord (fig 2.6). Although excision of most meningiomas is curative, even histologically benign meningiomas may penetrate the dura and infiltrate the surrounding bone. Rarely meningiomas occur as a diffuse plate like thickening of the meninges ("meningioma en plaque"). On occasion meningiomas may arise in the choroid plexus, presenting as an intraventricular mass. Anaplastic (malignant) meningiomas occur infrequently and, although these tend not to metastasise systemically, they demonstrate more aggressive local recurrence.

A wide range of other tumours may also be located in the meninges. Of particular note is the haemangiopericytoma which is essentially identical to the tumour of the same name occurring elsewhere in the body, being malignant in behaviour with the potential to metastasise systemically.

Malignant meningitis

Extensive involvement of the subarachnoid space by a malignant neoplasm may occur, with tumour cells spreading through the CSF. This situation may

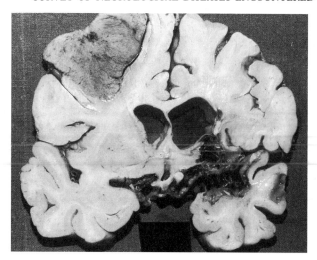

Fig 2.6 A meningioma arising from the meninges overlying the convexity of the left cerebral hemisphere. The tumour is well circumscribed and is indenting the surface of the brain

occur with both primary brain tumours (particularly PNET, ependymoma, glioblastoma, and germ cell tumours) and by metastatic spread of tumour from elsewhere in the body (for example, carcinoma and melanoma). Confirmation of the clinical suspicion of malignant meningitis can be made by cytological examination of a sample of CSF and identification of malignant cells. In many cases recognition of tumour cell antigens by immunocytochemistry can identify the nature of the tumour involving the meninges.

Lymphoma

Lymphoma can occur either as a primary tumour of the central nervous system or as a metastasis from a systemic lymphoma. Most primary neoplasms are non-Hodgkin's B cell lymphomas. These tumours have a particular tendency to occur in immunosuppressed patients, including those with AIDS, and there is evidence that they are increasing in incidence in many parts of the world. Primary CNS lymphomas may be single or multiple and sometimes occur with a periventricular distribution.

Germ cell tumours

Primary intracranial germ cell tumours occur most commonly in children and young adults, predominantly in the midline in the pineal and suprasellar regions. The histological appearance and the classification of these tumours are essentially identical to those occurring in the testis (germinoma, yolk sac

49

tumour, choriocarcinoma, and teratoma). Mixed germ cell tumours may occur and a small biopsy may not reveal the full spectrum of differentiation within a tumour. An important part of the investigation of germ cell tumours therefore involves examination of CSF and peripheral blood for substances which may be secreted by germ cell tumours (for example, α-fetoprotein and human chorionic gonadotrophin). Response to therapeutic regimens varies, with germinoma being particularly radiosensitive.

Cysts

A variety of cysts of presumed developmental origin may occur in different sites. The classification of these lesions is largely based on the histological appearance of the cyst lining and the anatomical location of the lesion. For example, Rathke cleft cysts are lined by an epithelium resembling that of the respiratory tract and arise in the pituitary fossa. Colloid cysts occur in the third ventricle and, as their name suggests, they contain gelatinous material. Epidermoid and dermoid cysts are lined by a stratified squamous epithelium which produces keratin. Enterogenous cysts are lined by epithelium resembling that of the gastrointestinal tract and occur in the spinal cord. Neuroglial cysts are lined by neuroglial tissue. Congenital arachnoidal cysts are mainly diagnosed on the occasion of an epileptic seizure. Generally they do not increase in size and in this case they should not be operated on. Only if there is evidence of midline structure shift is surgical evacuation or drainage indicated.

Tumours of the sellar region

Pituitary adenoma

These are benign tumours of the anterior pituitary gland and may secrete anterior pituitary gland hormones—growth hormone, prolactin, adrenocorticotrophic hormone (ACTH), luteinising hormone (LH), follicle stimulating hormone (FSH), or thyroid stimulating hormone (TSH), or commonly a combination of hormones. These secretory tumours most commonly present while small in size with endocrine disturbance (for example, acromegaly, Cushing's disease, or infertility). In contrast, non-secretory pituitary adenomas tend to present when they are larger and protrude upwards out of the pituitary fossa, compressing the optic chiasma from below.

Malignant tumours of the anterior pituitary gland (pituitary carcinoma) are exceptionally rare, but such tumours, with metastatic deposits, have been described.

Craniopharyngioma

This benign tumour is composed of epithelial cells and is located in the suprasellar region. Cysts within the tumour containing brown cholesterol laden fluid commonly occur. In spite of the histologically benign nature of this lesion, complete excision is often impossible as a result of tumour penetration or envelopment of vital structures at the base of the brain, and local recurrence is therefore common.

Extradural tumours

Primary tumours arising in the bone of the skull or spinal column may impinge on components of the nervous system. Of particular note is the chordoma which is a tumour arising from remnants of the primitive notochord, and occurs usually in the base of the skull or the sacrum. This tumour is of low grade malignancy and repeated local recurrence is common. Cartilaginous tumours, either benign (chondroma) or malignant (chondrosarcoma), may also arise in bone.

Metastatic tumours

Many malignant tumours arising in other organs may metastasise to involve the nervous system (fig 2.7). In neurosurgical centres metastatic tumours are usually encountered when, following neurological presentation, a single lesion is identified in the brain in the absence of a known systemic primary tumour. The tumour may then be removed or biopsied and the results indicate the likely source of origin of the metastasis. Pancranial radiotherapy should be considered. Metastatic deposits are typically well demarcated from the surrounding brain. Metastatic carcinomas often have

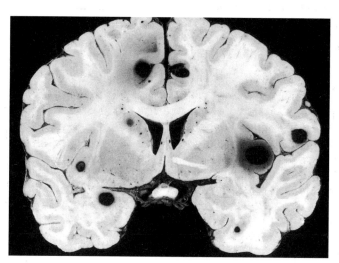

Fig 2.7 Numerous well circumscribed, deeply pigmented metastases from a cutaneous melanoma scattered throughout both cerebral hemispheres

51

necrotic centres, whereas metastatic melanoma may be pigmented and has a tendency to undergo haemorrhage. The most commonly encountered metastatic carcinomas arise from the bronchus, gastrointestinal tract, and breast.

Neurological complications in critically ill patients

So far we have addressed the neurological disorders that result in the need for intensive care support. Intensive care patients will often, however, develop various neurological problems as a consequence of critical illness. Encephalopathy and myelopathy may result from hypoxic–ischaemic insult, peripheral neuropathy may result in vitamin deficiency from drug usage or the Guillain–Barré syndrome occurring in a critically ill person, and finally there is increasing awareness of critical illness polyneuropathy. This condition affects at least 50% of patients who have been in an intensive care unit for a period in excess of two weeks, the first and occasionally the only sign being that of weakness of respiratory muscles which is manifested as difficulty in weaning from mechanical ventilation. Usually this is associated with some degree of limb weakness and tendon reflexes that cannot be elicited. Neurophysiological investigations demonstrate features suggestive of an axonal neuropathy. The mechanism for this condition is unknown, but a disorder of axonal transport systems is postulated which may be triggered by a septic syndrome. The neuropathy does not appear to have a nutritional basis and generally improves with the passage of time, although clearly it may hinder rehabilitation from a serious illness.[18]

Muscle wasting often accompanies prolonged sepsis and may again contribute towards respiratory weakness, even leading to respiratory failure. Whether this muscle weakness and wasting reflect a primary muscle disorder or whether they are a consequence of denervation atrophy remains uncertain.

Finally the term "septic encephalopathy" refers to altered brain function occurring as a consequence of overwhelming infection; this may have a complex metabolic explanation or, alternatively, may be the result of a secondarily acquired vasculitis.

Ischaemic brain damage

Irreversible ischaemic brain damage can occur whenever there is an insufficient supply of oxygen to nerve cells. It may, therefore, happen as a consequence of such diverse conditions as respiratory obstruction, shock, epilepsy, cardiac arrest, or an episode of severe hypotension, and is a potential hazard to any patient undergoing general anaesthesia. The clinical outcome will be determined by the severity and duration of the ischaemic insult and whether or not adequate resuscitation was started before brain damage became irreversible. Crises of this kind are not uncommon in clinical practice and yet the fundamental question as to what constitutes a critical insult, which represents the threshold between recovery and permanent brain damage in humans, remains uncertain. This is caused by a lack of adequate physiological information at the time of the emergency and the inadequate neuropathological examination of brains from fatal cases.

The final common pathway by which irreversible brain damage occurs is a reduction in the content of oxygen in the blood and reduced blood flow to the brain, often in combination. Each is provided by the functions of respiration and circulation, certain aspects of which need to be considered before the various patterns of ischaemic brain damage found in the neuroanaesthetic intensive care unit are described.

Circulation

The brain of the normal adult receives some 15% of the cardiac output. This represents a mean blood flow to the brain of about 50 ml/100 g per min in the adult and about twice as much in children aged six years. The important relationship between perfusion pressure and cerebral blood flow (CBF) is governed principally by the phenomenon of autoregulation, that is, CBF remains relatively constant in spite of moderate variations in perfusion pressure. Essentially it is an intrinsic phenomenon resulting from an interaction of metabolic and myogenic factors which may, however, be modified by extrinsic elements such as perivascular nerves in the cerebral vasculature.[19]

In humans, CBF remains constant within the pressure range 8·7–18·7 kPa (65–140 mm Hg). The autoregulatory mechanism fails (lower limit) below 8·7 kPa (65 mm Hg) when the vessels are dilated; the flow then falls together with decreasing pressure. The signs and symptoms of cerebral ischaemia do not develop immediately because the brain compensates by increasing its extraction of oxygen. At high levels of arterial pressure a point is reached where cerebral vasoconstriction cannot be sustained as CBF increases (upper limit of autoregulation).

Blood flow through the brain essentially depends on two main factors, namely the pressure difference between its arteries and veins (cerebral perfusion pressure or CPP) and the resistance of the intervening vessels (cerebrovascular resistance or CVR). CVR is determined by the ICP ($<0·67$ kPa or 5 mm Hg normally), the viscosity of the blood, and the tone of the smooth muscle in the walls of the blood vessel. This muscle tone is influenced by the intracranial pressure, the tension of oxygen and carbon dioxide in the blood, and also its pH. As the pressure inside the cerebral veins is very close to that of the CSF or ICP, the CPP is commonly regarded as the difference between the mean systemic arterial pressure (MAP) and the ICP. The interactions between these two pressures are complex and a critical point is reached when the ICP rises to within about 5·9 kPa (44 mm Hg) of the mean systemic arterial pressure after which CBF falls.

Any factor altering the ability of the cerebral vessels to constrict or dilate interferes with autoregulation. If perfusion pressure falls, vasodilatation is greatest in the anastomotic vessels along the arterial boundary zones, which is the first region in which blood flow is reduced to a critical level. Studies using positron emission tomography in patients with carotid artery occlusion have established a sequence of events that take place as local cerebral perfusion pressure falls.[20] When compensatory vasodilatation is maximal autoregulation fails and CBF starts to decline. Local cerebral oxygen metabolism is then maintained for a short time by increased extraction of available oxygen. Once extraction of oxygen becomes maximal the further decrease in local CBF will result in a disruption of normal cellular metabolism and function. In general the Pa_{O_2} remains normal and dysfunction first becomes evident after a 50% reduction in CBF.[21 22] Experimental work has shown that at levels of about 30% of normal, the EEG becomes isoelectric and the evoked potential is lost. At CBF values of about 12–15% of normal, there is an efflux of potassium and an influx of calcium, but it is not until the CBF has been reduced to levels of about 10% normal that irreversible brain damage occurs. There is therefore an upper threshold of electrical failure and a lower threshold of energy failure and ion pump failure, which in focal ischaemia characterises a ring of tissue—the penumbra—around the core of irreversibly damaged brain, in which energy failure and ion pump failure have developed. The tissue within the penumbra is therefore non-functioning but still viable and may recover fully using a variety of neuroprotective measures.[23]

Respiration

As a result of the close coupling between cerebral function and the production of adenosine triphosphate (ATP), the overall energy metabolism of the brain can be deduced from the amount of oxygen or glucose consumed. In many studies in normal adult resting subjects the cerebral metabolic rate of oxygen (CMR_{O_2}) is between 3·2 and 3·8 ml O_2/100 g per min with higher values in children.

The respiratory quotient (RQ or CO_2/O_2) of the brain is almost unity indicating that glucose is virtually the sole source of energy by oxidation. The oxygen content of blood falls from 19·6 ml/dl to 12·9 ml/dl while passing through the brain, and the carbon dioxide content rises from 48·2 ml/dl in arterial blood to 54·8 ml/dl in the internal jugular vein.

Various studies have shown that, if normal CBF is maintained, the metabolism and function of the brain are affected only when Pa_{O_2} falls below 6·7 kPa (50 mm Hg), when there is a rapid loss of critical judgment, progressive impairment of performance, and clouding of consciousness leading to unconsciousness at a Pa_{O_2} of about 4 kPa (30 mm Hg). It is not until the Pa_{O_2} is reduced to below 2·67 kPa (20 mm Hg) for at least eight minutes that the EEG becomes isoelectric and irreversible brain damage ensues.

54

Cerebral energy supply

Energy is produced in the brain almost entirely from the oxidative metabolism of glucose. The amount of glucose consumed is high (0·3 mml/min or 60 mg/min), reflecting the inability of the brain, unlike other organs, to make use of more complex substrates. The oxidative metabolism of glucose yields 38 molecules of ATP which are used in the synthesis of large molecules, in transport mechanisms, in the maintenance of membrane potentials, and in neurotransmitter metabolism.

Risk factors

Given that irreversible ischaemic brain damage results largely from a reduction in cerebral perfusion, it is important to have some appreciation of the types of factors that put particular categories of patients at risk. Either singly or in combination, many of these factors operate by altering cerebral autoregulation, not only in areas of acute intracerebral pathology but also diffusely, including areas remote from such a lesion in the so called healthy parts of the brain. Some of these remote effects, at least in part, are mediated by the development of complications such as oedema, epilepsy, and as a result of the distortion and internal herniation that develop as a consequence of raised ICP and the development of internal herniation.

Age

The incidence of "stroke" rises rapidly with increasing age, some 80% of cases occurring in patients over 65 years.[24]

There have been many studies which have shown that there is a decline in CBF and oxygen consumption with increasing age, particularly over the age of 70 years. Such evidence, however, needs to be treated with some caution because the investigations have been carried out in a wide spectrum of patients with various disorders, for example, diabetes mellitus and hypertension, many of whom have been treated. It is possible therefore that the changes in CBF and metabolism are not purely a consequence of age and that other causes, including drugs, are the reasons for the reductions observed in most studies.

Nevertheless, there are a number of conditions in which there is clear cut evidence of increased risk from developing cerebral ischaemia.

Hypertension

In addition to abnormal cerebrovascular physiology, hypertension produces pathological changes including aggravation of atheroma, hyaline arteriosclerosis, lacunae, multi-infarct dementia, hypertensive encephalopathology, and intracerebral haemorrhage.[26]

It is now well established that the absolute value for CBF is the same in hypertensive and normotensive subjects. Hypertensive patients, however, are more susceptible to cerebral ischaemia than normotensive patients because they are less able to compensate for a fall in blood pressure. This is because hypertension profoundly influences CBF autoregulation by shifting both the lower and upper limits towards higher pressures. Such adaptation, once established, can be attributed to hypertensive structural changes in blood vessels, which, in the short term, may be reversible. In long standing hypertension, however, the changes are more likely to be permanent as a result of small blood vessel disease.

Diabetes mellitus

Autoregulation of CBF may be chronically impaired in patients with long term diabetes mellitus. This is true even after allowing for other factors, including hypertension and atheroma, and can result, among other things, from an increase in plasma viscosity and a reduced deformability of red blood cells. In patients in diabetic coma it is possible to demonstrate a dissociation of CBF and oxygen consumption; such abnormalities are, however, reversible with appropriate insulin therapy. There is often a heterogeneous response and it is not wholly clear whether this can be attributed to the diabetes or to commonly associated vascular changes. In general, autoregulatory responses to hypotension are thought to be well maintained.

Head injury

Ischaemic brain damage is common (about 90%) in patients who die after a non-missile head injury.[27] Its pathogenesis is not yet fully understood but it was significantly more common in patients who sustained a known clinical episode of hypoxia and/or a high ICP during life. Comparisons of a cohort of patients who died between 1968–72 and 1981–2 have shown that the institution of measures to maintain adequate airway and blood gases, and the prompt correction of hypotension by replacement of blood volume, has reduced the number of cases with infarction in the arterial boundary zones. The critical importance of additional ischaemic insults to an already damaged brain is increasingly being recognised.[28 29]

There are marked changes in autoregulation of CBF in patients with severe head injury. The flow patterns are often complex comprising both hypoperfusion and hyperperfusion, and some correlation with changes in the ICP. For example, in patients with intact autoregulation ICP decreases in response to a blood pressure increase as a consequence of the autoregulatory cerebral vasoconstriction. In contrast ICP increases or remains unchanged in response to an increase in blood pressure in those patients with widely altered autoregulation.

Non-haemorrhagic cerebrovascular disease

Atheroma of the extracranial and intracranial arteries is the most important disease affecting the carotid and vertebrobasilar arterial systems, and there are geographical differences in the formation of atheroma in that there is greater intracranial disease in Afro-Caribbean female patients and in the Japanese, than in white patients from Europe and North America.

Thromboembolic occlusion of the internal carotid artery has been found in between 2% and 4% in an unselected group of postmortem examinations, and there is a strong association between carotid occlusion and cerebral infarction, the size of any cerebral infarct depending on the efficiency of the collateral circulation and whether the thrombus has extended into the blood vessels in the base of the skull.[26]

Permanent occlusion or major stenosis in one or more of the large arteries of the neck may be symptomless.[30] This has been shown even if both internal carotid arteries are occluded. This results in only a moderate reduction of local blood pressure distal to the occlusion and in these instances the local blood pressure may be at, or slightly below, the lower limit of autoregulation, and CBF may be normal or is slightly reduced in the resting state. These patients are, however, at particular risk because, with a drop in systemic blood pressure, the local blood pressure is further reduced resulting in focal CBF decrease; symptoms of ischaemia may be provoked from the territory of the artery that is no longer protected by autoregulation.

Loss of CBF autoregulation is a common and well known event in acute ischaemic stroke. For example, in the ischaemic areas distal to an arterial occlusion, pressure within the arterial bed will be below the normal lower limit of autoregulation. More generalised changes are also present, usually resulting from tissue acidosis, and it has been shown that autoregulation is also present in tissue being reperfused following recanalisation of a previously occluded blood vessel. Under these circumstances, rises in systemic blood pressure, which are a part of reperfusion injury, may aggravate the development of brain oedema and damage to the blood–brain barrier, thereby provoking haemorrhagic transformation of a previously ischaemic infarct or even frank haematoma formation.

The vascular bed distal to occlusion of a tight stenosis has become adapted to low pressure so that sudden revascularisation might then result in local blood pressure above the upper limit of autoregulation until readaptation has taken place. The vascular bed under these circumstances is therefore vulnerable to "hypertensive" damage. This condition, called a "hyperperfusion syndrome," has been ascribed to the lack of effective autoregulation in the revascularised area with the induction of a break through phenomenon (above upper limit of autoregulation).

Subarachnoid haemorrhage

Many patients die within the first day of the haemorrhage and the mortality rate during the first week after subarachnoid haemorrhage is about 30%; about 45% die within the first three months. The risk of a further haemorrhage within one month is about 33% and has a 42% mortality rate,

57

being greatest between the fifth and ninth days. The immediate intracranial complications of a ruptured saccular aneurysm are usually a combination of massive intraventricular haemorrhage, subarachnoid haemorrhage, and intracerebral haematoma. Late intracranial complications include cerebral infarction and hydrocephalus. Cerebral infarction is commonly found in patients who die as a result of a ruptured saccular aneurysm.[31] Although an operation for clipping aneurysms may contribute to the infarction, the condition is also found in patients who have not undergone surgery. The cause of infarction may be multiple factors including vasospasm, arterial compression by haematomas, effects of raised intracranial pressure, surgical retraction and resection, and induced systemic hypotension during the operation.

Between 5% and 20% of patients with subarachnoid haemorrhage develop delayed ischaemic neurological symptoms; these patients often show angiographic evidence of severe narrowing of the intracranial vessels, often close to the source of the bleeding and at the densest location of the subarachnoid blood. Techniques using computed tomography to estimate the thickness and extent of subarachnoid blood have now been derived for the prediction of delayed cerebral ischaemia.

CBF studies in patients after subarachnoid haemorrhage have shown both global reductions which do not appear to be related to angiographic vasospasm and regional reductions in the CBF within the territories of vasospastic arteries. It is considered that the global depression in flow does not result directly from spasm but rather is related to a depressed metabolic rate. Clinical studies have shown that the cerebrovascular response to both carbon dioxide and changes in blood pressure is altered, and remains impaired even one week after the onset of the subarachnoid haemorrhage. Such patients are therefore at risk from either induced hypertension or hypotension.[32 33] A further consequence of subarachnoid haemorrhage is a reduction in cerebral oxygen consumption which can be related directly to the degree of vasospasm.

Infections

CBF autoregulation may be impaired in patients with both encephalitis and bacterial meningitis. The impairment may be focal or diffuse, cerebral perfusion therefore being critically dependent on systemic blood pressure. This is probably not as widely appreciated as it might be, but there is no doubt that careful fluid management and ICP, and blood pressure monitoring in patients with bacterial meningitis is required to maintain an adequate CPP.

Brain tumours and other space occupying lesions

CBF autoregulation is impaired in intracranial tumours and other space occupying lesions such as intracerebral haematomas. This loss of autoregulation may be in the immediate vicinity of the lesion or more widely spread.

Raised intracranial pressure

Expanding lesions inside the skull result in shift and distortion of the brain and may result in internal herniae. Such herniae are the result of the anatomical arrangement of the dura mater within the skull and in the presence of the foramen magnum at the base of the skull.

It is generally accepted that vascular complications such as haemorrhage and necrosis are secondary to high ICP and are seen commonly in the brain stem and the anterior lobe of the pituitary gland. It is also appreciated that shift, distortion, and internal herniation of the brain are the causes of necrosis of structures supplied by the posterior cerebral, the anterior cerebral, the anterior choroidal, and the superior and posterior inferior cerebellar arteries. Such complications are particularly common when there is a unilateral space occupying lesion especially one in the supratentorial compartment.[34] The ICP may be raised after cardiac arrest, subarachnoid haemorrhage, and meningitis, but because the disease process is diffuse and, at least initially, does not generate pressure gradients, there will usually be no evidence of internal herniation and the attendant vascular complications.

Structural changes in the brain resulting from ischaemia

The different susceptibility of the various cellular elements in the nervous system to ischaemia has been known for many years. In general nerve cells are the most sensitive followed by oligodendroglia and astrocytes, whereas microglia and the cellular elements of the blood vessels are the least vulnerable. Following an episode of ischaemia, therefore, damage may be limited to nerve cells (selective neuronal necrosis) or may extend to involve glial and blood vessels (infarction).

The identification of irreversible damage in the human brain is made difficult because of the frequent occurrence of histological artefact. This artefact results partly from the autolysis that takes place between the onset of clinical brain stem death and the fulfilment of the second set of criteria, and between death and postmortem examination, partly from the slow penetration of the fixative in which the brain is immersed, and partly from shortcomings in the processing of the tissue.

If the patient dies immediately after the ischaemic event there will not be any identifiable histological abnormalities. If the patient lives between four and six hours under optimal conditions, however, it might be possible to identify the earliest changes, and certainly survivals greater than 12 hours are normally associated with readily identifiable histological abnormality. If the patient survives for more than 24–36 hours, more advanced changes occur and early reactive changes appear in astrocytes, microglia, and blood vessels. If irreversible damage is, however, limited to nerve cells then after a few days these will disappear and reactive changes will be minimal. In an area of infarction the reactive changes will become more intense with the formation of macrophages and, if survival is for more than a week or so, the damaged tissue becomes rarefied and there is a reactive astrocytosis.

Principal patterns of ischaemic brain damage

Diffuse

This is most commonly the result of either cardiac arrest or status epilepticus.

Cardiac arrest

This is often a complication of surgery under general anaesthesia at normal body temperature. Prognosis is good in patients who, after resuscitation, regain consciousness quickly with complete neurological recovery. If the cardiac arrest is of abrupt onset, however, and occurs in a patient at normal body temperature, complete clinical recovery is unlikely if the period of arrest is more than 5–7 minutes; many of the patients in fact die within 24 hours of the arrest.

The brain may appear normal externally and on section if death occurs within 24–36 hours of the arrest. Between 36 and 48 hours it may be possible to identify early necrosis within the depths of sulci in the posterior halves of the cerebral hemispheres and selective necrosis in the CA1 sector of Ammon's horn (fig 2.8). With increasing survival the true extent of the damage becomes evident, the cortex becoming thin, granular in texture, and often with a laminar distribution (fig 2.9). Changes may be seen in the basal ganglia. With increasing survival there is an appreciable reduction in the

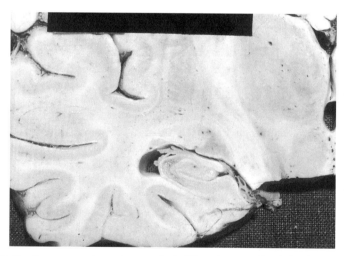

Fig 2.8 Cardiac arrest: three day survival. There is necrosis of the CA1 sector of the hippocampus

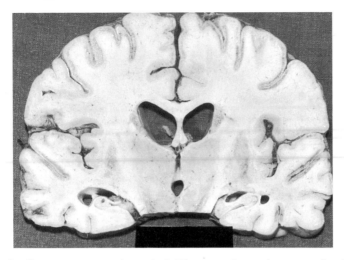

Fig 2.9 Cardiac arrest: two week survival. The cortex is greatly narrowed and there is enlargement of the ventricles; the hippocampi are small

weight of the brain as a result of atrophy and, on section, ventricular enlargement may be considerable (fig 2.10). The hippocampi may show the features of sclerosis of Ammon's horn and there may be diffuse atrophy of the cortex of the cerebellar hemispheres (fig 2.11).

Microscopy reveals a characteristic pattern of selective vulnerability with diffuse neuronal necrosis commonly maximal within the sides and depths of

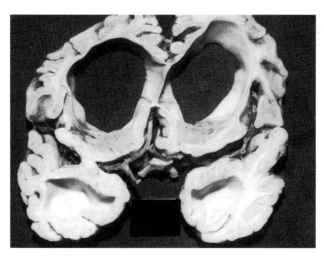

Fig 2.10 Cardiac arrest: four year survival. The neocortex is greatly narrowed and there is gross symmetrical enlargement of the ventricles

61

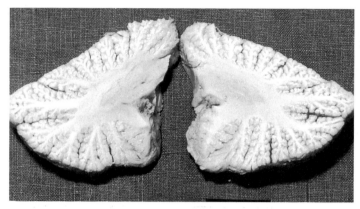

Fig 2.11 Cardiac arrest: four year survival. There is diffuse atrophy of the cerebellar cortex

sulci, rather than at the crests of gyri, and greatest in the third, fifth, and sixth layers of the parietal and occipital lobes. The CA1 and CA4 sectors are the most vulnerable in the hippocampus. The pattern of damage is variable within the basal ganglia and irreversible damage is common in the thalamus. Within the cerebellum there is diffuse loss of Purkinje cells. Damage in the brain stem tends to be limited to sensory nuclei and is more severe in infants and young children than in adults.

Status epilepticus

Although changes similar to those found in children can occur in the brains of adults who have died suddenly after status epilepticus, the frequency and amount of damage are less. If the seizures have been prolonged then one of three main patterns is possible:

1 Diffuse damage in the cortical ribbon, cerebellum, thalamus, and hippocampus
2 Cerebral hemiatrophy
3 Sclerosis of Ammon's horn.

In general there is a good correlation between the duration of the seizures and any subsequent brain damage.

Focal

Thromboembolic occlusion of artery—If the blood flow through an artery is arrested an infarct will develop within part or all of the distribution of the occluded vessel, and the size of the lesion and its distribution will depend on the efficiency of the collateral circulation. Thus, if there is no collateral circulation a massive lesion will result (fig 2.12). Occasionally the collateral circulation may be so efficient that the infarct is limited to the basal ganglia and the internal capsule.

Infarcts caused by thrombotic occlusion of an artery are usually "anaemic," whereas those resulting from embolic occlusion followed by fragmentation of the emboli and reperfusion of the ischaemic area are often haemorrhagic (fig 2.13) and if sufficiently large they constitute a space occupying mass within 24–48 hours, resulting in tentorial herniation with secondary haemorrhage into the brain stem.

The necrotic tissue is ultimately removed and replaced by a cystic scar, the boundaries of which are defined by glial and mesodermal tissue in which blood vessels may be seen. There will be compensatory enlargement of the related ventricular system (hydrocephalus *ex vacuo*) and the changes of wällerian degeneration will take place in tracts of white matter distal to the lesion (fig 2.14). With long survival this is readily seen in the brain stem which shows hemiatrophy as a result of loss within descending fibre tracts.

If blood flow through an artery, or one of its branches, is sufficiently impaired, usually as a result of a combination of systemic hypotension and narrowing of the blood vessel, then an infarct may result.

Factors that influence the size of an infarct include the functional efficiency in anastomotic blood vessels, the configuration of the circle of Willis, disease of the major neck arteries, and the level of systemic blood pressure. If all of these are normal then the cortical lesion will be small; if one or more are abnormal then the lesion will be larger. In general there are two important factors in the pathogenesis of cerebral infarction in humans, namely some impairment of cardiac function and some degree of stenotic and/or occlusive

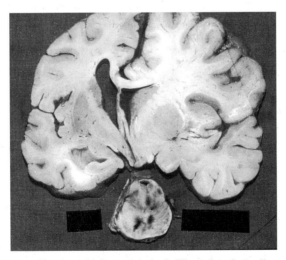

Fig 2.12 Cerebral infarction: 28 hour survival. There is a large "anaemic" swollen infarct in the territories supplied by the right anterior and middle cerebral arteries. Note the shift of the midline structures and the supracallosal hernia. There was a tentorial hernia and there is secondary haemorrhage into the brain stem

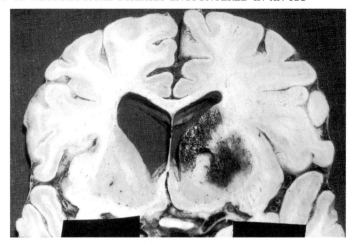

Fig 2.13 Cerebral infarction: three day survival. There is haemorrhagic transformation of an infarct in the right basal ganglia following temporary occlusion of the proximal part of the middle cerebral artery. The infarct is swollen and has encroached upon the body of the lateral ventricle

vascular disease. Cerebral infarction is therefore rarely the result of a single cause.

Lesion in the arterial boundary zones—Ischaemic brain damage may occur along the arterial boundary zones of the cerebral and cerebellar hemispheres as a result of a rapid and considerable reduction in CPP. They vary in size

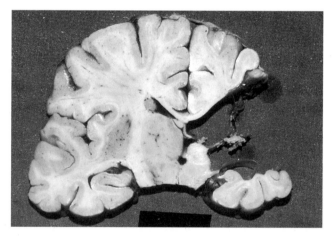

Fig 2.14 Cerebral infarction: survival of many years. There is a large defect in the lateral aspect of the right cerebral hemisphere in distribution of middle cerebral artery

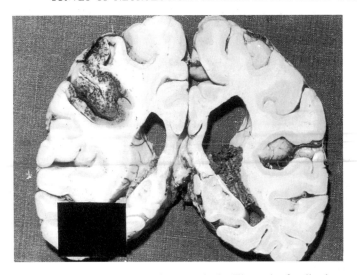

Fig 2.15 Cerebral infarction: six day survival. There is focally haemorrhagic infarction in the sides and depths of the left intraparietal sulcus, that is, in the boundary zone between the distributions of the anterior and middle cerebral arteries

from foci of necrosis in the cortex to large wedge shaped areas of damage that extend from the cortex almost to the angle of the lateral ventricle. Damage to the cortical ribbon is most frequent and severe in the parieto-occipital regions, that is, in the common boundary zone between the distributions of the anterior, middle, and posterior cerebral arteries; it decreases towards the frontal pole along the intraparietal and the superior frontal sulci, that is, between the distributions of the anterior and middle cerebral arteries (fig 2.15), and towards the temporal pole along the inferior temporal gyrus, that is, between the distributions of the middle and posterior cerebral arteries. The lesions are usually asymmetrical and may be unilateral, the pattern of damage often being determined by variations in the circle of Willis and by atheroma. In the cerebellum the boundary zone between the territories of the superior and posterior inferior cerebellar arteries lies just beneath the dorsal angle of each hemisphere. There is variable involvement of the basal ganglia whereas Ammon's horn and the brain stem are usually not involved.

This pattern of brain damage has been described in humans after dental anaesthesia in the semirecumbent position, after the overzealous treatment of malignant hypertension by antihypertensive agents, and in patients dying from non-missile head injuries.[25] The particular vulnerability of the arterial boundary zones is caused by the anatomy of the vascular supply to the cortex of the cerebrum and cerebellum, blood being delivered through large vessels in the neck, and ending in a system of small blood vessels that anastomose with their counterparts from the adjacent arterial fields. Once the capacity for autoregulation of blood flow is lost as a result of some combination of reduced perfusion pressure and hypoxaemia, oxygen falls to a critical level in those parts of each arterial territory that are most remote from the parent stems, that is, in the boundary zones.

Conclusions

Irreversible ischaemic brain damage may occur in diverse clinical situations where there is an inadequate supply of oxygen to nerve cells. Many patients who experience such an episode die within a few hours and the pathologist will be unable to identify any macroscopic abnormalities in the brain. If the patient survives for more than a few hours, however, varying degrees of damage are usually identified, particularly if the brain has been properly dissected after adequate fixation. Nevertheless, it is usually possible to establish whether a patient has experienced an episode of ischaemia that is sufficiently severe to produce damage by histological examination of the selectively vulnerable areas. In those patients who are under anaesthesia, or who have been treated with various neuroprotective agents, then the frequency and the distribution of the lesions may well have been modified.

1 Arnason BGW, Soliven B. Acute inflammatory demyelinating polyradiculopathies. In: Dyck PJ, Thoms PK, Lambert EH, Bunge R (Eds), *Peripheral neuropathy*, 3rd edn. Vol 2. Philadelphia: Saunders, 1993: 1437–97.
2 Dalakas MC. Polymyositis dermatomyositis and inclusion body myositis. *N Engl J Med* 1991; **325**: 1487–98.
3 Tandon R. Diseases of upper and lower motor neurones. In: Bradley WG, Daroff RB, Fenichel GM, Marsden CD (Eds). *Neurology in clinical practice*, Vol 2, Butterworth-Heinemann: 1990. 1687–717.
4 Howard R, Spencer G. Neurogenic respiratory failure. In: Greenwood R, Barnes MP, McMillan TM, Ward CD (Eds), *Neurological rehabilitation*. Edinburgh: Churchill-Livingston, 1993: 299–309.
5 Toyka KV, Mullges A. Myasthenia gravis and Lambert–Eaton syndrome. In: Hacke W (Ed.), Berlin: *Neurocritical care*. Berlin: Springer-Verlag, 1994: 806–15.
6 Caplan LR. Vertebrobasilar occlusive disease. In: Barnett HJM, Mohr JP, Stein BM, Yatsu FM (Eds), *Stroke. Pathophysiology, diagnosis and management*. Edinburgh: Churchill-Livingston, 1986: 549–621.
7 Bleck TP, Stefan H. Status epilepticus. In: Hacke W (Ed.), *Neurocritical care*. Berlin: Springer-Verlag, 1994: 765–9.
8 Lindsay KW, Bone I, Callander R. *Neurology and neurosurgery illustrated*. Edinburgh: Churchill Livingston, 1992.
9 Whitley R, Schlitt M. Encephalitis caused by Herpes virus. In: Schield WM, Whitley R (Eds), *Infections of the nervous system*. New York: Raven Press, 1991: 41–86.
10 Lambert HP. Meningitis. *J Neurol Neurosurg Psychiatry* 1994; **57**: 405–16.
11 Anderson M. Management of cerebral infection. *J Neurol Neurosurg Psychiatry* 1993; **56**: 1243–58.
12 Bolton CF, Young GB. Neurological complications in critically ill patients. In: Aminoff MJ (Ed.), *Neurology and general medicine*. Edinburgh: Churchill-Livingston, 1989: 713–31.
13 Kleihues P, Burger PC, Scheithauer BW. *Histological typing of tumours of the central nervous system*, 2nd edn. Berlin: Springer-Verlag, 1993.

14 Russell DS, Rubenstein LJ. *Pathology of tumours of the nervous system*, 5th edn. London: Edward Arnold, 1989.
15 Burger PC, Scheithauer BW. *Atlas of tumour pathology. Tumours of the central nervous system*, 3rd series, fascicle 10. Washington: Armed Forces Institute of Pathology, 1994.
16 Burger PC, Scheithauer BW, Vogil FS. *Surgical pathology of the nervous system and its coverings*, 3rd edn. New York: Churchill Livingston, 1991.
17 Okazaki H, Scheithauer BW. *Atlas of neuropathology*. New York: Gower Medical, 1988.
18 Thomas DGT, Graham DI. *Malignant brain tumours*. London: Springer-Verlag, 1995.
19 Edvinsson L, Mackenzie ET, McCulloch J. *Cerebral blood flow and metabolism*. New York: Raven Press, 1993.
20 Gibbs J, Wise R, Leenders KL, Jones T. Evaluation of cerebral perfusion reserve in patients with carotid artery occlusion. *Lancet* 1984; i: 310–14.
21 Baron JC, Rougemont D, Soussaline F, *et al*. Local interrelationships of cerebral oxygen consumption and glucose utilisation in normal subjects and ischemic stroke patients. A positron tomography study. *J Cereb Blood Flow Metab* 1984; **4**: 140–5.
22 Baron JC, Frackowiak RSJ, Herholz K, *et al*. Use of PET methods for measurements of cerebral energy, metabolism and hemodynomics in cerebrovascular disease. *J Cereb Blood Flow Metab* 1989; **9**: 723–42.
23 Nedergaard M. Neuronal injury in the infarct border: a neuropathological study in the rat. *Acta Neuropathol* 1987; **73**: 267–74.
24 Kannel WB. Epidemiology of cerebrovascular disease. In: Russell RWR (Ed.), *Cerebral arterial disease*. Edinburgh: Churchill-Livingstone, 1976: 1–23.
25 Leenders KL, Perani D, Lammertsma AA, *et al*. Cerebral blood flow, blood volume and oxygen utilisation. *Brain* 1990; **113**: 27–47.
26 Graham DI. Hypoxia and vascular disorder. In: Adams JH, Duchen LW (Eds), *Greenfield's neuropathology*, 5th edn. London: Edward Arnold, 1992: 153–268.
27 Graham DI, Ford I, Adams JH, *et al*. Ischaemic brain damage is still common in fatal non-missile head injury. *J Neurol Neurosurg Psychiatry* 1989; **52**: 346–50.
28 Chestnut R, Marshall L, Klauber M, *et al*. The role of secondary brain injury in determining outcome from severe head injury. *J Trauma* 1993; **34**: 216–22.
29 Jones PA, Andrews PJD, Midgley S, *et al*. Measuring the burden of secondary insults in head-injured patients during intensive care. *J Neurosurg Anesthesiol* 1994; **6**: 4–14.
30 Bone I, Mendelow AD, Graham DI. The management of carotid artery disease: application of new diagnostic techniques and their neuropathological significance. *Neuropathol Appl Neurobiol* 1993; **19**: 107–19.
31 Graham DI, Macpherson P, Pitts LH. Correlation between angiographic vasospasm, haematoma, and ischemic brain damage following SAH. *J Neurosurg* 1983; **59**: 223–30.
32 Pickard JD, Boisvert DPJ, Graham DI, Fitch W. Late effects of subarachnoid haemorrhage on the response of the primate cerebral circulation to drug-induced changes in arterial blood pressure. *J Neurol Neurosurg Psychiatry* 1979; **42**: 899–903.
33 Pickard JD, Matheson M, Patterson J, Wyper D. Prediction of late ischemic complications after cerebral aneurysm surgery by the intraoperative measurement of cerebral blood flow. *J Neurosurg* 1980; **53**: 305–8.
34 Graham DI, Lawrence AE, Adams JH, Doyle D, McLellan DR. Brain damage in non-missile head injury secondary to high intracranial pressure. *Neuropathol Appl Neurobiol* 1987; **13**: 209–17.

3: Radiological study of lesions of the central nervous system

G WILMS, C PLETS, AL BAERT

The brain

To give an overview of the actual trends in the radiological study of the brain, the following topics are studied:

1 The actual indications for plain radiographs of the skull, in both the traumatised and non-traumatised patient.
2 The relative value of computed tomography (CT) and magnetic resonance imaging (MRI) in the study of lesions of the brain.
3 The remaining indications for cerebral angiography.

Indications for plain radiographs of the skull

In most European countries, plain films of the skull still account for about 2·5–3% of the total budget for radiology. According to several studies this seems to be too high.

It was known before the advent of computed tomography that skull radiography has a low diagnostic yield in the evaluation of mild head trauma. In 1971 Bell and Loop,[1] based this on two observations: first, in patients with a clinically low yield, positive findings on skull radiography are extremely rare. Second, if positive, it mainly concerns clinically non-significant linear skull fractures. In 1987 Masters[2] repeated this study and came to the following conclusions:

1 In a "low risk group" the risk of missing an occult intracranial sequela or complicated skull fracture is three in 10 000 if no head imaging is requested.
2 Only 3% of trauma patients who have skull radiographs taken have skull fractures. In a low risk group, 0·7% of the patients will have fractures. Therefore the clinician who orders skull radiographs in low risk patients will receive a report of a normal finding in more than 99% of cases. The finding of an occasional skull fracture will be of no importance.
3 Of patients with skull fractures 91% do not have an associated intracranial injury.

4 Of patients with intracranial injury 51% do not have a skull fracture. Therefore, skull radiographs never rule out an intracranial lesion if they are negative (fig 3.1).

5 The information obtained from a plain skull radiograph affects clinical management of patients with head injury in less than 2% of cases.

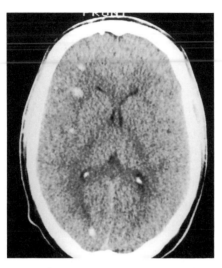

Fig 3.1 Shearing injuries: non-enhanced CT scan. Multiple focal areas of haemorrhage at the grey–white matter junction, pointing to shearing injuries. Note that a standard radiograph of the skull was negative

Some authors maintain the extreme standpoint that if radiological evaluation is not required in the low risk patient and, if the proper radiological evaluation of the high risk patient is performed with computed tomography, there are actually no indications for skull radiographs in head trauma.

Nevertheless, it has to be stressed that, in cases of depressed fractures, plain radiographs of the skull can offer very important information to the surgeon. In fact it is not always possible to determine on a CT scan whether a fracture crosses the superior sagittal or the transverse sinus. In these cases, plain radiographs are still indicated.

In spite of these very clear recommendations, the guidelines are rarely followed by clinicians, mainly for unclear medicolegal reasons or at the request of the patient. In a recent review David Hackney[3] found that skull radiographs were still taken, either frequently or always in almost 60% of all hospitals, and were used for the study of head trauma in 96% of the institutions studied. This increases both the health care cost and the radiation dose in the population. It is the role of the radiologist to educate those doctors who staff the accident and emergency rooms about this issue.

The following are the indications for plain skull radiograph in clinical practice:

1 Investigation of primary, mostly palpable, lesions of the skull bones, such as eosinophilic granuloma, epidermoid cyst, etc.
2 Investigation of conditions that frequently involve the skull bones, such as metastasis, Paget's disease, osteopetrosis, etc.
3 Search for foreign bodies in penetrating wounds as well as exclusion of ferromagnetic particles in the eye before magnetic resonance imaging.
4 Precise localisation of a depressed fracture.
5 Medicolegal purposes.

In children, a few more indications can be added:

1 Investigation of conditions involving the sutures.
2 Evaluation of craniofacial deformation, in addition to a CT scan of the skull base or the petrous bones.

Relative value of computed tomography and magnetic resonance imaging in the study of the brain

In the mid-1970s, the introduction of computed tomography revolutionised neuroradiological diagnosis. The direct visualisation of the brain parenchyma, ventricles, and cisternae, and of the pathological brain processes made invasive diagnostic procedures such as air encephalography, iodoventriculography, and meatocisternography obsolete and dramatically decreased the need for selective carotid or vertebral angiography.

The more recent use of magnetic resonance imaging (MRI) constitutes another important step forward in neuroradiological diagnosis.

The advantages of MRI are very well known[4] and include better intrinsic contrast of the images, higher sensitivity for pathological changes, especially on T2 weighted images, absence of artefacts from bone, especially in the posterior fossa and the pituitary region, possibility of multiplanar imaging, and the absence of known noxious effects.

Known disadvantages are the high cost and poor availability, the long examination time leading to image degradation by voluntary movement and respiration, the rather high percentage of patients with claustrophobia, and the incompatibility of the magnet's environment with metallic objects such as pacemakers, life support equipment, etc.

In recent years several papers have attempted to compare the results of computed tomography and MRI in different pathological fields. The choice between computed tomography and MRI is not only important for the individual patient but also has important economic implications. Below these findings are summarised for neurosurgical patients.

Traumatic lesions

The CT appearance of several traumatic lesions is typical and well described. Recent haemorrhage appears hyperdense, as a result of its high protein content. Subdural haematoma typically has a biconcave crescent like shape, and extends over the entire affected hemisphere. Epidural haematoma, on the other hand, is biconvex and usually more limited (fig 3.2). In children it is classically limited by the sutures. Contusions appear as inhomogeneous hyperdense areas, mostly localised in the temporal or frontal region. In case of deceleration or rotation injuries small hyperdensities are seen at the junction of the grey and white matter.

Over several weeks the density of the haematomas decreases, going through on isodense phase, and ending in hypodensity similar to that of cerebrospinal fluid (CSF).

With the exception of subarachnoid haemorrhage[5] MRI can demonstrate all acute traumatic lesions as well as or even better than computed tomography.[6 7] The degradation of haemoglobin causes a very typical sequence of changes in signal intensities, which differ on T1 and T2 weighted sequences. After 1 week the haemorrhage shows much more intensity on both sequences. Older haemorrhages show little intensity on T2 weighted sequences as a result of the presence of haemosiderin. It is therefore possible within certain limits to date the age of the haematoma. Nevertheless, patients with extensive skull and brain injuries or patients who have traumatic injuries in several different parts of the body are frequently unsuited for an MRI

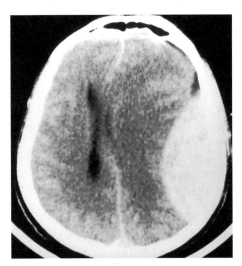

Fig 3.2 Epidural haematoma: non-enhanced CT scan. Lenticular shaped hyperdense collection in the left frontoparietal region. Note the midline shift and compression of the left lateral ventricle

71

study. In addition to the fact that comatose or subcomatose patients are too restless to undergo an MRI examination, they frequently need life support equipment, such as artificial respiration, and frequently have other abdominal or skeletal injuries, hindering transport on the MRI table.[4]

Brain oedema (fig 3.3) will be reflected by both computed tomography and MRI as a result of swelling of the brain with effacement of the superficial sulci and the basal subarachnoid cisternae. The cerebral ventricles appear small and compressed. The brain may show decreased grey–white matter differentiation.

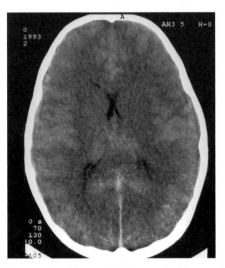

Fig 3.3 Brain oedema: non-enhanced CT scan. Evidence of "slit" ventricles and effacement of sulci and cisternae

Diffuse post-traumatic brain swelling can result from increased intravascular blood volume, increased brain water content, or both.[8] Differentiation of the conditions is not possible by simple imaging, although the treatment and prognosis are different.[9]

In the follow up of patients with head injury, MRI is clearly superior to computed tomography in two different conditions. The subacute subdural haematoma frequently appears isodense on CT scan, as a result of the progressive resorption of the blood degradation products. On MRI the presence of methaemoglobin will lead to shortening of T1 so that the lesion will appear to show more intensity in this sequence.[10]

In patients with severe post-traumatic cognitive disorders and negative CT scan, MRI will frequently show haemorrhagic lesions of the corpus callosum and the basal ganglia, known as diffuse axonal injury[7] (fig 3.4).

Computed tomography should be recommended as the primary diagnostic

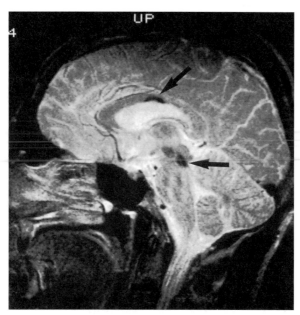

Fig 3.4 Diffuse axonal injury: midline sagittal T2 weighted (2000/90) MRI scan. Deposits of haemosiderin (indicated by arrow) in the corpus callosum and the midbrain, pointing to old haemorrhage

imaging method in the patient with acute head injury, especially if extensive calvarial fractures are present. MRI must be reserved for the study of patients with isodense subdural haematomas on CT scan and in the patients with unexplained severe post-traumatic cognitive disorders.

Infectious lesions

MRI is very sensitive to the early oedematous changes of parenchymal brain infection and gives a good demonstration of the development of the capsule bordering a liquefied abscess.[11] [12] As with computed tomography, the capsule enhances after contrast, pointing to its neovascularity.

MRI has particular advantages over computed tomography in the study of patients with herpes encephalitis[13] (fig 3.5). As a result of the absence of bony artefacts in the temporal fossa, MRI allows better detection of the affection of the temporal lobe, which is essential for the diagnosis. In the same way, subtle changes in the heterolateral temporal lobe can lead to early diagnosis of non-suspected bilateral disease. Finally, the ability of MRI to demonstrate haemorrhagic foci allows easy detection of petechial haemorrhage, which can be an important factor of differential diagnosis.

In some specific brain infections, such as cysticercosis,[14] the poor visualisation of calcification can be a drawback in the aetiological diagnosis of the disease, but the parenchymal cysts are well depicted.

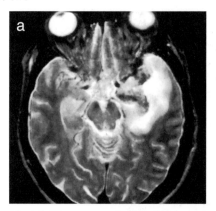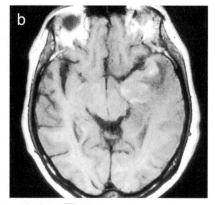

Fig 3.5 Herpes encephalitis: (a) transverse T2 weighted (2500/80) MRI scan. The left temporal lobe is smaller showing strong intensity and evidence of haemorrhage. (b) Transverse T1 weighted (600/15) MRI scan. Spots of greater intensity point to haemorrhage. Note the displacement of the brain stem

In patients with AIDS, MRI has shown dramatic advantages over computed tomography not only to select patients for antiviral treatment and to follow up the lesions under therapy, but especially for the selection of the most appropriate lesions for biopsy.

In about 50% of the patients with AIDS and neurological symptoms, MRI would reveal focal lesions that are not seen on a CT scan.[15] Problems remain, for example, the differential diagnosis between lymphoma and intercurrent infections such as toxoplasmosis.[16]

Haemorrhage

As mentioned above, as a result of paramagnetic effects of blood degradation products (deoxyhaemoglobin, methaemoglobin, haemosiderin, and ferritin), intraparenchymal haemorrhage displays a very typical sequence of signal alterations over time, allowing very precise dating of the bleeding.[17] Moreover, with sequences that emphasise magnetic susceptibility effects of small haemorrhages, such as the short flip angle gradient echo sequence, detection of a small haemorrhage is possible.[18]

Nevertheless, several disadvantages of MRI in the study of haemorrhagic lesions have to be mentioned. First of all, in fresh haemorrhage, a liquid collection of red blood cells containing oxyhaemoglobin is formed. As oxyhaemoglobin has no paramagnetic properties, prolongation of T1 and T2 relaxation times as a result of increased spin density will be non-specific and resemble any other focal oedematous process.[17] It can last for up to 24 hours before sufficient deoxyhaemoglobin is formed to cause magnetic susceptibility effects. Second, in acute subarachnoid haemorrhage, the paramagnetic effects of deoxyhaemoglobin are missed because of the very long T2 relaxation time of CSF and the pulsatile flow effects of CSF.[5] Therefore computed tomography is the method of choice when a subarachnoid haemorrhage is suspected. On the other hand, in the subacute stage the site of aneurysmal rupture may be indicated by the clot.[4] Finally, superficial siderosis of the brain stem and cisternae can be sequelae of a massive subarachnoid haemorrhage which is superbly demonstrated by MRI.

Vascular malformations such as the underlying cause of haemorrhage are seen on CT scans as enhancing clusters of abnormal vessels. The feeding arteries and drainage veins are enlarged and enhance strongly. On MRI (fig 3.6) they are detected by flow effects, such as flow void (absence of signal

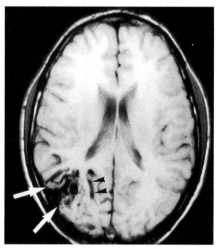

Fig 3.6 Right parietal arteriovenous malformation: transverse T1 weighted (680/20) MRI scan. Lesion (⇨) is recognised by the absence of signal (flow void). Nidus is fed by hypertrophic arteries and drained by hypertrophic veins (◄ ◄)

resulting from fast flow) in arterial feeders of brain arteriovenous malformation or even echo rephasing in venous anomalies with slow flow.[19] Aneurysms can be seen on CT scan as rounded structures that enhance, mostly located at the level of the circle of Willis. On MRI they are recognised as a result of their flow void. For both methods, however, 1 cm seems to be the inferior limit for detection, so angiography is still necessary. The MRI aspect of cavernous angiomas or cryptic arteriovenous malformations of the brain is pathognomonic[20] (fig 3.7). As a result of repeated, small, and often subclinical haemorrhages, a central small focus of high intensity, surrounded by a peripheral rim of very low intensity, is seen. Computed tomography is recommended in the first 24 hours to detect subarachnoid or parenchymal haemorrhage. For follow up of the haematoma and diagnosis of the underlying cause MRI is preferred.

75

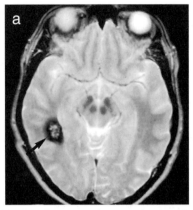 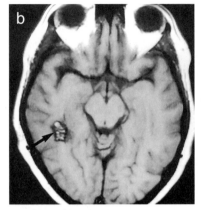

Fig 3.7 Cavernous haemangioma: (a) transverse T2 weighted (2500/90) MRI scan. Lesion ($\rightarrow$), surrounded by signal of low intensity, pointing to haemosiderin. (b) Transverse T1 weighted (600/15) MRI scan. The centre of the lesion ($\rightarrow$) shows strong intensity with multiple septations

Tumours

Tumours of the cerebral hemisphere are readily depicted on CT scans, so computed tomography remains the screening method for supratentorial neoplasms. It will show displacement of the midline and compression of the ventricles, as well as the tumoral mass itself. After administration of intravenous contrast, the type and degree of contrast enhancement can give valuable information about the vascularisation or nature of the tumour. In the posterior fossa, artefacts from bone frequently degrade the CT scans so that MRI is the preferred method for the diagnosis of these tumours. Once the tumour is detected, MRI can provide important additional information to the clinician.[4 21] Multiplanar imaging allows better determination of the exact position of the tumour, with regard to the rolandic fissure, the visual cortex, or the convexity. On T2 weighted images the nidus is separated from the surrounding oedema, allowing more accurate determination of tumour size.[21] Involvement of the corpus callosum by tumour is very well visualised on MRI as is the spread of tumour across the midline (fig 3.8). The knowledge that oedema associated with tumors does not spread into the corpus callosum can be of great value in the differential diagnosis. It has to be stressed that, in the postoperative period, after surgery for a brain tumour, the degree of residual brain oedema does not always show good correlation with the clinical condition of the patient. Therefore, unlike traumatic situations, severe postoperative brain oedema, even with huge mass effect, can be seen in patients who are conscious and functioning well.

Finally, MRI depicts more accurately the continuity of enhancing foci which appear as multiple enhancing nodules on computed tomography.[4]

In early experience with MRI, it was reported that meningiomas could easily be missed, as a result of having the same intensity as brain parenchyma[22] (fig 3.9). With high field MRI meningiomas are rarely of the same intensity on both (T1 and T2 weighted) sequences;[23] up to 45% of the lesions show much greater intensity on T2 weighted images. The presence of an enhancing dural tail after intravenous injection of gadolinium labelled diethylenetriaminepentaacetic acid (DTPA) can be a valuable differential diagnostic sign,[24] although it is found in a minority of superficial malignant tumours.[25]

In the study of cerebral metastases Gd enhanced MRI is superior to computed tomography in the detection of small lesions.[26] Moreover,

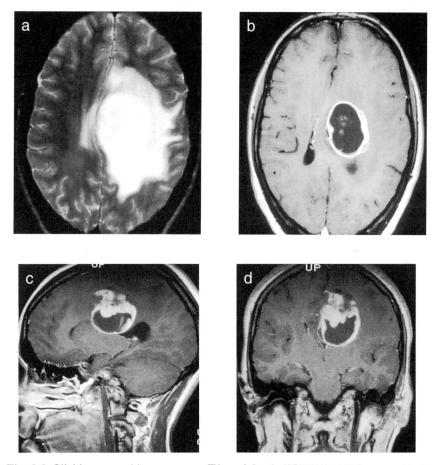

Fig 3.8 Glioblastoma: (a) transverse T2 weighted (2500/90) MRI scan. Oval inhomogeneous lesion showing hyperintensity. Note the surrounding oedema. (b) Transverse, (c) sagittal, and (d) Gd enhanced T1 weighted images. The lesion shows thick walled enhancement with evidence of focal mass enhancement in the superior part of the lesion. Note the invasion of the corpus callosum

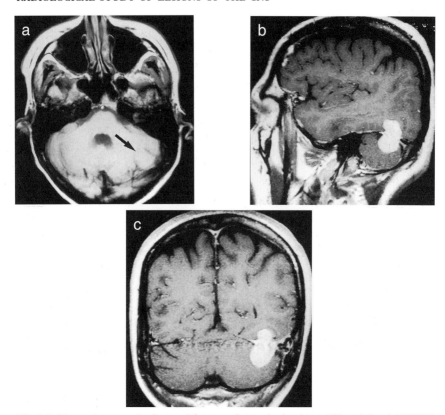

Fig 3.9 Tentorium meningioma: (a) non-enhanced transverse T1 weighted (650/20) MRI scan. Lesion (→) has the same intensity as grey matter. (b) Sagittal and (c) coronal Gd enhanced MRI scans. There is strong enhancement of the lesion and the neighbouring tentorium. Note the supratentorial and infratentorial extension

metastases of malignant melanoma show typical T1 and T2 shortening, caused by the presence of paramagnetic melanin in the lesion.[27] Other metastases, from mucinous adenocarcinomas of the gastrointestinal tract or from lung carcinomas, also exhibit low intensity on T2 weighted images although the reasons are not known.[4]

In the evaluation of a microadenoma of the pituitary gland, MRI is far superior to computed tomography, providing a meticulous technique is used. Thin section, high resolution, multiplanar imaging is necessary.[28] The exact pulse sequence and the dosage of Gd-DTPA[29][30] for study of the pituitary gland still need to be determined. In the diagnosis of small or purely intracanalicular acoustic neurinomas, the Gd enhanced lesions stand out against the low intensity CSF and the absent signal from the bone, allowing exact evaluation of the intracanalicular extension (fig. 3.10). Computed tomography can be used as a screening method for cerebral tumours,

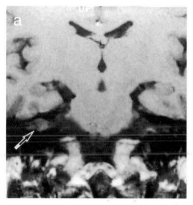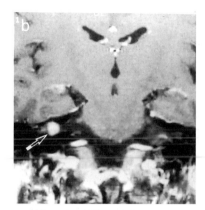

Fig 3.10 Small intracanalicular acoustic neuroma: (a) coronal T1 weighted (600/15) MRI scan. Note the small mass (→) within the petrous bone. (b) Enhanced image—note the strong enhancement (→)

especially if the symptoms point to a supratentorial lesion. MRI is recommended for the detection of tumours of the posterior fossa, the pituitary gland, and the cerebellopontine angle. It can be used to complete the preoperative set up of supratentorial tumours and for the diagnosis of small metastases.

Miscellaneous conditions

In both obstructive and communicating hydrocephalus, the degree of dilatation of the ventricular system is accurately measured and followed by computed tomography.

Sagittal MRI can provide additional information, for example, for the cause of hydrocephalus. Aqueductal stenosis is demonstrated directly by the narrowing of the sylvian aqueduct and indirectly by the absence of flow.[4 31]

The craniocervical junction is very well depicted by MRI. In patients with syringomyelia or meningomyelocele, the position of the cerebellar tonsils can be very accurately demonstrated, allowing easy diagnosis of the Chiari I malformation. In the Chiari II malformation the position of the fourth ventricle will be as low as the foramen magnum. The vermis is inferiorly displaced whereas the medulla forms a spur or a kink.

Indications for cerebral angiography

In spite of the development of alternative techniques for the demonstration of the intracerebral vasculature, such as magnetic resonance angiography (MRA) or spiral computed tomography, selective intra-arterial digital subtraction angiography remains the method of choice in the study of pure vascular lesions of the brain.[32]

The first indication concerns the study of cerebral aneurysms. Angiography will determine the presence of a lesion, the exact site and carrier vessel, the size of the neck, and the direction of the main axis of the aneurysm. Four vessel angiography is mandatory for exclusion of multiple aneurysms, present in up to 25% of the cases. Finally, in case of multiple aneurysms certain signs such as a "nipple" or a "dot" sign will indicate the lesion with recent haemorrhage.

In the study of cerebral arteriovenous malformations, angiography determines the origin, number, size, and course of the feeding arteries, the exact size and localisation of the nidus, and the number and course, either deep or superficial, of the draining veins.

In the same way, in dural arteriovenous fistula, the number of external carotid, internal carotid, and vertebral artery feeders can only be determined by angiography.

In carotid–cavernous fistula, angiography is the only technique able to demonstrate the exact site of the fistula.

On the other hand, the haemorrhagic complications of both aneurysms and arteriovenous malformations are better demonstrated with MRI and computed tomography.

In many centres, especially in Europe, angiography is still routinely used in the preoperative set up of intra-axial tumours, although it is considered by others that the required presurgical information is available on MRI. For most European neurosurgeons, however, angiography remains the method of choice for demonstrating the course of the afferent tumour vessels, to exclude encasement of large branches by the tumour, and to visualise the draining veins of the tumour. In extra-axial tumours, angiography is still widely used for the determination of the external carotid artery supply.

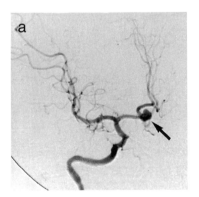 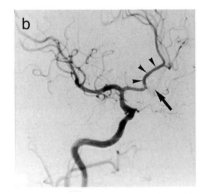

Fig 3.11 Embolisation of cerebral aneurysm with GDC coils: (a) selective right internal carotid angiogram before embolisation (right anterior oblique projection). Note the aneurysm (→) of the anterior communicating artery. (b) Selective right carotid angiogram after embolisation. The aneurysm is filled with coils (→) and excluded from the circulation; the anterior cerebral artery is patent (▶ ▶)

The exact value of MRA in the study of the cerebral vasculature is actually investigated in many centres.[34-37] Generally accepted indications for MRA are the follow up of arteriovenous malformations under or after treatment, and the study of the dural venous sinuses. Here, tumoral compression or intrinsic thrombosis can be very accurately demonstrated by MRA. The study of cerebral aneurysms, intracerebral vascular stenosis and collateral circulation, and cerebral tumours is possible, but actual resolution is insufficient to allow exact diagnosis or surgical decision making.

The treatment of choice for cerebral vascular malformations, including aneurysms, and for arteriovenous malformations is surgical. The neurosurgical treatment of aneurysms consists of surgical clipping or, in case of a broad neck, in wrapping of the lesion. In rare cases trapping of the lesion is performed by proximal and distal ligation of the feeding vessel.

Cerebral aneurysms can be inoperable as a result of either their location, such as some giant aneurysms of the basilar tip or the sinus cavernosus, or the absence of a surgical neck.[38] In these cases, endovascular treatment of the lesion can be considered. This treatment can be selective by the introduction of soft platinum coils (Guglielmi Detachable Coils or GDC coils) into the lesion[39] (fig 3.11). In other cases occlusion of the parental vessel with a detachable balloon is preferred.[38 40]

The neurosurgical treatment of cerebral arteriovenous malformations consists of total surgical removal of the nidus, with ligature of the feeding arteries and draining veins. If a lesion is too large or located in a surgically inaccessible location, such as the basal ganglia or the brain stem, or if the lesion is located in a highly functional area, such as the motor speech areas, endovascular treatment can be considered[41 42] (fig 3.12). With the use of microcatheters, the feeding arteries of arteriovenous malformations are catheterised as distally as possible, up to the nidus of the lesion, and embolised with a mixture of Lipiodol and acrylic glue. In this way the nidus of the lesion can be reduced considerably. The goal of the treatment is the total exclusion of the lesion or the reduction of its size so as to allow surgical removal or radiosurgery.[43]

Finally for the treatment of traumatic carotid–cavernous fistula, endovascular occlusion with balloons or GDC coils is the treatment of choice.[44]

The final decision for the treatment modalities of all these vascular lesions is made by multidisciplinary discussion between the teams involved in neurosurgery and neuroradiology.

The spinal canal

Degenerative disease of the spinal canal

For study of the bony spinal canal, plain films of the spine are still important. The form and height of the vertebrae are well visualised.

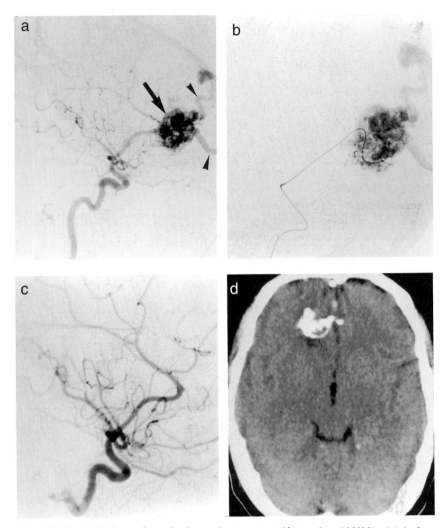

Fig 3.12 Embolisation of cerebral arteriovenous malformation (AVM): (a) before embolisation—right frontal AVM (→), fed by a hypertrophic frontopolar artery and drained by cortical veins (▶ ▶). (b) Superselective catheterisation of frontopolar artery. This artery supplies the entire malformation. (c) After embolisation (with histoacryl–Lipiodol)—the lesion is occluded. (d) CT scan after embolisation—note the embolic mixture in the lesion

Arthrotic changes such as facet joint hypertrophy and uncarthrosis are also well demonstrated. Plain films are irreplaceable if the mobility of the spine has to be evaluated by comparing the films taken in flexion, extension, or lateroflexion. Finally plain films can provide some information on the diameter of the spinal canal.

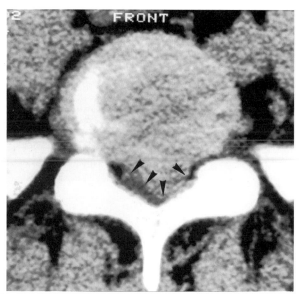

Fig 3.13 Disc herniation—CT scan: protrusion of huge fragment of disc material
(▶ ▶) within the spinal canal with compression of the dural sac

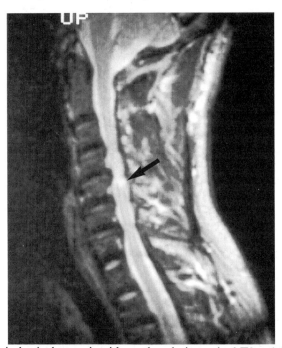

Fig 3.14 Cervical spinal stenosis with myelomalacia: sagittal T2 weighted (2500/90)
MRI scan. Uncodiscal narrowing of the spinal canal from C4 to C7. Note hyperin-
tense spot (→) in the cervical medulla at level C5, pointing to myelomalacia

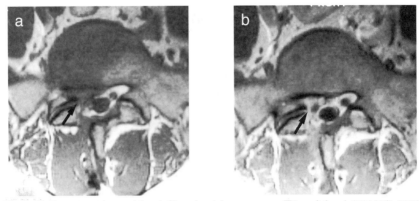

Fig 3.15 Postoperative epidural fibrosis: (a) transverse T1 weighted (600/15) MRI scan. Soft tissue mass in the right paramedian L5–S1 region, in a patient operated on for right disc herniation. (b) Gd enhanced image at the same level: strong enhancement of the tissue, surrounding the S1 nerve root (→). This enhancement points to dural fibrosis, rather than relapse of disc herniation

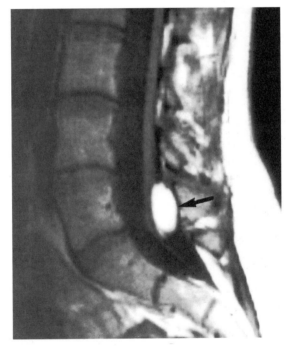

Fig 3.16 Tethered cord: sagittal T1 weighted (600/15) MRI scan. The cord is extending down to the L5–S1 junction. At this level a lipoma (→) can be seen

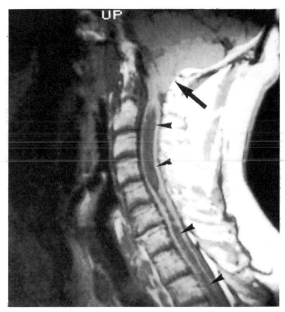

Fig 3.17 Syringomyelia: sagittal T1 weighted (600/15) MRI scan. Intramedullary cyst (▶ ▶) extending from C1 to the upper thoracic spinal cord. Note the low position of cerebellar tonsils (→) (Chiari I malformation)

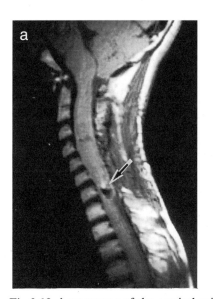
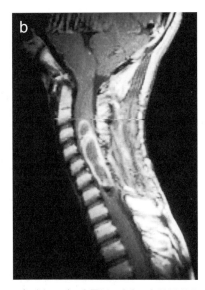

Fig 3.18 Astrocytoma of the cervical spinal cord: (a) sagittal T1 weighted (800/20) MRI scan. Diffuse enlargement of the cervical spinal cord from C1 to T1. Note the focal spot (→) of calcification or haemorrhage. (b) Sagittal T1 weighted MRI scan—irregular central enhancement of the lesion

85

For the diagnosis of disc herniation, computed tomography is the examination of choice[45][46] (fig 3.13). The herniation will be visible as a soft tissue mass, originating from the disc and presenting with the same density. The mass displaces the thecal sac or nerve root and effaces the epidural fat. Disc bulging is characterised by circumferential, broad based, and symmetrical protrusion of the disc beyond the vertebral end plate.

MRI can demonstrate disc herniation and bulging as well as computed tomography.[46] Through use of sagittal slices, MRI can study the relative position of disc and nerve root in the neuroforamen. Furthermore it can demonstrate additional tears of the annulus, which might predispose to disc degeneration or herniation.[47] The widespread use of MRI for these indications is limited by the poor availability of MRI equipment in most countries.

Spinal stenosis, either acquired or congenital, can be studied by computed tomography in the transverse direction.[48] Short pedicles, facet hypertrophy, hypertrophy of the ligamenta flava, posterior osteophytosis, or uncarthrosis are very well visualised. MRI can add valuable information in the sagittal direction by allowing exact evaluation of the anteroposterior diameter of the spinal canal.[49] Furthermore, atrophy or myelomalacic changes secondary to chronic cord compression can be demonstrated, frequently explaining the myelopathic symptoms of the patient[50] (fig 3.14).

MRI is of utmost importance in the diagnosis of spondylodiscitis when it shows both the affection of the disc and the vertebral end plates, as well as extension to the spinal canal.[51]

Finally MRI is of great value in the differential diagnosis of postoperative scar and recurrent disc herniation (fig 3.15). On MRI epidural scars show strong enhancement immediately after contrast enhancement. This feature is more prominent in the first year after operation.[52]

The actual role of myelography in the study of spinal degenerative disease remains controversial and there are strong differences between centres. The main advantage of myelography lies in the possibility of studying the entire spinal canal, the possibility of obtaining dynamic information in different positions, and the actual demonstration of nerve root compression. It certainly remains a method of choice if the findings on CT scan or MRI are equivocal, or do not correspond to the patient's complaints.[53]

Lesions of the spinal cord

Before the advent of MRI, the spinal cord could not be studied in a non-invasive way. Now it is possible to demonstrate the spinal cord directly, especially on sagittal scans, performed along the long axis of the cord. Therefore, MRI is the method of choice for patients presenting with spinal cord symptoms, such as weakness, impaired proprioception, paraparesis or tetraparesis, thermoanalgesia, cauda equina syndrome, etc.

MRI will demonstrate congenital anomalies such as diastomatomyelia or

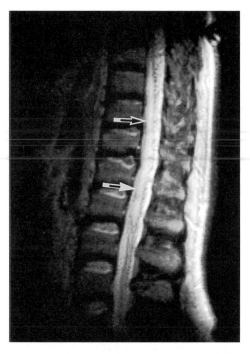

Fig 3.19 Spinal dural arteriovenous fistula with perimedullary venous drainage: sagittal T2 weighted (2500/80) MRI scan. Dilated retromedullary veins, presenting as serpiginous structures of low intensity. Note the aspect of the cord with greater intensity, pointing to oedema caused by venous hyperpression ($\rightarrow$)

tethered cord[54] (fig 3.16). In case of infections or demyelinating affections, the local oedema in the cord will be obvious. Enhancement can point to myelitis, on the basis of sarcoidosis, tuberculosis, Lyme disease, etc.[55]

In syringomyelia typically a large cyst is found reaching from the craniocervical junction to the conus terminalis (fig 3.17). The concomitant Chiari malformation is easily detected.[56]

MRI has proved to be a major step forward especially for the detection of tumours[57-59] (fig 3.18). MRI will detect the lesion, will show its exact craniocaudal and paravertebral extension, and will differentiate intramedullary, intradural and extradural tumours. Unfortunately it is impossible to make an exact anatomopathological diagnosis on the basis of the MRI characteristics of the tumour.

Finally, MRI is of invaluable help in the diagnosis of spinal cord arteriovenous malformations and fistulae[60] (fig 3.19). Dural and intradural arteriovenous malformations will present as focal areas of intramedullary flow voids. The enlarged veins will appear as tortuous, serpiginous foci of high velocity signal loss behind or around the spinal cord. Cord atrophy and high

87

signal intensity of the cord, pointing to venous hypertension, are commonly seen. The final diagnosis and therapeutic choice are based on selective spinal angiography.

1 Bell RS, Loop JW. The utility and futility of radiographic skull examination for trauma. *N Engl J Med* 1971; **284**: 236–9.
2 Masters SJ, McClean PhM, Arcarese JS, *et al.* Skull X-ray examinations after head trauma. *N Engl J Med* 1987; **316**(2): 84–91.
3 Hackney DB. Skull radiography in the evaluation of acute head trauma: a survey of current practice. *Radiology* 1991; **181**: 711–14.
4 Brant-Zawadzki M. MR imaging of the brain. *Radiology* 1988; **166**: 1–10.
5 Sato HS, Kadoya S. Magnetic resonance imaging of subarachnoid hemorrhage. *Neuroradiology* 1988; **30**: 361.
6 Wilberger J, Deeb Z, Rothfus W. Magnetic resonance imaging in cases of severe head injury. *Neurosurgery* 1987; **20**: 571–5.
7 Gentry LR, Thompson B, Godersky JC. Trauma to the corpus callosum: MR features. *AJNR* 1988; **9**: 1129–38.
8 Lobato RD, Sarabia R, Cordobes F, *et al.* Posttraumatic cerebral hemispheric swelling. *J Neurosurg* 1980; **68**: 417–23.
9 Aldrich EF, Eisberg HM, Saydjari C, *et al.* Diffuse brain swelling: severely head-injured children. *J Neurosurg* 1992; **76**: 450–4.
10 Wilms G, Marchal G, Geusens E, *et al.* Isodense subdural haematomas on CT: MRI findings. *Neuroradiology* 1992; **34**: 497–9.
11 Rauch RA, Jinkins JR. Infections of the central nervous system. *Curr Opin Radiol* 1991; **3**: 16–24.
12 Schroth G, Kretzschmar K, Gawehn J, Voigt K. Advantage of magnetic resonance imaging in the diagnosis of cerebral infections. *Neuroradiology* 1987; **29**: 120–6.
13 Demaerel Ph, Wilms G, Robberecht W, *et al.* MRI of herpes simplex encephalitis. *Neuroradiology* 1992; **34**: 490–3.
14 Chang KH, Lee HJ, Han MH, Han MC. The role of contrast-enhanced MR imaging in the diagnosis of neurocysticercosis. *AJNR* 1991; **12**: 509–12.
15 Ciricillo SF, Rosenblum ML. Use of CT and MR imaging to distinguish intracranial lesions and to define the need for biopsy in AIDS patients. *J Neurosurg* 1990; **73**: 720–4.
16 Dina TS. Primary central nervous system, lymphoma versus toxoplasmosis in AIDS. *Radiology* 1991; **179**: 823–8.
17 Gomori J, Grossman R, Goldberg H, Zimmerman RA, Bilaniuk L. Intracranial hematomas: imaging by high-field MR. *Radiology* 1985; **157**: 89–93.
18 Atlas SW, Mark AS, Grossman RI, Gomori JM. Intracranial hemorrhage: gradient-echo MR imaging at 1.5T: comparison with spin-echo imaging and clinical applications. *Radiology* 1988; **168**: 803.
19 Nüssel F, Wegmüller H, Huber P. Comparison of magnetic resonance angiography, magnetic resonance imaging and conventional angiography in cerebral arteriovenous malformations. *Neuroradiology* 1991; **33**: 56.
20 Lemme-Plaghos L, Kucharczyk W, Brant-Zawadzki M, *et al.* MR imaging of angiographically occult vascular malformations. *AJNR* 1986; **7**: 217–22.
21 Zimmerman RA. Imaging of adult central nervous system primary malignant gliomas: staging and follow-up. *Cancer* 1991; **67**: 1278–83.
22 Schubeus P, Schorner W, Rottacker C, Sander B. Intracranial meningiomas: how frequent are indicative findings in CT and MRI? *Neuroradiology* 1990; **32**: 467–73.
23 Demaerel P, Wilms G, Lammens M, *et al.* Intracranial meningiomas: correlation between MR imaging and histology in fifty patients. *J Comput Assist Tomogr* 1991; **15**: 45–51.
24 Aoki S, Sasaki Y, Machida T, Tanioka H. Contrast-enhanced MR images in patients with meningioma: importance of enhancement of the dura adjacent to the tumor. *AJNR* 1990; **11**: 935–8.
25 Wilms G, Lammens M, Marchal G, *et al.* Prominent dural enhancement adjacent to nonmeningiomatous malignant lesions on contrast-enhanced MR-images. *AJNR* 1991; **12**: 761–4.

26 Sze G, Shin J, Krol G, Johnson G, Liu D, Deck MDF. Intraparenchymal brain metastases: MR imaging versus contrast enhanced CT. *Radiology* 1988; **168**: 187.

27 Atlas S, Grossman R, Gomori J, *et al*. MR imaging of intracranial metastatic melanoma. *J Comput Assist Tomogr* 1987; **11**: 577–82.

28 Stadnik T, Stevenaert A, Beckers A, Luypaert R, Buisseret T, Osteaux M. Pituitary microadenomas: diagnosis with two- and three-dimensional MR imaging at 1.5 T before and after injection of gadolinium. *Radiology* 1990; **176**: 419–28.

29 Sakamoto Y, Takahashi M, Korogi Y, Bussaka H, Ushio Y. Normal and abnormal pituitary glands: gadopentolate dimeglumine-enhanced MR imaging. *Radiology* 1991; **178**: 441–5.

30 Davis KA, Joseph GJ, Petermans SP, *et al*. Pituitary adenoma: correlation of half dose gadolinium-enhanced MR imaging with signal findings in 26 patients. *Radiology* 1991; **180**: 779.

31 Bradley W, Kortman K, Burgoyne B. Flowing cerebrospinal fluid in normal and hydrocephalic states: appearance on MR images. *Radiology* 1986; **159**: 611–15.

32 Elster AD, Chen MYM. Chiari I malformations: clinical and radiologic reappraisal. *Radiology* 1992; **183**: 347–53.

33 Osborn AG. Intracranial vascular malformations. In: *Introduction to cerebral angiography*. St Louis: Mosby-Year Book, 1991: 85–91.

34 Marchal G, Bosmans H, Van fraeyenhoven L, *et al*. Intracranial vascular lesions: optimization and clinical evaluation of three-dimensional time-of-flight MR angiography. *Radiology* 1990; **175**: 443.

35 Sevick RJ, Tsuruda JS, Schmalbrock P. Three-dimensional time-of-flight MR angiography in the evaluation of cerebral aneurysms. *J Comp Assist Tomogr* 1990; **14**: 874–81.

36 Blatter DD, Parker DL, Robinson R. Cerebral MR angiography with multiple overlapping thin slab acquisition. Part I: quantitative analysis of vessel visibility. *Radiology* 1991; **179**: 805–11.

37 Marchal G, Michiels J, Bosmans H, Van Hecke P. Contrast enhanced MRA of the brain. Technique and first clinical results. *J Comput Assist Tomogr* 1992; **16**: 25–9.

38 Fox AJ, Vinuela F, Pelz DM, *et al*. Use of detachable balloons for proximal artery occlusion in the treatment of unclippable cerebral aneurysms. *J Neurosurg* 1987; **66**: 40.

39 Guglielmi G, Vinuela F, Dion J, *et al*. Electrothrombosis of saccular aneurysms via endovascular approach. Part 2: Preliminary clinical experience. *J Neurosurg* 1991; **75**: 8.

40 Halbach VV, Higashida RT, Hieshima GB, *et al*. Aneurysms of the petrous portion of the internal carotid artery: results of treatment with endovascular or surgical occlusion. *AJNR* 1990; **11**: 253.

41 Vinuela F, Dion J, Lylyk P, Duckwiler G. Update on interventional neuroradiology. *AJR* 1989; **153**: 23–33.

42 Fox AJ, Pelz DM, Lee DH. Arteriovenous malformations of the brain: recent results of endovascular therapy. *Radiology* 1990; **177**: 51–7,

43 Pelz DM, Fox AJ, Vinuela F, Drake CC, Ferguson GG. Preoperative embolisation of brain AVM's with isobutyl-2-cyanoacrylate. *AJNR* 1988; **9**: 757–64.

44 Debrun G, Lacour P, Vinuela F, Fox A, Drake CG, Caron JP. Treatment of 54 traumatic carotid–cavernous fistulas. *J Neurosurg* 1981; **55**: 678–92.

45 Thornbury JR, Fryback DG, Turski PA, *et al*. Disk-caused nerve compression in patients with acute low-back pain: diagnosis with MR, CT myelography, and plain CT. *Radiology* 1993; **186**: 731–8.

46 Williams AL, Haughton VM. Disc herniation and degenerative disc disease. In Newton TH, Potts DG (Eds), *Modern neuroradiology*, vol 1, *Computed tomography of the spine and spinal cord*. St Louis: CV Mosby, 1983: 231–49.

47 Yu S, Sether LA, Ho PSP, *et al*. Tears of the anulus fibrosus: correlation between MR and pathologic findings in cadavers. *AJNR* 1988; **9**: 367–70.

48 Kent DL, Haynor DR, Larson EB, Deyo RA. Diagnosis of lumbar spinal stenosis in adults: a metaanalysis of the accuracy of CT, MR, and myelography. *AJR* 1992; **158**: 1135–44.

49 Mehalic TF, Pezzuti RT, Applebaum BI. Magnetic resonance imaging and cervical spondylitic myelopathy. *Neurosurgery* 1990; **26**: 216–27.

50 Takahashi M, Yamashita Y, Sakamoto Y, Kojima R. Chronic cervical cord compression: clinical significance of increased signal intensity on MR images. *Radiology* 1989; **173**: 219–24.

51 Smith AS, Weinstein MA, Mizushima A, *et al*. MR imaging of characteristics of tuberculosis spondylitis vs. vertebral osteomyelitis. *AJNR* 1989; **10**: 619–25.
52 Bundschuh CV, Stein L, Slusser JH, *et al*. Distinguishing between scar and recurrent herniated disk in postoperative patients: value of contrast-enhanced CT and MR imaging. *AJNR* 1990; **11**: 949–58.
53 Lutz JD, Smith RR, Jones HM. CT myelography of a fragment of a lumbar disk sequestered posterior to the thecal scar. *AJNR* 1990; **11**: 610–11.
54 Byrd SE, Darling CF, McLone DG. Developmental disorders of the pediatric spine. *Radiol Clin N Am* 1991; **29**: 711.
55 Gero B, Sze G, Sharif H. MR imaging of intradural inflammatory disease of the spine. *AJNR* 1991; **28**: 809.
56 Sze G. MR imaging of the spinal cord: current status and future advances. *AJR* 1992; **159**: 149–59.
57 Li MH, Holtas S. MR imaging of spinal intramedullary tumors. *Acta Radiol* 1991; **32**: 505.
58 Parizel PM, Balériaux D, Rodesch G, *et al*. Gd-DTPA-enhanced MR imaging of spinal tumors. *AJNR* 1989; **10**: 249–58.
59 Sze G. Magnetic resonance imaging in the evaluation of spinal tumors. *Cancer* 1991; **67**: 1229–41.
60 Tomlinson FH, Rufenacht DA, Sundt TM, *et al*. Arteriovenous fistulas of the brain and spinal cord. *J Neurosurg* 1993; **79**: 16–27.

4: Anaesthetic agents: total intravenous and inhalational anaesthesia

H VAN AKEN

Understanding the effects of anaesthesia on cerebral physiology is of major importance. Todd and co-workers[1] found equally satisfactory operative conditions with isoflurane, high dose fentanyl, or propofol–fentanyl, but, after total intravenous anaesthesia with propofol and alfentanil, Van Hemelrijck *et al*[2] demonstrated that the time taken to return to normal orientation and concentration was shorter and more predictable than with a more commonly used technique based on thiopentone (thiopental) sodium, nitrous oxide (N_2O), fentanyl, and isoflurane (fig 4.1).

Operative conditions depend on the interrelationship of several factors to which the anaesthetic agents make only a modest contribution. The specific cerebral effects of anaesthetic agents, which can be convincingly demonstrated in the laboratory or under well controlled clinical conditions, can also be easily manipulated by co-administration of other agents, ventilatory changes, the position of the patient, drainage of cerebrospinal fluid (CSF), and other pharmacological or physiological interventions. Although both inhalational and intravenous anaesthesia may lead to very similar operative conditions and outcomes, it cannot be denied that both techniques are characterised by specific benefits and problems. Those characteristics that plead in favour of inhalational agents are of more general kind, whereas those in favour of intravenous anaesthesia relate more to the cerebral effects of the agents. With the exceptions of N_2O and ketamine, inhalational anaesthetic and intravenous hypnotic agents decrease the cerebral metabolic rate (CMR). In contrast to intravenous hypnotic agents, which produce a decrease in cerebral blood flow (CBF) secondary to the decrease in CMR, inhalational agents are cerebral vasodilators. Although these cerebral effects may not be equally important in every patient, they can become critical in the management of those with severely compromised intracranial compliance.

Intravenous agents

Pharmacokinetic properties

When choosing drugs for intravenous anaesthesia, the question of their

91

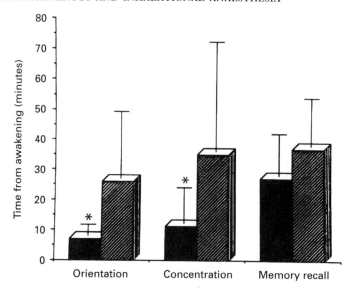

Fig 4.1 Effect of anaesthetic technique on behaviour: recovery times for orientation, concentration, and short memory tests. The times from the patients' initial responses to commands to the correct performance of the tests are indicated. ■ Propofol–alfentanil; ▨ thiopentone–fentanyl–isoflurane–N_2O. Values are mean $\pm$ SD; $*p < 0.05$ N_2O = nitrous oxide. (Reproduced from Van Hemelrijck et al[2] with permission)

pharmacokinetic properties arises. Recovery after neurosurgery should be reliably short. Evidence based on computer simulations of drug infusions suggests that the rate of decline in concentration at the effect site is more important to the recovery characteristics than the drug's terminal half life.[3][4] Fig 4.2 shows simulations of the time required for the concentration of thiopentone and propofol at the effect site to decline by 50%;[5] the simulations are based on the pharmacokinetics of each drug and the rate of equilibration between plasma and effect site, and the figure relates the increasing time required for recovery to increase in duration of infusion. When the infusion is stopped, the concentration of propofol at the effect site decreases by 50% far more rapidly than that of thiopentone, and the time required for that decline increases far more with the duration of infusion for thiopentone than for propofol. This is consistent with the clinical experience that, using thiopentone for maintenance of anaesthesia, recovery may be unacceptably slow. By contrast, even after a 6 hour infusion of propofol, only 15 minutes are required for a 50% decrease in concentration. Of course, if the drug is precisely titrated so that the percentage decrease required for recovery is less than 50%, the time required will be less than that shown in fig 4.2 and will asymptotically approach zero for a 0% decrease. In view of these facts, it is not surprising that propofol is, for the moment, the most suitable hypnotic for total intravenous anaesthesia (TIVA).

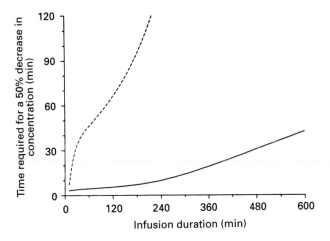

Fig 4.2 Recovery curves showing time required for a 50% decrease in propofol (——) and thiopentone (– – –) concentration following discontinuation of continuous infusion. (Reproduced from Shafer *et al*[5] with permission)

This effect has also been demonstrated for opioids.[6] Although alfentanil has a shorter terminal half life than sufentanil, the time to reach a 50% decrease in concentration at the effect site, for infusion times of up to eight hours, is actually shorter for sufentanil than for alfentanil, presumably because of the higher lipophilicity of alfentanil. Propofol infusions are often

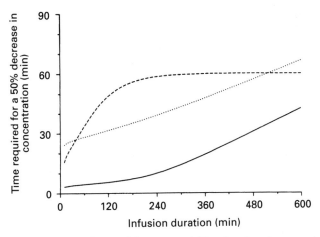

Fig 4.3 Recovery curves of propofol versus opioids, showing time required for 50% decrease in propofol (——), alfentanil (– – –), and sufentanil (· · ·) concentration following discontinuation of continuous infusion. (Reproduced from Shafer *et al*[5] with permission)

Table 4.1   TIVA dosing guidelines for propofol and opioids

Induction

Propofol 1·5–2 mg/kg in 60–120 s

Alfentanil 10–20 μg/kg

or

Sufentanil 0·3–1 μg/kg

Maintenance

Propofol infusion

150–200 μg/kg per min for 10 min

120–150 μg/kg per min for 10 min

100–120 μg/kg per min until closure of the skull

Turn off the propofol infusion about 10 min before the desired time of emergence from anaesthesia. Give 10–20 mg boluses of propofol as needed to keep the patient unconscious until the desired time

Alfentanil infusion

1·5–2 μg/kg per min until the dura is open

0·3–1 μg/kg per min until the dura is closed

Turn off the alfentanil infusion about 30 min before the desired time of emergency from anaesthesia

Sufentanil infusion

0·5–1 μg/kg per h until the dura is open

0·15–0·5 μg/kg per h until the dura is closed

Caveats for propofol dosing

Induction

Even small boluses (10–20 mg) may cause apnoea, especially after premedication

Reduce doses of propofol by 40% for elderly or very ill patients, or after heavy premedication

Anticipate that the blood pressure will drop after induction with propofol/opioid; it usually returns promptly on intubation

Maintenance

Check repeatedly that the infusion is running; if it stops for more than a few minutes, the patient will wake up during the operation

Propofol is not amnestic, so patients must be kept completely unconscious with propofol to prevent intraoperative awareness

If the patient is too deep, turn off the propofol for a minute or two, but remember to turn it back on or the patient will wake up. If your patient is too light, give a 10–40 mg bolus of propofol and increase the infusion rate

Once the infusion is stopped, be prepared to give 10–20 mg boluses of propofol if there are signs of light anaesthesia. This allows assessment of the depth of anaesthesia, and thus facilitates rapid emergence from its effects at the end of surgery

---

combined with opioid infusions during anaesthesia. Fig 4.3 compares the relationship between duration of infusion and recovery time for propofol (as also shown in fig 4.2) with that for alfentanil and sufentanil, based on the published pharmacokinetics of alfentanil[7] and sufentanil.[8] As the decline in propofol concentration is considerably faster than the decline in opioid concentrations, it makes pharmacokinetic sense to stop the infusion of the opioid 30–60 minutes before the end of anaesthesia. Table 4.1 gives clinical guidelines on dosing for TIVA combining propofol and alfentanil[9] and propofol and sufentanil.[5]

Cerebral effects

A second consideration when choosing drugs for intravenous use is their

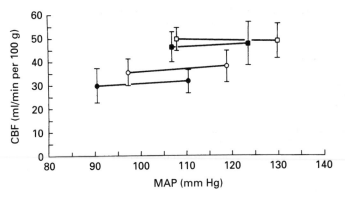

Fig 4.4 Cerebral blood flow (CBF) before and during acute increases in systemic arterial pressure. Cerebral blood flow was measured before and during an acute increase in MAP produced by intravenous infusion of angiotensin II amide in the absence of propofol and during infusion of propofol at rates of 3, 6, and 12 mg/kg per hour. □ Baseline conditions; ■ propofol 3 mg/kg per hour; ○ propofol 6 mg/kg per hour; ● propofol 12 mg/kg per hour. Values are mean ± SD. (Reproduced from Van Hemelrijck et al[10] with permission)

cerebral effects. Intravenous anaesthetic agents in general cause a decrease in CBF and cerebral metabolic rate for oxygen (CMR_{O_2}), but they may not be vasoconstrictors in a strict sense, because barbiturates, for example, dilate

Terms	
CBF	cerebral blood flow
CBV	cerebral blood volume
CMR	cerebral metabolic rate
CMR_{O_2}	cerebral metabolic rate for oxygen
CMRglu	cerebral metabolic rate for glucose
CPP	cerebral perfusion pressure
CSFP	pressure in the cerebrospinal fluid
CVR	cerebrovascular resistance
ICP	intracranial pressure
MABP	mean arterial blood pressure
MAC	minimum alveolar concentration of an anaesthetic
MAP	mean blood pressure
P_{CO_2}	carbon dioxide tension or partial pressure
TIVA	total intravenous anaesthesia

isolated cerebral vessels in vitro. The decrease in CBF induced by most intravenous anaesthetics appears to be the result of decreased metabolism secondary to cerebral functional depression. Among the intravenous anaesthetics, ketamine may be unique because it produces an increase in both CBF and CMR_{O_2}.

Hypnotics

Propofol

Although the effect of propofol on cerebral perfusion pressure (CPP) caused concern when the drug was first introduced into clinical practice, it has been convincingly demonstrated that undesirable, pronounced, haemodynamic effects can be prevented by avoiding high peak concentrations.[8 9] The effects of propofol on CMR and CBF are very similar to those of barbiturates. In baboons, propofol produced a dose dependent decrease in CBF and CMR, and autoregulation was preserved[10] (fig 4.4); similar results were obtained in dogs.[11] In another study in dogs, a decrease in cerebrospinal fluid (CSF) pressure, and dose dependent changes in CBF, CMR, and the electroencephalogram (EEG) were demonstrated, but autoregulation and reactivity to CO_2 were unaffected.[12] A dose related decrease in CBF and CMR was also found in rabbits.[13] In early investigations in humans, it was shown that propofol decreased CBF and CMR.[14 15] In patients with brain injury, anaesthesia with propofol decreased CPP, intracranial pressure (ICP), and CBF.[16] The difference in arteriobulbar oxygen content was unaltered. Preservation of the reactivity of cerebral perfusion to CO_2 during propofol anaesthesia has been demonstrated in patients.[14 17 18]

Although N_2O can be avoided by using TIVA, its use might be considered in combination with intravenous anaesthetics because its analgesic and amnestic effects are beneficial. N_2O given during intravenous anaesthesia with propofol decreases the requirements for propofol and provides more stable haemodynamic conditions during maintenance of anaesthesia.[19] In contrast to volatile anaesthetics, propofol appears to abolish the cerebrostimulatory effects of N_2O. In baboons the effects of different infusion rates of propofol on CBF and CMR were identical with and without N_2O.[10] These findings have been confirmed in patients; the addition of N_2O to propofol did not alter blood flow velocity in the middle cerebral artery or the CO_2 response curve.[18] Although there has been some controversy over the effect of propofol on corticol synthesis, it was recently demonstrated that anaesthesia using propofol does not inhibit the ability of the adrenal cortex to synthesise cortisol in response to adrenocorticotrophic hormone (ACTH).[20]

Barbiturates

Barbiturates have been used since 1937 to reduce the ICP.[21] Pierce et al[22] demonstrated that thiopentone is a pronounced and dose dependent cerebral vasoconstrictor. During anaesthesia with barbiturate, CMR_{O_2} is reduced in proportion to the depth of anaesthesia. At the point of EEG isoelectricity, there is no further reduction in CMR_{O_2} even if the babiturate dose is increased further.[23] CBF appears to follow these changes in metabolic rate, so that the greatest reduction in flow is with the deepest anaesthesia.[24] The maximal decrease in CMR_{O_2} induced by thiopentone is 55–60%. Thus, with barbiturates, functional depression appears to be coupled with the reduction in CBF and CMR_{O_2}, which suggests that barbiturates also reduce the metabolic components linked to brain function and produce only minimal effects on metabolic function related to the maintenance of cellular integrity.

A similar reduction in blood flow in the spinal cord, with the formation of a plateau, was found with high doses of thiopentone in dogs.[25] Continuous administration of thiopentone has been successfully employed for neurosurgical procedures using, on average, a total dose of 1230 mg; it is a useful adjunct to balanced anaesthesia for such operations.[26 27] The ICP is reduced by barbiturates, possibly as a result of the reduction in CBF and CBV. This effect is used during treatment of raised ICP in patients with head injuries, although this is controversial,[28] as well as during neurosurgical procedures for stopping or transiently controlling acute waves of increased ICP.[29] Barbiturates attenuate the cerebral vasodilatation produced by N_2O and ketamine and thus are useful as supplemental anaesthetics.[30 31]

Etomidate
Etomidate is a non-barbiturate imidazole compound which has some beneficial effects because it produces little, if any, cardiovascular depression in healthy individuals. Even in the presence of cardiovascular disease, etomidate depresses the cardiovascular system minimally. It may have advantages for poor risk patients and where preservation of a normal systemic arterial pressure is crucial. Enthusiasm for etomidate has been eroded by the frequent occurrence of involuntary muscle activity and by the recognition that it suppresses adrenocortical function. The increased mortality in critically ill patients sedated with an etomidate infusion[32] was attributed to its effect on cortisol synthesis. Etomidate inhibits the activity of the 17α-hydroxylase and 11β-hydroxylase enzymes necessary for the synthesis of cortisol, aldosterone, 17-hydroxyprogesterone, and corticosterone; even after an induction dosage, adrenal suppression persists for 5–8 hours.[33 34] The clinical effect of any short term blockade of cortisol synthesis can, however, probably be ignored.

A cerebral metabolic effect of etomidate, similar to that of barbiturates, was found in experiments on dogs;[35] during the infusion, CMR_{O_2} decreased progressively until an isoelectric EEG appeared, but as with thiopentone, increasing the doses of etomidate after flattening of the EEG did not produce a further reduction in CMR_{O_2}, and brain energy metabolism remained normal. Unlike the CMR_{O_2}, the CBF decreased precipitously with the start of the infusion, and achieved a maximal decrease before the CMR_{O_2}. This might suggest that etomidate causes vasoconstriction by a different mechanism (possibly by direct action) from that of the barbiturates. A parallel decrease in ICP and CBF was observed.

In humans, etomidate reportedly induced almost parallel reductions in CBF and CMR_{O_2}; with clinical doses, they were both decreased by about 30–50%. Reactivity to CO_2 is preserved during anaesthesia with etomidate.[36 37]

Etomidate effectively decreases ICP[38] without decreasing CPP.[39] In patients with severe head injuries, etomidate decreased ICP while electrocortical activity was present but was not effective when that activity was already maximally suppressed.[40] This indicates that the decrease in ICP may be caused by the reduction of CBF which is induced by functional (metabolic) depressant effects of etomidate.

Ketamine

Ketamine is a derivative of phencyclidine. Phencyclidine was introduced as a general anaesthetic in 1957 but never received approval for human use, although it is commonly used as a hypnotic in animals. Increases in CBF and CMR_{O_2} have been reported with ketamine in animals;[41–43] pre-treatment with thiopentone completely blocks these effects.[42] Vasodilatation caused by ketamine has been attributed, in part, to metabolic stimulation. It also has a direct dilating effect on cerebral arteries caused, in part, by interference with the transmembrane influx of Ca^{2+}.[43] Ketamine induced increases in CBF are blocked by hyoscine (scopolamine) and enhanced by CO_2 or physostigmine;[44] thus it may increase CBF by a cholinergic mechanism. In goats, ketamine had no significant influence on CBF.[45] Whether these discrepant effects are caused by differences in the background anaesthesia (N_2O) or are a species difference is not clear. Cerebral metabolic effects of ketamine appear to vary among the various brain structures.

In humans, intravenous ketamine 3 mg/kg increases CBF by about 60% and reduces cerebrovascular resistance (CVR) but CMR_{O_2} does not change significantly.[46] The increases in regional CBF in the frontal and parieto-occipital areas are remarkable and might be associated with the dreams or hallucinations peculiar to ketamine. It has been suggested that metabolic regulatory mechanisms are involved in the cerebrovascular response to ketamine.[47]

Ketamine markedly increases ICP;[48–50] such increases can be blocked or attenuated by induced hypocapnia[49] or by the administration of thiopentone or a benzodiazepine,[48 49] but there are some reports of failure to block them with quinalbarbitone (secobarbital), droperidol, diazepam, or midazolam.[51] All the available evidence suggests that ketamine should not be used during anaesthesia for neurosurgery or neuroradiology, especially in patients with elevated ICP or decreased intracranial compliance.

Benzodiazepines

The benzodiazepines are considered receptor specific, which accounts for their unique cerebral effects and for the development of specific antagonists. With the introduction of the water soluble compound midazolam, its use for inducing anaesthesia has gained in popularity whereas the other benzodiazepines are now administered primarily for providing sedation and amnesia only. Midazolam produces a parallel reduction in CBF and $CMRo_2$.[52][53] Metabolic suppression is less with midazolam than with barbiturates. In dogs, the infusion of midazolam produces parallel decreases in CBF and $CMRo_2$ to a maximum of 25%; increasing the dose produces no further decreases and this plateau may reflect saturation of the benzodiazepine receptors.

In humans, midazolam 0·15 mg/kg decreases CBF by about 30%[54][55] with a concomitant reduction in $CMRo_2$;[55] this effect is completely blocked by the specific benzodiazepine antagonist flumazenil.[56]

Midazolam reportedly produced either a decrease[54] or no change[57] in ICP. In patients with brain tumours the induction of anaesthesia with midazolam 0·25 mg/kg had no apparent effect on ICP, and this was comparable with the actions of thiopentone,[57] although these negative results may result from the presence of a normal ICP before administration of the drugs. In patients with elevated ICP, anaesthetised with fentanyl and N_2O, midazolam 0·2 mg/kg decreased ICP, although it had no significant effect in those with normal ICP.[54] Midazolam appears to maintain better haemodynamic stability than thipentone when given to patients with brain tumours; there is a smaller fall in mean arterial blood pressure (MABP) and CPP tends not to decrease.

The effects of diazepam on CBF and $CMRo_2$ are variable and species dependent. Moderate decreases in both were found in dogs; intravenous diazepam 0·25 mg/kg decreased them by about 15%, accompanied by the slowing of the EEG.[58] In rats, diazepam decreased CBF by 30% with minimal change in $CMRo_2$, but the combination of diazepam and N_2O (70%) decreased $CMRo_2$ (and CBF) by about 40%, suggesting a synergy between these two agents.[59] In dogs, the decrease in $CMRo_2$ after diazepam was not attenuated by the addition of N_2O.[60]

In normal humans, diazepam in combination with fentanyl and N_2O produces parallel decreases in CBF and $CMRo_2$; CO_2 reactivity is preserved.[61] In patients with head injuries, diazepam produced a 25% decrease in CBF and $CMRo_2$.[62] Contrary to the assumption that ICP would be decreased because of a lower CBF, diazepam 0·25 mg/kg did not change ICP.[63] Lorazepam, triazolam, and flurazepam seem to have similar effects to those of diazepam and midazolam.

As a specific receptor antagonist is now available, benzodiazepine derivatives are useful as induction or supplemental drugs during neuroanaesthesia, but it must be recognised that the competitive antagonist, flumazenil, also antagonises the effects of midazolam on CBF, $CMRo_2$, and ICP.[64][65] Thus

99

this drug must be used cautiously when reversing benzodiazepine induced sedation in patients with impaired intracranial compliance.

Opioids

The literature on the cerebral effects of opioids is marked by apparently controversial findings. Many of the controversies can, however, be resolved by considering the background anaesthetic used in the various experiments. When a vasodilating agent is used, such as volatile anaesthetics or N_2O, opioids usually cause cerebral vasoconstriction and a decrease in CBF. Conversely, when the background anaesthetic causes vasoconstriction (for example, barbiturates) or when opioids are used without adding another agent, there is no or only a very slight effect on CBF as long as the carbon dioxide tension (P_{CO_2}) is kept within normal limits.[65] Opioids do not influence cerebral autoregulation or CO_2 reactivity.[66-69]

The effect on cerebral metabolism is also influenced by the associated anaesthetic. Together with N_2O, opioids cause a definite decrease in cerebral metabolism, but when used as a sole agent there is no such clear effect.

Opioids do not offer cerebral protection; fentanyl induced decrease in cerebral metabolism did not have the same positive effect on the postischaemic metabolic state as a similar decrease caused by barbiturates and hypothermia.[70] On the other hand, there is no demonstrably negative effect.

Morphine

An early study found that morphine increased CBF, but this may have been due to an increase in arterial P_{CO_2} (Pa_{CO_2}), secondary to respiratory depression.[71] In more recent studies, incremental doses of morphine caused a progressive and parallel decrease in CBF and CMR_{O_2} in normocapnic dogs anaesthetised with N_2O. A metabolic depressive effect which accompanied the decreased CBF was antagonised by nalorphine (N-allylnormorphine).[72] Several reports demonstrate that morphine does not significantly affect CBF, CMR_{O_2}, and CMRglu (cerebral metabolic rate of glucose).

When non-anaesthetised individuals were given 60 mg morphine, Moyer et al[73] found a significant reduction in CMR_{O_2} with no change in CBF. In normocapnic human volunteers, morphine–N_2O anaesthesia did not significantly affect CBF, CMR_{O_2}, or cerebral autoregulation;[74 75] possibly the vasoconstrictive effect of morphine is counteracted by the vasodilating effect of N_2O. Recently it was demonstrated that low dose morphine, when given postoperatively, causes a rise in P_{CO_2} in spontaneously breathing patients; this in turn caused an increase in CBF and the formation of oedema.[71]

Fentanyl, alfentanil, sufentanil

In dogs and rats, fentanyl, when given with N_2O as the background anaesthetic, causes a decrease in CBF and CMR_{O_2}.[66 76-78] In unanaesthetised newborn lambs, fentanyl in doses as high as 4·4 mg/kg did not alter CBF or CMR_{O_2}.[79] Increases in CBF and CMR_{O_2} occurred in rats when seizures were induced with high doses of fentanyl,[76 78] but the increases in CBF were not comparable with those in CMR_{O_2}.[76] Whether the disproportionate increase in metabolism causes ischaemic brain damage has not yet been determined. In recent publications there has been much controversy about the cerebral effects of sufentanil and alfentanil. First in the study on dogs by Newberg *et al*,[80] they showed that sufentanil causes a significant increase ($40 \pm 8\%$) in CBF,[80] but this increase was accompanied by a decrease in cerebral metabolism and a stable ICP. The same investigators later found a similar temporary increase with alfentanil 0·3 μg/kg bolus in dogs, followed by a decrease of metabolism and flow.[81]

These animal studies were followed by the human studies of Marx *et al*,[82] who compared the effects of fentanyl, alfentanil, and sufentanil on the pressure in the cerebrospinal fluid (CSFP) and on cerebral perfusion pressure (CPP), with CPP being the difference between mean arterial pressure (MAP) and CSFP. Fentanyl 5 μg/kg did not influence the CSFP and decreased the CPP by only $14 \pm 3\%$. Alfentanil 50 μg/kg (followed by an infusion of 1 μg/kg per min) and sufentanil 1 μg/kg caused increases in CSFP of $22 \pm 5\%$ ($p < 0·01$) and $89 \pm 31\%$ ($p < 0·05$), respectively. The CPP decreased by $25 \pm 5\%$ after sufentanil and by $37 \pm 3\%$ after alfentanil. Marx *et al* warned against the use of alfentanil and sufentanil in patients with reduced intracranial compliance. Their results for fentanyl and alfentanil were confirmed in a subsequent study.[83] If one considers the absolute value of the increased CSFP, however, it appears that the proportional increase caused by sufentanil ($89 \pm 31\%$) accounted for only $2·7 \pm 0·9$ mm Hg of the pressure. It must be remembered that the CSFP is only an approximation of the ICP. Albanese *et al*[84] found a rise in ICP secondary to a bolus of sufentanil (1 μg/kg every 6 min) caused by a significant increase in CBF; the rise caused a decrease in CPP below 45 mm Hg, a value that could cause cerebral ischaemia. During infusion (0·005 μg/kg per min) the ICP returned to baseline and the CPP rose to a normal value of 55 mm Hg.[84] The critical rise in ICP is probably the result of indirect vasodilatation caused by systemic hypotension, possibly secondary to the large initial dose. This problem can be avoided by administering sufentanil slowly and preventing systemic hypotension.

Sperry *et al*[85] recently demonstrated that both fentanyl 3 μg/kg and sufentanil 0·6 μg/kg can cause an increase in ICP (8 ± 2 and 6 ± 1 mm Hg, respectively) in patients with cerebral trauma. Both opioids decreased MAP by 10–11 mm Hg.[85] Numerous other investigators have produced different results. In 1985, Keykhah *et al*[86] showed that sufentanil caused a decrease in CBF and cerebral metabolism in rats. Werner *et al*[87] described a 35–40% decrease in cerebral metabolism and blood flow in dogs treated with sufentanil 20 μg/kg; there was no change in ICP.

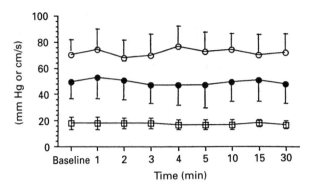

Fig 4.5 Cerebral perfusion pressure ($\ominus$, CPP, mm Hg), intracranial pressure ($\boxminus$, ICP, mm Hg), and middle cerebral artery mean blood flow velocity ($\bullet$, V_{mean}, cm/s) before and 1–20 min after intravenous sufentanil 3 µg/kg in patients with severe brain injury ($n = 14$). Values are mean ± SD. V_{mean} and ICP did not change significantly as CPP was maintained. (Reproduced from Werner et al[94] with permission)

Using a different background anaesthetic, Van Hemelrijck et al[88] found no changes in ICP when sufentanil was given to dogs with a normal or artificially elevated ICP. Sheehan et al[89] looked at ICP changes in rabbits after cryogenic brain injuries. In this model the cerebrovascular effects of fentanyl and sufentanil were compared with those in a control group; the CPP decreased in all three groups, which was a logical effect of the artificially raised ICP, but the blood flow did not change significantly. There were no differences between fentanyl and sufentanil as far as an influence on MAP, ICP, and CBF was concerned. Stephan et al[68] found a decrease of cerebral metabolism and blood flow when patients were given sufentanil 10 µg/kg followed by an infusion ($0\cdot15$ µg/kg per min); the CO_2 reactivity of the CBF was maintained. Herrick et al[90] found no changes in pressure under the brain retractors and observed similar decreases in CPP when fentanyl, alfentanil, or sufentanil was used; they concluded that all three opioids are safe for intraoperative use. Weinstanbl et al[91] found no changes in ICP when sufentanil was administered to patients with increased ICP (>20 mm Hg) in the presence of a decrease in MAP; theoretically this could have caused cerebral vasodilatation secondary to ischaemia, but their technique for measurement of ICP is less accurate than intraventricular measurements. In a clinical study by Cuillerier et al,[92] no difference was found when comparing the effects of the three opioids on the CPP. In a double blind study in neurosurgical patients, From et al[93] could not demonstrate differences in the clinical effects of fentanyl, alfentanil, and sufentanil.

In an open study, Werner et al[94] examined patients for 30 minutes after a bolus of sufentanil 3 µg/kg with a P_{CO_2} of $3\cdot99$ kPa (30 mm Hg); they found no charges in mean CBF and ICP (fig 4.5), findings that are consistent with those of earlier studies in dogs. Mahla et al[95] used transcranial Doppler to study the influence of sufentanil on blood flow in the mid-cerebral artery, comparing patients with and without intracranial pathology; in both groups sufentanil 1 μg/kg did not influence this blood flow, either with or without hyperventilation, and it was concluded that it does not cause cerebral vasodilatation. Similar findings were obtained by Cheng et al[96] comparing sufentanil with midazolam; sufentanil (0·1 and 0·2 μg/kg) had no effect on CBF and midazolam decreased it (15–25%).

In a dose–response study Slee et al[97] studied the influence of sufentanil (0·5 and 1 μg/kg) on CBF and ICP with a P_{CO_2} of 3·72–4·26 kPa (28–32 mm Hg). It did not cause direct cerebral vasodilatation, and the ICP increased only with a high dose, apparently secondary to indirect vasodilatation caused by an autoregulatory response to systemic hypotension. The absolute increase was modest and not clinically relevant.

In conclusion, it appears that alfentanil and sufentanil are successfully used in neuroanaesthesia as the main anaesthetic.[98–101] The safety of fentanyl, alfentanil, and sufentanil in combination with hypnotics is also established.[8 93 102 103] All three are considered equally reliable.

Remifentanil

Remifentanil, a new agent, appears to qualify as an ideal short acting opioid.[104–106] In most respects, its pharmacodynamic profile is staightforward. It is a typical opioid agonist selective for μ receptors. As with alfentanil, it can produce intense analgesia with an extremely rapid onset of action, and the initial clinical studies showed that it has an analgesic potency similar to that of fentanyl.[107] It also appears to produce other typical opioid effects such as respiratory depression, bradycardia, and hypertonus of skeletal muscle. The acute effects are reversed or prevented by the administration of naloxone. At the time of writing, remifentanil is undergoing phase II clinical investigation.

Clearly, the novel aspect of this new opioid lies in the ester linkage that makes it susceptible to rapid hydrolysis by circulating and tissue non-specific esterases. (The β-adrenergic blocker esmolol is metabolised by similar enzymatic machinery.) The β half life is only about 10–20 min in most individuals and the clearance is an impressive 3–4 l/min. Almost 90% of the drug is recovered in the urine as an acid metabolite, G190291, which in animals has only 1/300th to 1/1000th of the analgesic potency of the parent compound, but this has not yet been confirmed in humans.

Both Egan et al[105] and Westmoreland et al[106] use the same computer simulation to show that the duration of a remifentanil infusion should have almost no influence on the time required for a 50% decrease in its concentration in plasma or at the effect site. It appears that no major adjustments of dosage will be required for patient age, gender, or body weight. Within limits, the recovery time should not be greatly influenced by the dose.

103

Hoffman *et al*[108] report on the cerebrovascular and EEG effects of remifentanil; its short duration of action is readily seen in their data. When remifentanil and alfentanil were infused to equivalent EEG end points in isoflurane anaesthetised dogs, both produced essentially identical reductions in CBF, but neither significantly reduced CMR_{O_2}.[109] After 60 min, the drug infusions were abruptly stopped, and recovery was monitored for a further 30 min, during which, in the alfentanil group, neither the CBF nor the EEG recovered whereas in the remifentanil group the CBF and quantitative EEG patterns both quickly returned to their preinfusion baselines.

The clinical utility of this new opioid remains undefined because human trials are in their infancy. Obviously, questions remain, particularly about long term use. Will accumulation of the metabolite slow recovery, or will rapid disappearance of opioid effects have any unexpected consequences (withdrawal)? The data presented by Hoffmann *et al*[108] suggest that this drug may find an important niche in the anaesthetic armamentarium.

Neuromuscular blocking agents

Depolarising neuromuscular blocking agents

Suxamethonium There is little doubt that suxamethonium (succinylcholine) can increase ICP in humans.[110][111] In early work, the changes in ICP could not be separated from those caused by laryngoscopy or changes in ventilation, but more recent studies indicate that suxamethonium has effects on ICP that are distinctly independent of other events.[110–112] In animal studies these changes were associated with increased CBF and may be related to increases in muscle spindle afferent activity.[110–112] These effects on ICP can be completely blocked by prior paralysis or "precurarisation" with pancuronium or metocurine, indicating that the peripheral neuromuscular junctions play some part.

It has also been reported that suxamethonium induced ventricular fibrillation in patients with subarachnoid haemorrhage, an effect possibly caused by elevation of serum K^+, although some have demonstrated that such an elevation is not significant if patients receive the drug at a relatively early stage (within 4 days).[113] Does this mean that suxamethonium is contraindicated in neurosurgery? Probably not. The changes in ICP are modest and transient. There seems little reason to avoid the drug where very rapid paralysis is needed. This does not apply to most elective conditions, but in an emergency the consequences of an unsecured airway and hypoxia/hypercapnia are far worse than any changes that might occur with suxamethonium. In such cases, small doses of non-depolarising neuromuscular blocking agents should be given before the suxamethonium. Lignocaine (lidocaine) may also be helpful.

Non-depolarising neuromuscular blocking agents

There have been many studies of the effects on CBF/ICP of the non-depolarising neuromuscular blocking agents. These drugs are quite safe; the only suggestion of a detrimental effect is that following the administration of large boluses of d-tubocurarine, where histamine release can increase both cerebral blood volume (CBV) and ICP,[114] but in most Western countries tubocurarine is no longer on the market.

There is one practical concern about non-depolarising neuromuscular blocking agents in neurosurgical patients. Case reports and clinical studies have demonstrated that medication with phenytoin (and possibly carbamazepine) increases the dose requirements for all such agents;[115 116] the dose–response curves for most of them are shifted to the right and the duration of effects is markedly reduced;[115] the mechanism is, however, unknown. The fact that the acute administration of phenytoin to a patient receiving vecuronium will enhance the blockade is confusing.

One other factor, the presence of local neurological deficits, particularly hemiplegia, occasionally complicates the use of non-depolarising neuromuscular blocking agents in neurosurgery. It has been long known that paretic/plegic extremities are relatively resistant to the action of these agents.[117] Titration of these drugs in response to twitch monitoring of such extremities can lead to relative overdosage and difficulties with reversal. This can pose certain unique problems during intracranial surgery if the non-paretic extremity is not easily accessible for monitoring of neuromuscular function.

Pancuronium   Pancuronium does not produce an increase in CBF, $CMRo_2$ or ICP in dogs anaesthetised with 1 MAC (minimum alveolar concentration) of halothane.[118] Pancuronium frequently induces an increase in blood pressure and heart rate, however, which could be disadvantageous for certain patients, such as those with hypertension, especially if they have disturbed autoregulation; in such patients a substantial elevation of ICP could occur.

Atracurium   In animals, atracurium seems to have no significant effect on CBF, $CMRo_2$,[118] or ICP.[118 119] Its metabolite, laudanosine, can readily cross the blood–brain barrier and cause seizures. The serum concentration of laudanosine after clinical doses of atracurium should not, however, have undesirable consequences.[120 121] Lanier et al[118] found no significant differences between the seizure thresholds for lignocaine in cats paralysed with atracurium, pancuronium, or vecuronium. High doses of atracurium are able to release histamine, but this potential is considerably less than that of d-tubocurarine.[122] In humans, atracurium had no effect on ICP.[123 124]

Vecuronium   Vecuronium does not induce the release of histamine or change blood pressure or heart rate. In cats with elevated ICP, it did not induce a further rise in ICP.[125] In patients with brain tumours, vecuronium had no or only a minimal effect on ICP.[126 127]

Pipecuronium   Pipecuronium, a new, long acting, non-depolarising, neuromuscular blocking agent, reportedly has no significant effect on ICP or CPP in patients with intracranial tumours when their ICP is not raised at the time of administration.[128]

Summary When non-depolarising neuromuscular blocking agents are used, changes in CBF and ICP are minimal in most clinical states, if respiration is well controlled and an increase in Pa_{CO_2} avoided.

Inhalational anaesthetics

Effects on cerebral physiology

Nitrous oxide

The fact that N_2O has long been considered a benign drug with minor effects on cerebral physiology is surprising, because in 1963 McDowall *et al*[129] observed a reversible decrease in CBF when air replaced N_2O during halothane anaesthesia, and in 1968 Theye and Michenfelder[130] demonstrated that N_2O produced an increase in cerebral metabolism in dogs. The underestimation of these cerebral effects has caused much confusion in research on anaesthesia and cerebral physiology. The contradictions in the observed cerebral effects in early investigations on animals can at least partly be explained by the interspecies differences in MAC for N_2O. When comparing the effects of identical inspired concentrations of this gas among different species, the effects of very different MAC equivalents are being compared. There are numerous investigations, both in animals and in humans, which confirm that N_2O produces cerebral vasodilatation in excess of its stimulatory effects on metabolism. An increase in cerebral metabolism was shown in rats,[131] goats,[132] and dogs.[130 133] Hoffman *et al*[134] found that the addition of N_2O partly offset the effect of midazolam on CMR in rats.[134] A cerebral vasodilatory effect was recorded in rabbits,[135 136] cats,[137] rats,[138] dogs,[31 133] pigs,[139] and human volunteers.[140] In the study of volunteers by Deutsch and Samra,[140] analysis of regional CBF revealed heterogeneous changes in CBF, with a tendency to increase in the anterior and decrease in the posterior cortical regions. This anterior–posterior gradient differs from the changes produced by other vasodilators such as CO_2, which causes a uniform increase in CBF in all cortical areas.[141] The increase in CBF with N_2O is most evident during inhalational anaesthesia. Sakabe *et al*[141] found an increase in CBF when N_2O was added to anaesthesia with halothane. Hansen *et al*[138] studied the effects of combining N_2O with isoflurane or halothane on CBF in rats; the combination produced a higher CBF than simply increasing the concentration of isoflurane or halothane to obtain an equal MAC. Interestingly, CBF during 1 MAC isoflurane combined with N_2O was higher than with 1 MAC halothane combined with N_2O, although the opposite relationship was observed with 1 MAC of the volatile agents without N_2O. These findings have now been confirmed during isoflurane anaesthesia in humans.[142]

Theoretically, the changes in CBF with N_2O could either be secondary to changes in CMR or the result of a direct effect on the cerebral vessels. Reasoner and co-workers[131] demonstrated that an increase in anaesthetic depth from 0·5 to 1 MAC, achieved with isoflurane alone, caused a significant reduction in CMRglu, whereas the addition of 70% N_2O (0·5 MAC) to 0·5 MAC isoflurane (1 MAC total) left CMRglu unchanged. The absence of any change in CMR when 0·5 MAC N_2O was added to 0·5 MAC isoflurane, in contrast to the associated increase in CBF, appears to indicate that the effect of N_2O on CBF is, at least partly, direct and mediated by factors other than changes in cerebral metabolism.

Although CO_2 reactivity remains intact during the administration of N_2O,[137] hyperventilation did not blunt the cerebral vasodilatation when N_2O was added to an inhalational anaesthetic in the rabbit.[143] Although N_2O clearly increases CBF and CMR, these effects may be different when it is given with intravenous hypnotics. Investigating the effects of propofol infusions in baboons Van Hemelrijck *et al*[10] found that the substitution of air in the respiratory mixture with 60% N_2O had no effect on CBF or CMR; these findings have been confirmed in patients.[144] Recently, Lam *et al*[145] demonstrated that N_2O is a more potent cerebral vasodilator than isoflurane in humans. Accordingly, Jung *et al*[146] found that the impact of N_2O on CSFP in patients with brain tumours is more important than the effect of an equipotent concentration of isoflurane (fig 4.6).[146] As early as 1974, N_2O was reported to increase ICP in patients with reduced cerebral compliance.[147] An influence of N_2O on autoregulation has never been demonstrated.

The classic inhalational anaesthetics: halothane, enflurane, isoflurane

The conventional concept is that anaesthetics alter neuronal function, thereby altering the metabolic demands and, secondary to this, the transport of oxygen and glucose to the brain. In other words, function drives metabolism and metabolism drives flow. Inhalational anaesthetics (except N_2O) produce a decrease in CMR, which is maximal when the functional activity of the brain cells stops, that is, when the EEG is isoelectric. Newberg *et al*[148] demonstrated that progressive metabolic depression occurs with concentrations of isoflurane greater than 1 MAC until the EEG becomes isoelectric; this metabolic depression by isoflurane appears to be more extensive than that by equipotent concentrations of halothane.[149]

In 1972 Smith and Wollmann[150] showed that inhalational anaesthetics have the unique characteristic of uncoupling the close relationship that normally exists between CBF and CMR_{O_2}. Although such anaesthetics decrease CMR, they increase CBF, and the magnitude of this uncoupling effect is dose dependent. This traditional concept was challenged by Hansen *et al*:[151] during halothane and isoflurane anaesthesia in rats, they demonstrated a strong correlation between CMR and CBF within individual anatomical

107

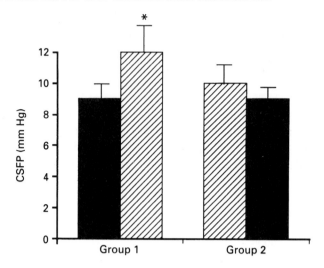

Fig 4.6 Change in cerebrospinal fluid pressure (CSFP) in patients with brain tumours ($n = 20$) when 0.68 ± 0.01 vol% isoflurane was replaced with $65 \pm 1\%$ nitrous oxide (group 1), or when $68 \pm 1\%$ nitrous oxide was replaced with 0.71 ± 0.01 vol% isoflurane (group 2). Values are mean $\pm$ SEM. $\star p < 0.05$ versus value at initial situation. CSFP increased significantly when isoflurane was replaced with nitrous oxide, but not when nitrous oxide was replaced with isoflurane. (■) Isoflurane; (▨) N_2O. (Reproduced from Jung et al[146] with permission)

regions and over a wide range of metabolic values. In addition, for an identical CMRglu, CBF was higher during isoflurane than during halothane anaesthesia. These findings suggested that the coupling between CBF and CMR remained intact. When autoradiological techniques were used to determine regional and global CBF, it appeared that isoflurane and halothane produce distinctly different patterns of flow distribution within the brain; although the greatest effect of halothane on blood flow was in the cortex, the values for subcortical flow were greater with isoflurane.[152] The seemingly contradictory findings on the coupling of flow and metabolism can be explained by the use of different methods to determine CBF and CMR. Only with techniques that measure local CBF and CMR is it possible to prove that the coupling is preserved. However, the notion that inhalational anaesthetics appear to change the relationship between global CBF and global CMR remains useful in explaining the clinical observations when these agents are used in neurosurgical patients.

The effects of anaesthetics on cerebrovascular tone are the sum of direct and indirect effects. An indirect effect occurs when flow is altered secondary to a metabolic effect. Thus, an increase in CBF results from an increase in CMR, and a decrease in CBF is the result of a decrease in CMR. Volatile anaesthetics cause cerebral vasodilatation by direct action, and therefore tend to increase CBF; on the other hand, volatile anaesthetics decrease CMR, resulting in a reduction in flow by an indirect effect. The net effect is the result of the balance between these two opposite actions. During the administration of increasing concentrations of halothane or isoflurane in the cat, a dose related decrease in $CMRo_2$ was demonstrated;[149] the decrease was always greater with isoflurane. This probably explains the difference between the effects of isoflurane and halothane on CBF: isoflurane causes less vasodilatation than halothane as a result of the greater decrease in CMR. In experiments on rabbits, Drummond et al[153] proved the validity of this hypothesis. Under anaesthesia with morphine and N_2O, isoflurane produced a larger decrease in $CMRo_2$ than halothane, resulting in a decrease in CBF with isoflurane and an increase with halothane. However, under pentobarbitone (pentobarbital) anaesthesia, neither agent produced any change in CMR, but both resulted in a small and identical increase in CBF. The different degree of metabolic depression with isoflurane and halothane at lower inspired concentrations also explains why the CBF did not change during the administration of up to 1 MAC of isoflurane, but only up to 0·375% of halothane in two similar experiments in baboons.[154 155]

The fact that inhalational anaesthetics are cerebral vasodilators explains why they may increase ICP, especially when intracranial compliance is reduced. Although the greatest reduction in CVR is produced by halothane, this response can be blunted by first establishing hyperventilation.[156] The increase in ICP produced by isoflurane in patients with brain tumour can be blocked by the simultaneous introduction of hyperventilation;[157 158] the increase in ICP appears to parallel the expected changes in CBF.[158] Patients with a midline shift on computed tomography (severely reduced cerebral compliance) are more likely to have an elevation of the ICP.[159]

Low concentrations of inhalational anaesthetics attenuate the efficacy of autoregulation, which is finally abolished at high concentrations. In experiments in baboons, Van Aken et al[154] demonstrated that autoregulation remained intact with concentrations of isoflurane below 1 MAC, but was impaired with higher concentrations (fig 4.7); these findings have been confirmed in humans[160 161] and in dogs.[162] Recently, Hoffman et al[163] showed in experiments on rats that the loss of autoregulation with isoflurane was not only dose dependent but also regionally specific. During halothane anaesthesia in cats, autoregulation was even lost with concentrations below 1 MAC.[149] These findings were confirmed in experiments on baboons by Brüssel et al[155] (fig 4.8).

The CO_2 reactivity of CBF appears normal during inhalational anaesthesia.[164–166] When high concentrations of isoflurane were given to rats, however, and the MAP decreased below the limits of autoregulation, Ringaert et al[167] demonstrated that CO_2 reactivity was lost. Nevertheless, by hyperventilation it appears possible to blunt, abolish, or even reverse the cerebral vasodilatation that occurs when volatile anaesthetics are adminis-

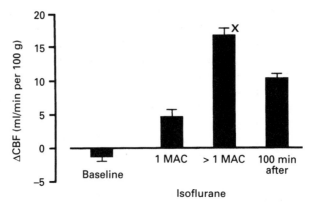

Fig 4.7 Change in cerebral blood flow (ΔCBF) associated with an acute increase in mean arterial blood pressure (MAP) before, during 1 MAC and over 1·5 MAC isoflurane, and 100 min after administration of isoflurane. When the cerebral autoregulation is intact, this increase in MAP does nto change the CBF. Autoregulation was intact before and during 1 MAC isoflurane, but it was impaired significantly by higher concentrations of isoflurane. Even 100 min after withdrawal of isoflurane, changes in CBF were elevated but not significant. Values are mean ± SD. X indicates $p \leqslant 0.05$. (Reproduced from Van Aken et al[154] with permission)

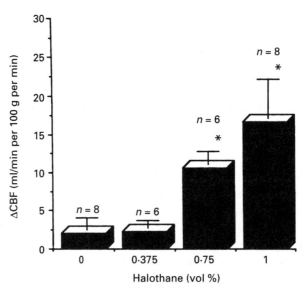

Fig 4.8 Change in cerebral blood flow (ΔCBF) associated with an acute increase in mean arterial blood pressure before halothane and during 0·375, 0·75, and 1·0 vol% of halothane. Values are mean ± SD. $\star p < 0.05$. (Reproduced from Brussel et al[155] with permission)

tered. It must be emphasised that this only applies predictably to the normal brain and may not be so in the presence of intracranial pathology. Following a cryogenic brain injury in rabbits, for example, ICP increased during both halothane and isoflurane anaesthesia, and the increase could not be prevented by hyperventilation.[168] In the presence of brain oedema, Shah et al[169] found that the response to hypocapnia was preserved with fentanyl but not with supplemental isoflurane. This is clinically important, because it means that hyperventilation will be far more effective in reducing brain volume and/or ICP during a fentanyl based anaesthesia than with an isoflurane supplemented anaesthetic in patients with space occupying lesions and significant brain oedema.

By what mechanism do volatile anaesthetics dilate cerebral vessels?

Halothane and isoflurane alter the tension of isolated cerebral vascular smooth muscle, a response that is further modulated by the CO_2 tension.[170] These direct effects on cerebral vessels may explain the disturbed relationship between flow and metabolism. Since the discovery of the endothelial modulation of vascular reactivity in 1981, almost every effect of anaesthetics on the vessels is believed to be mediated by the endothelium. The vasodilatory action of halothane is thought by some to involve nitric oxide (NO)[171] but by others to be independent of it.[172] Indeed, halothane reduces the vasodilatory effect of NO,[172 173] an effect that ought to attenuate the vasodilatation. In contrast to the conflicting results about the role of NO, it is generally agreed that halothane depletes intracellular (sarcoplasmic) Ca^{2+} stores; this effect is less pronounced during isoflurane, enflurane, and sevoflurane anaesthesia.[174 175] Another interesting finding is that volatile anaesthetics produce hyperpolarisation in snail neurons;[176] if this is also the case in cerebral vascular smooth muscle, it could be a plausible explanation for the reduced effect of halothane and isoflurane during K^+ stimulated compared with prostaglandin $F_{2\alpha}$ ($PGF_{2\alpha}$) stimulated contraction.[170] This notion is based on the fact that a hyperpolarisation is not attainable in K^+ stimulated arteries.

The new inhalational agents: desflurane and sevoflurane

Both desflurane and sevoflurane have a low blood gas solubility and their pharmacokinetics are therefore characterised by a more rapid cerebral wash in and wash out than with the currently available volatile agents. As a result, both favour rapid recovery from anaesthesia, a feature that could be of benefit in neuroanaesthesia. The available evidence, although still relatively limited, points, however, to a pattern of cerebral effects rather similar to that of isoflurane.

Desflurane

Lutz et al[177] examined the effects of desflurane in dogs: it produced a dose dependent decrease in CMR_{O_2} and, as with the older volatile agents, it appeared to be a cerebral vasodilator, causing a dose dependent decrease in CVR. As a result the CBF increased at concentrations of desflurane above 1 MAC, if the blood pressure was supported with a phenylephrine infusion; however, if MAP was allowed to decrease below the limits of autoregulation the CBF decreased. The changes in ICP were minimal. It must be emphasised that the dogs in this study had no intracranial pathology and their ICP was not experimentally increased.

In another study on dogs, CO_2 reactivity was preserved at 1, 1·5, and 2 MAC of desflurane.[178] Milde and Milde[179] studied the cerebral effects of desflurane induced hypotension in dogs: 2·2 and 2·4 MAC of desflurane were needed to reduce the MAP to 50 and 40 mm Hg and decrease the CBF by 36% and 60%, respectively, whereas the CMR_{O_2} was decreased by 20%. Cerebral concentrations of ATP, phosphocreatinine, and lactate remained within normal limits, indicating that global perfusion was adequate for the metabolic demands. CBF decreased at these high concentrations of desflurane, as a result of the fall in the CPP below the lower limit of autoregulation. The decrease in CMR_{O_2} was limited to 20%; this was probably because maximal metabolic depression was achieved at a concentration of more than 2 MAC. The changes in CBF and CMR produced by desflurane in both studies were comparable with those produced by equivalent concentrations of isoflurane in methodologically similar investigations.

Ornstein *et al*[180] compared the effects on CBF of 1·0 and 1·5 MAC isoflurane and desflurane in an air–oxygen mixture in hyperventilated patients undergoing craniotomy for tumour; both agents had similar effects and normal CO_2 reactivity was preserved. The effects of desflurane on CSFP were studied using lumbar spinal fluid catheters;[181] in spite of hyperventilation a sustained increase in CSFP from 11 ± 4 mm Hg to 19 ± 6 mm Hg ($p < 0.002$) was observed when 1 MAC of desflurane in oxygen was given to these patients. The same investigators found no increase in CSFP when 0·5 MAC of isoflurane or desflurane in 50% nitrous oxide was administered.[182] It is not clear if the increase in CSFP with 1 MAC of desflurane was the result of a decrease in arteriolar tone causing an increase in CBF, or of an increase in CBV caused by venodilatation.

Sevoflurane

In isocapnic pigs 1 MAC of sevoflurane produced a moderate decrease in blood flow in all regions of the brain;[183] when the concentration was increased to 1·5 MAC, no further increase in flow occurred in the cerebrum but in the cerebellum flow returned to control values owing to a decrease in CVR. Cortical CMR_{O_2} was decreased by 50% and 52% compared with awake values using 1 and 1·5 MAC of sevoflurane; the fall exceeded that in CBF. These results suggest that the cerebral effects of sevoflurane are similar to those of isoflurane.

Scheller *et al*[184] compared the cerebral effects when 0·5 and 1 MAC of sevoflurane or isoflurane were added to N_2O/morphine background anaesthesia in rabbits. CBF remained unchanged with both supplemental anaesthetics when compared with baseline measurements for morphine/N_2O alone. The CMR_{O_2} decreased to the same extent (50% at 1 MAC, $p < 0.05$). A similar, small, but statistically significant increase in ICP was observed. In dogs, isoflurane and sevoflurane produced a significant fall in CMR_{O_2},[185] but CBF was identical with 0·5, 1·5, or 2·15 MAC of isoflurane or sevoflurane. The measurements of CBF in this investigation may have been influenced by the significant decrease in MAP produced by the higher concentrations of both agents. Rats anaesthetised with sevoflurane showed a dose related increase in the diameter of cerebral vessels and an increase in CBF.[186] Nevertheless, the same investigators demonstrated that sevoflurane was a less potent vasodilator than isoflurane;[187] the changes in vessel diameter and flow in single pial arterioles were significantly more pronounced under isoflurane than under sevoflurane anaesthesia and, accordingly, the changes in ICP were more pronounced with isoflurane.

Adjuvant drugs

Sedation, analgesia, and anaesthesia are often accompanied by a reduction in arterial pressure, cardiac output, systemic vascular resistance, and heart rate. This cardiovascular depression may be advantageous as long as it is controlled to levels consistent with adequate perfusion of vital tissues. When haemodynamic variables are recorded continuously throughout neurosurgical operations, they reveal disturbing fluctuations and stimulus–response phenomena. Hypertensive episodes may occur during the anaesthesia but are most likely to be stimulated during laryngoscopy and intubation, at the time of skin incision and during extubation.[188 189]

Autoregulation of CBF may be disturbed in patients who have undergone neurosurgery, and compensation by cerebral vasoconstriction for sudden increases in arterial blood pressure may be difficult.[190 191] Under these conditions, an increase in arterial blood pressure may lead to a sudden elevation in CBF and ICP. Every hypertensive reaction may initiate a breakdown of the blood–brain barrier and a transudation of fluid causing cerebral oedema or intracerebral haemorrhage, or both.[192 193] Normally, an increase in intracranial volume is compensated for by displacement of CBF from the cranium. In patients with space occupying lesions, however, this mechanism may be insufficient and the ICP may increase dramatically. This can happen when the initial ICP is normal if the intracranial compliance is reduced. Here the mechanisms for compensation are already exhausted, and sudden increases in arterial pressure in the perioperative period should therefore be assiduously avoided.

Catecholamines are the principal mediators of such intraoperative hypertensive reactions. There are two options available to the anaesthetist:

1 Attempt to suppress this response after it has occurred
2 Prevent its occurrence at the outset.

Treatment of hypertension often relies on agents that relax vascular smooth muscle. In patients with compromised intracranial compliance, however, cerebral vasodilatation must be avoided because it leads to an increase in CBV. This, in turn, may raise ICP and result either in herniation of brain contents or a decrease in cerebral perfusion leading to brain ischaemia. Different pharmacological means of preventing or suppressing such intraoperative hypertensive reactions will now be reviewed. Many of the drugs produce adverse effects that could preclude their use in patients with reduced intracranial compliance; α-adrenergic and β-adrenergic receptor blockers can safely be used with such patients.[194]

Lignocaine

Many reports on the prevention of hypertension during intubation have centred on the use of lignocaine, either topically or intravenously, to block the afferent or efferent limb of the reflexes responsible.[195][196] Anaesthesia of the pharynx, larynx, and trachea by topical application of lignocaine has been investigated by several workers. It is time consuming and may induce coughing with its contraindicated effects on blood pressure; it is also frequently ineffective in preventing intracranial hypertension during laryngoscopy and intubation.[196] Nevertheless, lignocaine has been used for years to facilitate such procedures, even though it does not have much proven effect on the stress response. Previous intravenous administration of lignocaine can attenuate but not prevent increases in blood pressure during intubation and extubation. Hamill et al[196] showed that intravenous administration of lignocaine 1·5–2 mg/kg prevents the increase in ICP associated with endotracheal intubation of patients with brain tumours.

Antihypertensive drugs

Different antihypertensive drugs have been suggested for the prevention and treatment of hypertensive reactions.

Sodium nitroprusside

Sodium nitroprusside is a vasodilating drug most commonly used to induce hypotension during surgery; its onset of action is rapid, and its action short and readily controllable. Nitroprusside acts primarily on arteriolar tone; only 65–70% of arterial sodium nitroprusside is recovered in venous plasma.[197] Accurate knowledge of dose, rate of administration, and total dose given is a prerequisite to its use. The recommended maximum dosages of 1.5 μg/kg for acute administration and 0.5 mg/kg per h (8 μg/kg per min) for chronic administration appear to be safe.[198]

Data on the effects of sodium nitroprusside on CBF during controlled hypotension are inconsistent. Some studies report no change in CBF from baseline;[199–201] others state that the CBF decreased[202–204] or, along with ICP, increased (in animals and neurosurgical patients).[205 206] The reasons for these conflicting results are not easily determined; differences in species, anaesthetic technique, and baseline conditions might be involved. Delay in measurement of CBF after the start of sodium nitroprusside may explain why early changes in flow were not observed.

One study showed the importance of the degree of hypotension induced by sodium nitroprusside on CBF.[207] Initially, when nitroprusside was given to decrease MAP moderately, CBF also increased, but as larger doses were given to decrease MAP further, the CBF remained close to its baseline until MAP reached 65 mm Hg; when MAP fell below this, the pressure–flow relationship was linear.

Impairment or loss of autoregulation of CBF is a primary concern when hypotensive agents are used in neurosurgical anaesthesia. Clearly, sodium nitroprusside impairs autoregulation in normal animals.[207] Such impairment precludes any modulation of CBF in response to acute alterations in systemic arterial blood pressure. Under these circumstances, the intracranial contents not only are subjected to the specific pharmacological activity of the hypertensive agents but will also closely reflect changes in the systemic circulation. Marsh et al[208] found that the magnitude of the change in ICP was related to the speed of onset of the drug effect. When the dose of sodium nitroprusside was gradually increased over many minutes no changes in ICP were seen, so presumably this approach allowed time for spatial compensation.

Glyceryl trinitrate

Glyceryl trinitrate (nitroglycerin) directly dilates venous capacitance vessels;[209] it has a short half life and no clinically significant toxic metabolites. As with sodium nitroprusside, low intracranial compliance contraindicates the use of glyceryl trinitrate before opening of the dura mater.[210] Even when the dura has been opened, both nitrates incur some risk of increased CBV and significant brain swelling.[211] Differences between sodium nitroprusside and glyceryl trinitrate clearly exist; although both are able to decrease arterial blood pressure, the effect of sodium nitroprusside is more rapid and consistent.

Hydralazine

Hydralazine, a smooth muscle blocking agent, effectively induces hypotension when low concentrations of enflurane are administered; rebound hypertension does not occur and ICP increases significantly.[212] On the other hand, hydralazine given slowly has been used widely and safely in neurosurgical practices; presumably this technique allows time for spatial compensation.

Purine derivates

A natural substance that produces hypotension would be an attractive alternative to the previously discussed drugs; both ATP and adenosine meet this criterion.[213] Similar degrees of hypotension can be achieved as with sodium nitroprusside, but recovery is more rapid and there is no rebound hypertension.[214 215] Unfortunately, ATP and adenosine dilate cerebral vessels, increase CBF, increase ICP when intracranial compliance is low, and impair cerebral autoregulation.[215–217]

Urapidil

Urapidil, an antihypertensive drug not available in the United States of America, has two mechanisms of action: antagonism of peripheral α-adrenergic receptors and interaction with the hydroxytryptamine (serotonin) 5-HT_{1A} receptors in the brain. This pharmacological profile explains the vasodilatation and lack of significant sympathetic activation observed during the administration of urapidil.[218] ICP and intracranial compliance were not affected in animals or patients given urapidil.[219 220] The CBF of baboons did not change when MAP was decreased from 107 ± 13 to 70 ± 13 mm Hg with urapidil;[221] greater degree of hypotension could not be achieved by increasing the dose and rebound hypertension did not occur. Urapidil seems to be a suitable agent for the induction of moderate degrees of hypotension (MAP = 70 mm Hg). Administration of urapidil with isoflurane for induced hypotension in animals attenuated the undesirable effects and diminished the required concentration of the volatile anaesthetic (fig 4.9);[222] this technique is often used in clinical practice in Europe.

Esmolol

Esmolol is a short acting, cardioselective, intravenous, β-adrenergic receptor blocking drug with a very rapid onset of action.[223] It has been used by itself to decrease blood pressure[224–226] or in combination with other drugs.[227]

Labetalol

Labetalol produces hypotension by blocking both α_1-receptors and β_1-receptors; it also blocks β_2-receptors. As a result of decreases in cardiac output and peripheral vascular resistance, blood pressure decreases promptly after intravenous administration of labetalol. An important advantage of this drug is the absence of any increase in ICP, even when intracranial compliance is reduced.[228] Experiments in rats showed that blood flow to vital organs was

116

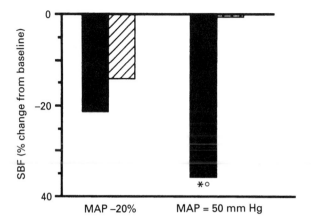

Fig 4.9 Changes in splanchnic blood flow from baseline during deliberate hypotension at a 20% decrement of mean arterial pressure and a mean arterial pressure of 50 mm Hg. ▨ IVA; ■ ISO. Values are mean ± SEM. *$p < 0.05$ between groups; ○ $p < 0.05$ as compared with baseline. IVA = intravenous anaesthesia; ISO = isoflurane; SBF = splanchnic blood flow. (Reproduced from Kick et al[222] with permission)

significantly better when the hypotensive agent was isoflurane combined with labetalol rather than isoflurane alone.[229]

Convulsant and anticonvulsant effects of anaesthetics

The proconvulsant and anticonvulsant effects of anaesthetics have been extensively reviewed by Modica et al.[230] In humans, propofol produced excitatory activity (for example, movements, myoclonus, muscle tremors, and hiccoughs) during induction of anaesthesia.[231] There is a recent report of anticonvulsant activity by propofol in experimental status epilepticus in rabbits.[232] Propofol, when compared with methohexitone (methohexital) as an anaesthetic for electroconvulsive therapy, was associated with less seizure activity,[233] and it was also successfully used to control resistant status epilepticus.[234–236] In patients without a history of seizures, low doses of thiopentone and methohexitone can elicit EEG activity; with increasing doses of these sedative–hypnotic drugs, slower waveforms of higher amplitude appear, which progress to burst suppression at high doses.[237] EEG or clinical seizure activity has not been reported in non-epileptic patients treated with these ultrashort acting barbiturates, but excitatory phenomena such as abnormal muscle movements, hiccoughing, and tremor may occur with both thiopentone and methohexitone, more commonly with the second.[238]

The tendency of methohexitone to provoke convulsions during intravenous induction (0·5–1 mg/kg) in patients with a history of epilepsy is well

117

known.[239] In one series of more than 900 patients with unspecified types of epilepsy, the frequency of epileptiform activity during induction with methohexitone was much less than in previous sleep and conscious EEGs.[240] Methohexitone has never been shown to provoke either EEG or clinical seizure activity in patients with generalised convulsive disorders.[237]

Thiopentone has well known anticonvulsant properties in humans. After an initial intravenous injection of 250–1000 mg given slowly until cessation of seizures, continuous thiopentone infusions (80–120 mg/h) for as long as 13 days have been used successfully in intubated and ventilated patients to control status epilepticus refractory to more conventional anticonvulsant drugs.[241 242] The infusions were titrated to produce a burst suppression EEG pattern. Interestingly, the seizures did not recur after discontinuation of the infusion. Thus, although the epileptogenic effects of methohexitone in patients with psychomotor epilepsy are well established,[243] the ultrashort acting barbiturates are predominantly potent anticonvulsants.

The EEG patterns produced by etomidate are similar to those associated with thiopentone;[244 245] the main difference between equipotent doses of the hypnotics etomidate ($0\cdot3$ mg/kg) and thiopentone ($3\cdot5$ mg/kg) is a lack of β activity during "light stages" of etomidate anaesthesia. Higher doses of etomidate produce burst suppression patterns analogous to those seen with the barbiturates. Involuntary myoclonic movements are common during induction with etomidate and occasionally resemble generalised convulsive seizures.[244 246] Surface EEG studies on patients without a history of epilepsy given etomidate did not reveal spiking during these myoclonic movements,[244 245] but such studies in patients with a history of epilepsy do reveal its proconvulsant effects.[247] Etomidate appears also to possess anticonvulsant properties in both humans and animals. The drug increased the threshold for opioid induced EEG seizures in dogs.[248] In humans, administering etomidate successfully ended status epilepticus recorded on EEG.[249] Overall, etomidate has both proconvulsant and anticonvulsant effects on EEG.

In patients without a history of seizures, cortical EEG recordings 1–2 min after intravenous ketamine 1–3 mg/kg are characterised by the initial appearance of fast β activity at 30–40 Hz, which is followed by moderate voltage θ activity mixed with high voltage δ waves recurring at 3–4 second intervals.[250] Higher doses of intravenous ketamine (>2 mg/kg) produce a burst suppression pattern.

EEG seizure activity has not been reported in non-epileptic patients during ketamine administration. Myoclonic and seizure-like motor activity has, however, been observed clinically in non-epileptic children and adults after intravenous (2 mg/kg) or intramuscular (10–12 mg/kg) ketamine.[251 252] These movements occurred soon after induction[251] and later after additional incremental doses, but unfortunately, simultaneous EEG recordings were not available. It is well established that ketamine will activate epileptogenic foci in patients with known seizure disorders.[253 254] The available evidence indicates that ketamine primarily possesses potent cerebral stimulatory properties, especially in patients with seizure disorders, in whom the drug activates subcortical seizure activity.

After intravenous diazepam 10–20 mg an increase in EEG amplitude can be seen in the β band between 12 and 22 Hz; this is probably related to the major clinical effects of the benzodiazepines—sedation and amnesia.[255] EEG or clinical seizure activity has not been reported in non-epileptic patients treated with benzodiazepines. In patients with the Lennox–Gastaut syndrome, a form of secondary generalised epilepsy,[256] benzodiazepines used in anaesthetic practice possess potent anticonvulsant properties. Intramuscular midazolam 15 mg is as effective as intravenous diazepam 20 mg in abolishing interictal spikes.[257] Although intravenous diazepam (or midazolam) is often regarded as the drug of choice in emergency therapy of generalised seizure disorders, it appears that intramuscular midazolam is an acceptable alternative where it is not possible to establish intravenous access.[257] Overall, the benzodiazepines are effective in controlling status epilepticus in more than 90% of patients with generalised seizure disorders. Also, they are effective in about 60% of cases of status epilepticus in partial epilepsy.

High dose morphine causes seizures in animals,[248] but this has never been shown in humans, even with large doses.[258] There are rare reports of epileptic problems associated with epidural and intrathecal morphine but causation was never proved.[259]

Pethidine (meperidine) has neuroexcitatory activity, mainly resulting from its metabolite norpethidine (normeperidine).[260] The possibility of seizures increases with chronic oral intake, as a result of an important first pass effect which enhances the production of norpethidine. Even after intramuscular administration, seizures have been reported, and with intravenous administration the concentrations of norpethidine can become raised because of the prolonged elimination half life (14–21 h).

In rodents, high dose fentanyl, sufentanil, or alfentanil, also caused seizures,[248] but this was not shown in EEG studies on humans.[261 262] Fentanyl, alfentanil, or sufentanil causes muscle rigidity during induction which resembles myoclonic seizure activity. Although the exact reason is not clear, most clinical and EEG findings do not suggest epileptic effects and the extreme muscle rigidity is probably secondary to a neurochemical process in the striatonigral pathway.[263] Muscle rigidity can cause a rise in ICP; to prevent this, the administration of neuromuscular blocking agents is recommended when cerebral compliance is limited.

In conclusion, morphine and pethidine seem to cause some seizure activity, but this is not a problem with fentanyl, sufentanil, and alfentanil, where the only possible effect is muscle rigidity, which can be prevented with neuromuscular blocking agents.

N_2O is the oldest and most widely used general anaesthetic and has a long standing record of safety. There are only a few reported cases of convulsions in which N_2O may have played a part.[264 265] Withdrawal convulsions have been observed in mice[266] and volunteers exposed to hyperbaric N_2O exhibited muscle rigidity and jerking movements.[267] EEG studies have not, however, revealed any seizure activity during the administration of N_2O to patients.[268] N_2O has no anticonvulsant properties. In spite of its known "cerebral stimulatory" effects, its epileptogenic potential appears to be extremely low and it is not contraindicated in epileptic patients. In both normal and epileptic patients, clinical and EEG seizure activity have been observed when enflurane was administered.[269-271] High concentrations of enflurane (3–6%) generate high voltage spike and dome activity with intermittent periods of burst suppression. The ability of enflurane to produce seizures is influenced by its concentration and is enhanced at low Pa_{CO_2}.[272] As a result of its propensity for inducing epileptic activity and the availability of otherwise equivalent inhalational agents, the use of enflurane is relatively contraindicated in neuroanaesthesia.

There are only a few early reports of seizures in patients receiving halothane,[264 273] and these also received N_2O at the same time. EEG studies have never revealed any epileptogenic activity of halothane, which actually possesses distinct anticonvulsant effects.[274]

Induction of anaesthesia with isoflurane is characterised by low voltage, fast wave EEG activity which progresses towards high voltage, slow wave activity at 1 MAC; at 1·5 MAC a burst suppression pattern is noted, followed by an isoelectric EEG at ±2 MAC.[275] In older patients these EEG changes are more prominent at lower concentrations of isoflurane.[276] There are a few reports of clinical seizure like activity when isoflurane was administered together with N_2O, but it is not clear if these myoclonic movements were the result of real epileptic phenomena.[277] One report concerns spiking activity associated with clinical seizures that appeared during induction with N_2O and isoflurane but did not continue during maintenance.[265] Seizure like movements have not been reported during isoflurane anaesthesia in epileptic patients. In fact, isoflurane has potent anticonvulsant properties and has been used for the treatment of refractory status epilepticus,[278 279] although 50% of the patients' seizure activity resumed when isoflurane was discontinued.

Knowledge of the EEG effects of the newer inhalational anaesthetics, desflurane and sevoflurane, is still limited. In pigs and in humans the EEG changes produced by desflurane appeared to be similar to those with equipotent concentrations of isoflurane, with no indication of any convulsant activity.[280 281] In rabbits the EEG pattern produced by sevoflurane was identical to that with equipotent concentrations of isoflurane.[184] No epileptic activity was observed when up to 2·25 MAC of sevoflurane was given to dogs, with or without hyperventilation, but enflurane did produce sustained EEG and motor evidence of seizure activity induced by auditory stimuli at concentrations above 1 MAC.[185] In human volunteers, the EEG under sevoflurane anaesthesia differed from that with halothane or isoflurane;[282] anaesthetic concentrations of sevoflurane appeared to produce a characteristic EEG activity of 10–14 Hz, and at higher inspired concentrations the 5–8 Hz activity increased with persistence of the 10–14 Hz activity. There is no EEG or clinical evidence for seizure activity with desflurane or sevoflurane in epileptic patients. Further studies are needed to determine if these agents have anticonvulsant properties. In conclusion, except for enflurane all inhalational anaesthetics seem to be safe with regard to their possible epileptogenic properties, although there are some reservations concerning sevoflurane and desflurane in view of the limited experience with these new drugs.

1 Todd MM, Warner DS, Sokoll MD, et al. A prospective, comparative trial of three anesthetics for elective supratentorial craniotomy Anesthesiology 1993; 78: 1005–20.
2 Van Hemelrijck J, Van Aken H, Merckx L, Mulier J. Anesthesia for craniotomy: total intravenous anesthesia with propofol and alfentanil compared to anesthesia with thiopental, isoflurane, fentanyl, and nitrous oxide. J Clin Anesth 1991; 3: 131–5.
3 Hughes MA, Glass PSA, Jacobs JR. Context-sensitive half-time in multicompartment pharmacokinetic models for intravenous anesthetic drugs. Anesthesiology 1991; 76: 334–41.
4 Shafer SL, Stanski DR. Improving the clinical utility of anesthetic drug pharmacokinetics. Anesthesiology 1992; 76: 327–30.
5 Shafer L. Advances in propofol. Phamacokinetics and pharmacodynamics. J Clin Anesth 1993; 5: 14S–21S.
6 Shafer SL, Varvel JR. Pharmacokinetics, pharmacodynamics, and rational opioid selection. Anesthesiology 1991; 74: 53–63.
7 Scott JC, Stanski DR. Decreased fentanyl and alfentanil dose requirements with age. A simultaneous pharmacokinetic and pharmacodynamic evaluation. J Pharmacol Exp Ther 1987; 240: 159–66.
8 Hudson RJ, Bergstrom RG, Thomson IR, Sabourin MA, Rosenbloom M, Strunin L. Pharmacokinetics of sufentanil in patients undergoing abdominal aortic surgery. Anesthesiology 1989; 70: 426–31.
9 Ravussin P, Guinard JP, Ralley F, Thorin D. Effect of propofol in cerebrospinal fluid pressure and cerebral perfusion pressure in patients undergoing craniotomy. Anaesthesia 1988; 43: 37–41.
10 Van Hemelrijck J, Fitch W, Mattheussen M, Van Aken H, Plets C, Lauwers T. The effect of propofol on the cerebral circulation and autoregulation in the baboon. Anesth Analg 1991; 71: 49–54.
11 Werner C, Hoffman WE, Kochs E, Albrecht RF, Schulte am Esch J. The effects of propofol on cerebral blood flow in correlation to cerebral blood flow velocity in dogs. J Neurosurg Anesthesiol 1992; 4: 41–6.
12 Artru AA, Shapira Y, Bowdle TA. Electroencephalogram, cerebral metabolic, and vascular responses to propofol anesthesia in dogs. J Neurosurg Anesthesiol 1992; 4: 99–109.
13 Ramani R, Todd MM, Warner DS. A dose–response study of the influence of propofol on cerebral blood flow, metabolism and the electroencephalogram in the rabbit. J Neurosurg Anesthesiol 1992; 4: 110–19.
14 Stephan H, Sonntag H, Schenk HD, Kohlshausen S. Einfluss van Disoprivan (Propofol) auf die Durchblutung und den Sauerstoffverbrauch des Gehirns und die CO_2-Reaktivität der Hirngefässe beim Menschen. Anaesthesist 1987; 36: 60–5.
15 Vandesteene A, Trempont V, Engelman E, et al. Effect of propofol on cerebral blood flow and metabolism in man. Anaesthesia 1988; 43: 42–3.
16 Pinaud M, Lelausque JN, Chetanneau A, Fauchoux N, Ménégalli D, Souron R. Effects of propofol on cerebral hemodynamics and metabolism in patients with brain trauma. Anesthesiology 1990; 73: 404–9.
17 Fox J, Gelb AW, Enns J, Murkin JM, Farrar JK, Manninen PH. The responsiveness of

cerebral blood flow to changes in arterial carbon dioxide is maintained during propofol–nitrous oxide anesthesia in humans. *Anesthesiology* 1992; **77**: 453–6.

18 Eng C, Lam AM, Slee Mayberg T, Lee C, Mathisen T. The influence of propofol with and without nitrous oxide on cerebral blood flow velocity and CO_2 reactivity in humans. *Anesthesiology* 1992; **77**: 872–9.

19 Van Hemelrijck J, Tempelhoff R, White PF, Jellish WS. EEG-assisted titration of propofol infusion during neuroanesthesia: effect of nitrous oxide. *J Neurosurg Anesthesiol* 1992; **4**: 11–20.

20 Van Hemelrijck J, Weekers F, Van Aken H, Bouillon R, Heyns W. Propofol anesthesia does not inhibit stimulation of cortisol synthesis. *Anesth Analg* 1995; **80**: 573–6.

21 Horsley JS. The intracranial pressure during barbital narcosis. *Lancet* 1937; **i**: 141.

22 Pierce EC, Jr, Lambertsen CJ, Deutsch S, *et al.* Cerebral circulation and metabolism during thiopental anesthesia and hyperventilation in man. *J Clin Invest* 1962; **41**: 1664–71.

23 Michenfelder JD. The interdependency of cerebral functional and metabolic effects following massive doses of thiopental in the dog. *Anesthesiology* 1974; **41**: 231–6.

24 McDowall DG. The effects of general anaesthetics on cerebral blood flow and cerebral metabolism. *Br J Anaesth* 1965; **37**: 236–45.

25 Hitchon PW, Kassell NF, Hill TR, Gerk MK, Sokoll MD. The response of spinal cord blood flow to high-dose barbiturates. *Spine* 1982; **7**: 41–5.

26 Hunter AR. Synergism between halothane and labetalol. *Br J Anaesth* 1972; **44**: 506–10.

27 Grundy BL, Yanas H, Diven W, Procapio P, Snyder J, Wingard L. Thiopentone infusion in neuroanaesthesia: blood concentrations and E.E.G. correlates. *Br J Anaesth* 1981; **53**: 303P.

28 Ward JD, Becker DP, Miller JD, *et al.* Failure of prophylactic barbiturate coma in the treatment of severe head injury. *J Neurosurg* 1985; **62**: 383–8.

29 Shapiro HM, Galindo A, Wyte SR. Rapid intraoperative reduction of intracranial pressure with thiopentone. *Br J Anaesth* 1973; **45**: 1057–62.

30 Sakabe T, Kuramoto T, Inoue S, Takeshita H. Cerebral effects of nitrous oxide in the dog. *Anesthesiology* 1978; **48**: 195–200.

31 Dawson B, Michenfelder JD, Theye RA. Effect of ketamine on canine cerebral blood flow and metabolism: modification by prior administration and thiopental. *Anesth Analg* 1971; **50**: 443–7.

32 Ledingham IM, Watt I. Influence of sedation on mortality in critically ill multiple trauma patients. *Lancet* 1983; **i**: 1270.

33 Vanacker B, Wiebalck A, Van Aken H, Sermeus L, Bouillon R, Amery A. Induktionsqualität und Nebennierenrindenfunktion. Ein klinischer Vergleich von Etomidat-Lipuro® und Hypnomidate®. *Anaesthesist* 1993; **42**: 81–9.

34 Crozier TA, Beck D, Schlaeger M, Wuttke W, Kettler D. Endocrinological changes following etomidate, midazolam, or methohexital for minor surgery. *Anesthesiology* 1987; **66**: 628–35.

35 Milde LN, Milde JH, Michenfelder JD. Cerebral functional, metabolic, and hemodynamic effects of etomidate in dogs. *Anesthesiology* 1985; **63**: 371–7.

36 Cold GE, Ekskesen V, Eriksen H, Amtoft O, Madsen JB. CBF and $CMRO_2$ during continuous etomidate infusion supplemented with N_2O and fentanyl in patients with supratentorial cerebral tumors. A dose–response study. *Acta Anaesthesiol Scand* 1985; **29**: 490–4.

37 Renou AM, Vernhiet J, Macrez P, *et al.* Cerebral blood flow and metabolism during etomidate anaesthesia in man. *Br J Anaesth* 1978; **50**: 1047–51.

38 Prior JGL, Hings CJ, Williams J, Prior PF. The use of etomidate in the management of severe head injury. *Intensive Care Med* 1983; **9**: 313–20.

39 Dearden NM, McDowall DG. Comparison of etomidate and althesin in the reduction of increased intracranial pressure after head injury. *Br J Anaesth* 1985; **57**: 361–8.

40 Bingham RM, Procaccio F, Prior PF, Hinds CJ. Cerebral electrical activity influences the effects of etomidate on cerebral perfusion pressure in traumatic coma. *Br J Anaesth* 1985; **57**: 843–8.

41 Cavazzuti M, Porro CA, Biral GP, Benassi C, Barbieri GC. Ketamine effects on local cerebral blood flow and metabolism in the rat. *J Cereb Blood Flow Metab* 1987; **7**: 806–11.

42 Davis DW, Mans AM, Biebuyck JF, Hawkins RA. The influence of ketamine on regional brain glucose use. *Anesthesiology* 1988; **69**: 199–205.

43 Fukuda S, Murakawa T, Takeshita H, Toda N. Direct effects of ketamine on isolated canine cerebral and mesenteric arteries. *Anesth Analg* 1983; **62**: 553–8.

44 Reicher D, Bohalla P, Rubinstein EH. Cholinergic cerebral vasodilation effect of ketamine in rabbits. *Stroke* 1987; **18**: 445–9.

45 Schwedler M, Miletich DJ, Albrecht RF. Cerebral blood flow and metabolism following ketamine administration. *Can Anaesth Soc J* 1982; **29**: 222–6.

46 Takeshita H, Okuda Y, Sari A. The effects of ketamine on cerebral circulation and metabolism in man. *Anesthesiology* 1972; **36**: 69–75.

47 Hougaard K, Hansen A, Brodersen P. The effect of ketamine on regional cerebral blood flow in man. *Anesthesiology* 1974; **41**: 562–7.

48 Artru AA, Katz RA. Cerebral blood volume and CSF pressure following administration of ketamine in dogs; modification by pre- or post-treatment with hypocapnia or diazepam. *J Neurosurg Anesthesiol* 1989; **1**: 8–15.

49 Sari A, Okuda Y, Takeshita H. The effect of ketamine on cerebrospinal fluid pressure. *Anesth Analg* 1972; **51**: 560–5.

50 Wyte SR, Shapiro HM, Turner P, Harris AB. Ketamine-induced intracranial hypertension. *Anesthesiology* 1972; **36**: 174–6.

51 Belapavovic M, Buchthal A. Modification of ketamine-induced intracranial hypertension in neurosurgical patients by pretreatment with midazolam. *Acta Anaesth Scand* 1982; **26**: 458–62.

52 Hoffman WE, Miletich DJ, Albrecht RF. The effects of midazolam on cerebral blood flow and oxygen consumption and its interaction with nitrous oxide. *Anesth Analg* 1986; **65**: 729–33.

53 Fleischer JE, Milde JH, Moyer TP, Michenfelder JD. Cerebral effects of high-dose midazolam and subsequent reversal with RO 15-1788 in dogs. *Anesthesiology* 1988; **68**: 234–42.

54 Larsen R, Hilfiker O, Radle J, Sonntag H. The effects of midazolam on the general circulation, the cerebral blood flow and cerebral oxygen consumption in man. *Anaesthetist* 1981; **30**: 18–21.

55 Forster A, Juge O, Morel D. Effects of midazolam on cerebral blood flow in human volunteers. *Anesthesiology* 1982; **56**: 453–5.

56 Forster A, Juge O, Louis M, Nahory A. Effects of a specific benzodiazepine antagonist (RO15-1788) on cerebral blood flow. *Anesth Analg* 1987; **66**: 309–13.

57 Giffin JP, Cottrell JE, Shwiry B, Hartung J, Epstein J, Lim K. Intracranial pressure, mean arterial pressure, and heart rate following midazolam or thiopental in humans with brain tumors. *Anesthesiology* 1984; **60**: 491–4.

58 Maekawa T, Sakabe T, Takeshita H. Diazepam blocks cerebral metabolic and circulatory responses to local anesthetic-induced seizures. *Anesthesiology* 1974; **41**: 389–91.

59 Carlsson C, Hägerdal M, Kaasik AE, Siesjö BK. The effects of diazepam on cerebral blood flow and oxygen consumption in rats and its synergistic ineraction with nitrous oxide. *Anesthesiology* 1976; **45**: 319–25.

60 Roald OK, Steen PA, Milde JH, Michenfelder JD. Reversal of the cerebral effects of diazepam in the dog by the benzodiazepine antagonist RO15-1788. *Acta Anaesthesiol Scand* 1986; **30**: 341–5.

61 Vernhiet J, Renou AM, Orgogozo JM, Constant P, Caille JM. Effects of a diazepam-fentanyl mixture on cerebral blood flow and oxygen consumption in man. *Br J Anaesth* 1978; **50**: 165–9.

62 Cotev S, Shalit Mn. Effects of diazepam on cerebral blood flow and oxygen uptake after head injury. *Anesthesiology* 1975; **43**: 117–22.

63 Tateiski A, Maekawa T, Takeshita H, Wakuta K. Diazepam and intracranial pressure. *Anesthesiology* 1981; **54**: 335–7.

64 Artru AA. Flumazenil reversal of midazolam in dogs: dose-related changes in cerebral blood flow, metabolism, EEG and CSF pressure. *J Neurosurg Anesthesiol* 1989; **1**: 46–55.

65 Cold GE, Christensen KSJ, Nordentoft J, Engberg M, Bach Pedersen M. Cerebral blood flow, cerebral metabolic rate of oxygen and relative CO_2 reactivity during neuroleptanaes-

thesia in patients subjected to craniotomy for supratentorial cerebral tumors. *Acta Anaesthesiol Scand* 1988; **32**: 310–15.

66 McPherson RW, Traystman RJ. Fentanyl and cerebral vascular responsivity in dogs. *Anesthesiology* 1984; **60**: 180–6.

67 McPherson RW, Krempasanka E, Eimerl D, Traystman RJ. Effects of alfentanil on cerebral vascular reactivity in dogs. *Br J Anaesth* 1985; **57**: 1232–8.

68 Stephan H, Gröger P, Weyland A, Hoeft A, Sonntag H. Einfluss von Sufentanil auf Hirndurchblutung. Hirnstoffwechsel und die CO_2-Reaktivität der menschlichen Hirngefässe. *Anaesthesist* 1991; **40**: 153–60.

69 Shah N, Long C, Marx W, *et al.* Cerebrovascular response to CO_2 in edermatous brain during either fentanyl or isoflurane anesthesia. *J Neurosurg Anesthesiol* 1990; **2**: 11–15.

70 Keykhah MM, Smith DS, O'Neil J, Harp J. The influence of fentanyl upon cerebral high energy metabolites, lactate and glucose during severe hypoxia in the rat. *Anesthesiology* 1988; **69**: 566–70.

71 Cold GE, Felding M. Even small doses of morphine might provoke "Luxury Perfusion" in the postoperative period after craniotomy. *Neurosurgery* 1993; **32**: 327.

72 Takeshita H, Michenfelder JD, Theye RA. The effects of morphine and N-allylnormorphine on canine cerebral metabolism and circulation. *Anesthesiology* 1972; **37**: 605–12.

73 Moyer JH, Pontius R, Morris G, Hershberger R. Effect of morphine and n-allylnormorphine on cerebral hemodynamics and oxygen metabolism. *Circulation* 1957; **15**: 379–84.

74 Jobes DR, Kennell E, Bitner R, Swenson E, Wollman H. Effects of morphine–nitrous oxide anesthesia on cerebral autoregulation. *Anesthesiology* 1975; **42**: 30–4.

75 Jobes DR, Kennell E, Bush GL, *et al.* Cerebral blood flow and metabolism during morphine–nitrous oxide anesthesia in man. *Anesthesiology* 1977; **47**: 16–18.

76 Carlsson C, Smith DS, Keykhah MN, Englebach I, Harp JR. The effects of high dose fentanyl on cerebral circulation and metabolism in rats. *Anesthesiology* 1982; **57**: 375–80.

77 Michenfelder JD, Theye RA. Effects of fentanyl, droperidol and innovar on canine cerebral metabolism and blood flow. *Br J Anaesth* 1971; **43**: 630–6.

78 Safo Y, Young ML, Smith DS, Greenberg J, Carlsson C, Reivich M. Effects of fentanyl on local cerebral blood flow in the rat. *Acta Anaesthesiol Scand* 1985; **29**: 594–8.

79 Yaster M, Koehler RC, Traystman RJ. Effects of fentanyl on peripheral and cerebral hemodynamics in neonatal lambs. *Anesthesiology* 1987; **66**: 524–30.

80 Newberg ML, Milde JH, Gallagher WJ. Effects of sufentanil on cerebral circulation and metabolism in dogs. *Anesth Analg* 1990; **70**: 138–46.

81 Lutz LJ, Milde J, Newberg Milde L. Effects of alfentanil in dogs with reduced intracranial compliance. *J Neurosurg Anesthesiol* 1989; **1**: 169–70.

82 Marx W, Shah H, Long C, *et al.* Sufentanil, alfentanil and fentanyl impact on CSF pressure in patients with brain tumors. *J Neurosurg Anesthesiol* 1989; **1**: 3–7.

83 Jung R, Shah N, Reinsel R, *et al.* Cerebrospinal fluid pressure in patients with brain tumors: impact of fentanyl versus alfentanil during nitrous oxide anesthesia. *Anesth Analg* 1990; **71**: 419–22.

84 Albanese J, Durbic O, Viviand X, Potie F, Alliez B, Martin C. Sufentanil increases intracranial pressure in patients with head trauma. *Anesthesiology* 1993; **79**: 493–7.

85 Sperry RJ, Bailey RL, Reichman MV, Peterson JC, Petersen PB, Pace NL. Fentanyl and sufentanil on cerebral metabolism and circulation in the rat. *Anesthesiology* 1992; **77**: 416–20.

86 Keykhah M, Smith D, Carlsson C, Yaw S, Engleback J, Harp J. Influence of sufentanil on cerebral metabolism and circulation in the rat. *Anesthesiology* 1985; **63**: 274–7.

87 Werner C, Hoffman WE, Baughman VL, Albrecht RF, Schulte am Esch J. Effects of sufentanil on cerebral blood flow, cerebral blood flow velocity and metabolism in dogs. *Anesth Analg* 1991; **72**: 177–81.

88 Van Hemelrijck J, Mattheussen M, Wüsten R, Lauwers T, Van Aken H. The effect of sufentanil on intracranial pressure (ICP) in anesthetized dogs. *Acta Anaesth Belg* 1989; **40**: 239–45.

89 Sheehan PB, Zornow MH, Scheller MS, Peterson BM. The effects of fentanyl and

sufentanil on intracranial pressure and cerebral blood flow in rabbits with an acute cryogenic brain injury. *J Neurosurg Anesthesiol* 1992; **4**: 261–7.

90 Herrick IA, Gelb AW, Manninen PH, Reichman H, Lownie S. Effects of fentanyl, sufentanil and alfentanil on brain retractor pressure. *Anesth Analg* 1991; **72**: 359–63.

91 Weinstabl C, Mayer N, Richling B, Czech T, Spiss CK. Effects of sufentanil on intracranial pressure in neurosurgical patients. *Anaesthesia* 1991; **46**: 437–40.

92 Cuillerier DJ, Manninen PH, Gelg AW. Alfentanil, sufentanil and fentanyl: effect on cerebral perfusion pressure. *J Neurosurg Anesthesiol* 1990; **2**: S8.

93 From RP, Warner DS, Todd MM, Sokoll M. Anesthesia for craniotomy: a double-blind comparison of alfentanil, fentanyl and sufentanil. *Anesthesiology* 1990; **73**: 896–904.

94 Werner C, Kochs E, Bause H, Bischoff P, Schulte am Esch J. The effects of sufentanil on cerebral hemodynamics in patients following severe brain injury. *Anesthesiology* 1992; **77**: A203.

95 Mahla ME, Totten JA, Clark RK, Choi SJ. Sufentanil does not cause cerebral vasodilation in humans. *Anesthesiology* 1992; **77**: A166.

96 Cheng MA, Hoffman WE, Baughman VL. The effects of midazolam or sufentanil sedation on middle cerebral artery blood flow velocity in awake patients [abstracts]. *Anesth Analg* 1993; **76**: S1–476.

97 Slee TA, Lam AM, Winn HR. Cerebral blood flow velocity and intracranial pressure response study. *Anesthesiology* 1990; **73**: A176.

98 McKay RD, Varner PD, Hendrickx PL, Adams ML, Harsh CR. The evaluation of sufentanil N_2O-O_2 vs. fentanyl N_2O-O_2 anesthesia for craniotomy. *Anesth Analg* 1984; **63**: 250–5.

99 Shupack RC, Harp JR. High dose sufentanil vs fentanyl anaesthesia in neurosurgery. *Br J Anaesth* 1985; **57**: 375–81.

100 Welling EC, Donegan J. Neuroleptanalgesia using alfentanil for awake craniotomy. *Anesth Analg* 1989; **68**: 57–60.

101 Dubois M, Hatendi A, Kaufman J, Schwartz S. Alfentanil infusion in neurosurgical patients. *J Neurosurg Anesthesiol* 1989; **1**: 328–32.

102 Jansen GFA, Kedaria M, Zuurmond WWA. Total intravenous anesthesia during intracranial surgery. Continuous propofol infusion in combination with either fentanyl or sufentanil. *Can J Anaesth* 1990; **37**: S128.

103 Bristow A, Shalev D, Rice B, Lipton JM, Giesecke AH. Low-dose synthetic narcotic infusions for cerebral relaxation during craniotomies. *Anesth Analg* 1987; **66**: 413–16.

104 Rosow C. Editorial: Remifentanil: a unique opioid analgesic. *Anesthesiology* 1993; **79**: 875–6.

105 Egan TD, Lemmens HJM, Fiset P, *et al.* The pharmacokinetics of the new short-acting opioid remifentanil (G187084B) in healthy adult male volunteers. *Anesthesiology* 1993; **79**: 881–92.

106 Westmoreland CL, Hoke JF, Sebel PS, Hug CC Jr, Muir KT. Pharmacokinetics of remifentanil (G187084B) and its major metabolite (G190291) in patients undergoing elective inpatient surgery. *Anesthesiology* 1993; **79**: 893–903.

107 Marton JP, Hardman HD, Kamiyama Y, Donn KH, Glass PSA. Analgesic efficacy of single escalating doses of G187084B administered intravenously to healthy adult male volunteers [abstract]. *Anesthesiology* 1991; **75**: A378.

108 Hoffman WE, Cunningham F, James MK, Baughman VL, Albrecht RF. Effects of remifentanil, a new short-acting opioid, on cerebral blood flow, brain electrical activity, and intracranial pressure in dogs anesthetized with isoflurane and nitrous oxide. *Anesthesiology* 1993; **79**: 107–13.

109 Drumond J, Todd M. Are the data missing? *Anesthesiology* 1993; **79**: 1451.

110 Minton MD, Grosslight K, Stirt JA, Bedford RF. Increases in intracranial pressure from succinylcholine: prevention by prior nondepolarizing blockade. *Anesthesiology* 1986; **65**: 165–9.

111 Stirt JA, Grosslight KR, Bedford RF, Vollmer D. "Defasciculation" with metocurine prevents succinylcholine-induced increases in intracranial pressure. *Anesthesiology* 1987; **67**: 50–3.

112 Lanier WL, Iaizzo PA, Milde JH. Cerebral function and muscle afferent activity following

intravenous succinylcholine in dogs anesthetized with halothane: effects of pretreatment with a defasciculating dose of pancuronium. *Anesthesiology* 1989; **71**: 87–95.

113 Manninen PH, Mahendran B, Gelb AW, Merchant R. The effects of succinylcholine on serum potassium in patients with acutely ruptured cerebral aneurysms. *Anesth Analg* 1989; **68**: S180.

114 Tarkkanen L, Laitinen L, Johansson G. Effects of *d*-tubocurarine on intracranial pressure and thalamic electrical impedance. *Anesthesiology* 1974; **40**: 247–51.

115 Ornstein E, Matteo RS, Young WL, Diaz J. Resistance to metocurine-induced neuromuscular blockade in patients receiving phenytoin. *Anesthesiology* 1985; **63**: 294–8.

116 Ornstein E, Matteo RS, Schwartz AE, Silverberg PA, Young WL, Diaz J. The effect of phenytoin on the magnitude and duration of neuromuscular block following atracurium or vecuronium. *Anesthesiology* 1987; **67**: 191–6.

117 Moorthy SS, Hildenberg JC. Resistance to nondepolarizing muscle relaxants in paretic upper extremities of patients with residual hemiplegia. *Anesth Analg* 1980; **59**: 624–9.

118 Lanier WL, Sharbrough FW, Michenfelder JD. Effects of atracurium, vecuronium or pancuronium pretreatment on lignocaine seizure thresholds in cats. *Br J Anaesth* 1988; **60**: 74–80.

119 Giffin JP, Litwak B, Cottrell JE, Hartung J, Capuano C. Intracranial pressure, mean arterial pressure and heart rate after rapid paralysis with atracurium in cats. *Can Anaesth Soc J* 1985; **32**: 618–21.

120 Chapple DJ, Miller AA, Ward JB, Wheatley PL. Cardiovascular and neurological effects of laudanosine. *Br J Anaesth* 1987; **59**: 218–25.

121 Tateishi A, Zornow MH, Scheller MS, Canfell PC. Electroencephalographic effects of laudanosine in an animal model of epilepsy. *Br J Anesth* 1989; **62**: 548–52.

122 Basta SJ, Savarese JJ, Ali HH, Moss J, Gionfriddo M. Histamine-releasing potencies of atracurium, dimethyl tubocurarine and tubocurarine. *Br J Anaesth* 1983; **55**: 105S–6S.

123 Minton MD, Stirt JA, Bedford RF, Haworth C. Intracranial pressure after atracurium in neurosurgical patients. *Anesth Analg* 1985; **64**: 1113–16.

124 Rosa G, Orfei P, Sanfilippo M, Vilardi V, Gasparetto A. The effects of atracurium besylate (Tracrium) on intracranial pressure and cerebral perfusion pressure. *Anesth Analg* 1986; **65**: 381–4.

125 Giffin JP, Hartung J, Cottrell JE, Capuano C, Shwiry B. Effects of vecuronium on intracranial pressure, mean arterial pressure and heart rate in cats. *Br J Anaesth* 1986; **58**: 441–3.

126 Rosa G, Sanfilippo M, Viardi V, Orfei P, Gasparetto A. Effects of vecuronium bromide on intracranial pressure and cerebral perfusion pressure. *Br J Anaesth* 1986; **58**: 437–40.

127 Stirt JA, Maggio W, Haworth C, Minton MD, Bedford RF. Vecuronium: effect on intracranial pressure and hemodynamics in neurosurgical patients. *Anesthesiology* 1987, **67**: 570–3.

128 Rosa G, Sanfilippo M, Orfei P, *et al*. The effects of pipecuronium bromide on intracranial pressure and cerebral perfusion pressure. *J Neurosurg Anesthesiol* 1991; **3**: 253–7.

129 McDowall DG, Harper AM, Jacobson I. Cerebral blood flow during halothane anaesthesia. *Br J Anaesth* 1963; **35**: 394–402.

130 Theye RA, Michenfelder JD. The effect of nitrous oxide on canine cerebral metabolism. *Anesthesiology* 1968; **29**: 1119–24.

131 Reasoner DK, Warner DS, Todd MM, MacAllister A. Effects of nitrous oxide on cerebral metabolic rate in rats anaesthetized with isoflurane. *Br J Anaesth* 1990; **65**: 210–15.

132 Pelligrino DA, Miletich DJ, Hoffman WE, Albrecht RF. Nitrous oxide markedly increases cerebral cortical metabolic rate and blood flow in the goat. *Anesthesiology* 1984; **60**: 405–12.

133 Oshita S, Ishikawa T, Tokutsu Y, Takeshita H. Cerebral circulatory and metabolic stimulation with nitrous oxide in the dog. *Acta Anaesthesiol Scand* 1979; **23**: 177–81.

134 Hoffman WE, Miletich DJ, Albrecht F. The effect of midazolam on cerebral blood flow and oxygen consumption and its interaction with nitrous oxide. *Anesth Analg* 1986; **65**: 729–33.

135 Drummond JC, Scheller MS, Todd MM. The effect of nitrous oxide on cortical blood flow during anesthesia with halothane and isoflurane, with and without morphine, in the rabbit. *Anesth Analg* 1987; **66**: 1083–9.

136 Kaieda R, Todd MM, Cook LN, Warner DS. The effects of anesthetics and $PaCO_2$ on the

cerebrovascular, metabolic, and electroencephalographic responses to nitrous oxide in the rabbit. *Anesth Analg* 1989; **68**: 135–43.

137 Drummond JC, Todd MM. The response of the feline cerebral circulation to P_aCo_2 during anesthesia with isoflurane and halothane and during sedation with nitrous oxide. *Anesthesiology* 1985; **62**: 268–73.

138 Hansen TD, Warner DS, Todd MM, Vust LJ. Effects of nitrous oxide and volatile anaesthetics on cerebral blood flow. *Br J Anaesth* 1989; **63**: 290–5.

139 Manohar M, Parks C. Regional distribution of brain and myocardial perfusion in swine while awake and during 1.0 and 1.5 MAC isoflurane anesthesia produced without or with 50% nitrous oxide. *Cardiovasc Res* 1984; **18**: 344–53.

140 Deutsch G, Samra SK. Effects of nitrous oxide on global and regional cortical blood flow. *Stoke* 1990; **21**: 1293–8.

141 Sakabe T, Kuramoto T, Kumagae S, Takeshita H. Cerebral responses to the addition of nitrous oxide to halothane in humans. *Br J Anaesth* 1976; **48**: 957–61.

142 Algoston L, Messeter K, Rosen I, Holmin T. Effects of nitrous oxide on cerebral haemodynamics and metabolism during isoflurane anaesthesia in man. *Acta Anaesthesiol Scand* 1992; **36**: 46–52.

143 Todd MM. The effects of P_aCO_2 on the cerebrovascular response to nitrous oxide in the halothane-anesthetized rabbit. *Anesth Analg* 1987; **66**: 1090–5.

144 Eng C, Lam AM, Mayberg TS, Lee C, Mathisen T. The influence of propofol with and without nitrous oxide on cerebral blood flow velocity and CO_2 reactivity in humans. *Anesthesiology* 1992; **77**: 872–9.

145 Lam AM, Slee TA, Cooper JO, Bachenberg KL, Mathisen TL. Nitrous oxide is a more potent cerebrovasodilator than isoflurane in humans. *Anesthesiology* 1991; **75**: A168.

146 Jung R, Reinsel R, Marx W, Galicich J, Bedford R. Isoflurane and nitrous oxide: comparative impact on cerebrospinal fluid pressure in patients with brain tumors. *Anesth Analg* 1992; **75**: 724–8.

147 Missfeldt BBM, Jorgensen PB, Rishoi M. The effect of nitrous oxide and halothane upon the intracranial pressure in hypocapnic patients with intracranial disorders. *Br J Anaesth* 1974; **39**: 781–5.

148 Newberg LA, Milde JH, Michenfelder JD. The cerebral metabolic effects of isoflurane at and above concentrations that suppress cortical electrical activity. *Anesthesiology* 1983; **59**: 23–8.

149 Todd MM, Drummond JC. A comparison of the cerebrovascular and metabolic effects of halothane and isoflurane in the cat. *Anesthesiology* 1984; **60**: 276–82.

150 Smith AL, Wollmann H. Cerebral blood flow and metabolism: effects of anaesthetic drugs and techniques. *Anesthesiology* 1972; **36**: 378–400.

151 Hansen TD, Warner DS, Todd MM, Vust LJ. The role of cerebral metabolism in determining the local cerebral blood flow effects of volatile anesthetics: evidence of persistent flow-metabolism coupling. *J Cereb Blood Flow Metab* 1989; **9**: 323–8.

152 Hansen TD, Warner DS, Todd MM, Vust LJ, Trawick BS. Distribution of cerebral blood flow during halothane versus isoflurane anaesthesia in rats. *Anesthesiology* 1988; **69**: 332–7.

153 Drummond JC, Todd MM, Scheller MS, Shapiro HM. A comparison of the direct cerebral vasodilating potencies of halothane and isoflurane in the New Zealand white rabbit. *Anesthesiology* 1986; **65**: 462–7.

154 Van Aken H, Fitch W, Graham DI, Brüssel T, Themann H. Cardiovascular and cerebrovascular effects of isoflurane-induced hypotension in the baboon. *Anesth Analg* 1986; **65**: 565–74.

155 Brüssel T, Fitch W, Brodner G, Arendt I, Van Aken H. Effects of halothane in low concentrations on cerebral blood flow, cerebral metabolism, and cerebrovascular autoregulation in the baboon. *Anesth Analg* 1991; **73**: 758–64.

156 Adams RW, Gronert GA, Sundt TM, Michenfelder JD. Halothane, hypocapnia, and cerebrospinal fluid pressure in neurosurgery. *Anesthesiology* 1972; **37**: 510–14.

157 Adams RW, Cucchiara RF, Gronert GA, Messick JM, Michenfelder JD. Isoflurane and cerebrospinal fluid pressure in neurosurgical patients. *Anesthesiology* 1981; **54**: 97–102.

158 Gomez Sainz JJ, Elexpuru Camiruaga JA, Fernandez Cano F, De la Herran JL. Effects of isoflurane on intraventricular pressure in neurosurgical patients. *Br J Anaesth* 1988; **61**: 347–9.

159 Grosslight K, Foster R, Colohan AR, Bedford RF. Isoflurane for neuroanesthesia: risk factors for increases in intracranial pressure. *Anesthesiology* 1985; **63**: 533–6.

160 Madsen JB, Cold GE, Hansen ES, Bardrum B. The effect of isoflurane on cerebral blood flow and metabolism in humans during craniotomy for small supratentorial tumors. *Anesthesiology* 1987; **66**: 332–6.

161 Madsen JB, Cold GE, Hansen ES, Bardrum B, Kruse-Larsen C. Cerebral blood flow and metabolism during isoflurane-induced hypotension in patients subjected to surgery for cerebral aneurysms. *Br J Anaesth* 1987; **59**: 1204–7.

162 McPherson RW, Traystman RJ. Effects of isoflurane on cerebral autoregulation. *Anesthesiology* 1988; **69**: 493–9.

163 Hoffman WE, Edelman G, Kochs E, Werner Ch, Segil L, Albrecht RF. Cerebral autoregulation in awake versus isoflurane-anesthetized rats. *Anesth Analg* 1991; **73**: 753–7.

164 Miletich DJ, Ivankovich AD, Albrecht RF, Reimann CR, Rosenberg R, McKissic E. Absence of autoregulation of cerebral blood flow during halothane and enflurane. *Anesth Analg* 1976; **55**: 100–9.

165 McPherson RW, Brian JE, Traystman RJ. Cerebrovascular responsiveness to carbon dioxide in dogs with 1.4% and 2.8% isoflurane. *Anesthesiology* 1989; **10**: 843–850.

166 Young WL, Prohovnik I, Correl JW, Ostapkovich N, Ornstein E, Quest DO. A comparison of cerebral blood flow reactivity to CO_2 during halothane versus isoflurane anesthesia for carotid endarterectomy. *Anesth Analg* 1991; **73**: 416–21.

167 Ringaert KRA, Mutch WAC, Malo LA. Regional cerebral blood flow and response to carbon dioxide during controlled hypotension with isoflurane anesthesia in the rat. *Anesth Analg* 1988; **67**: 383–8.

168 Scheller MS, Todd MM, Drummond JC, Zornow MH. The intracranial pressure effects of isoflurane and halothane administered following cryogenic brain injury in rabbits. *Anesthesiology* 1987; **67**: 507–12.

169 Shah N, Long C, Marx W, *et al.* Cerebrovascular response to CO_2 in edematous brain during either fentanyl or isoflurane anesthesia. *J Neurosurg Anesthesiol* 1990; **2**: 11–15.

170 Reinstrup P, Uski T, Messeter K. Influence of halothane and isoflurane on the contractile response to potassium and prostaglandin F_{2a} in isolated human pial arteries. *Br J Anaesth* 1994; **72**: in press.

171 Koenig HM, Pelligrino DA, Albrecht RF. Halothane vasodilation and nitric oxide in rat pial vessels. *J Neurosurg Anesthesiol* 1993; **5**: 264–71.

172 Hart J, Jing M, Bina S, Freas W, van Dyke RA, Muldoon SM. Effects of halothane on EDRF/cGMP-mediated vascular smooth muscle relaxation. *Anesthesiology* 1992; **79**: 323–31.

173 Jing M, Bina S, Freas W, van Dyke RA, Muldoon SM. Interaction of halothane and LY-63583 on nitric oxide induced relaxation of blood vessels. *Anesthesiology* 1993; **79**: A398.

174 Yamamoto M, Kakuyama M, Nskamura K, Tachibana T, Hatano Y. Effects of halothane, isoflurane and sevoflurane on sarcoplasmic reticulum of vascular smooth muscle in dog mesenteric artery. *Anesthesiology* 1993; **79**: A603.

175 Wheeler DM, Katz A, Rice T, Hansford RG. Volatile anesthetic effects on sarcoplasmic reticulum Ca^{2+} content and sarcolemmal Ca^{2+} flux in isolated rat cardiac cell suspension. *Anesthesiology* 1994; **80**: 372–82.

176 Yost S, Owens DF, Wingegar B, Forsayeth JM, Mayeri E. Concentration-dependent hyperpolarization of identified aplasia neurons by volatile anesthetics. *Anesthesiology* 1993; **79**: A396.

177 Lutz LJ, Milde JH, Milde LN. The cerebral functional, metabolic, and hemodynamic effects of desflurane in dogs. *Anesthesiology* 1990; **73**: 125–31.

178 Lutz LJ, Milde JH, Milde LN. The response of the canine cerebral circulation to hyperventilation during anesthesia with desflurane. *Anesthesiology* 1991; **74**: 504–7.

179 Milde LN, Milde JH. The cerebral and systemic hemodynamic and metabolic effects of desflurane-induced hypotension in dogs. *Anesthesiology* 1991; **74**: 513–18.

180 Ornstein E, Young WL, Ostapkovich N, Prohovnik I, Stein BM. Comparative effects of desflurane and isoflurane on cerebral blood flow. *Anesthesiology* 1991; **75**: A209.

181 Muzzi D, Daltner C, Losasso T, Weglinski M, Milde L. The effect of desflurane and

isoflurane with N_2O on cerebrospinal fluid pressure in patients with supratentorial mass lesions. *Anesthesiology* 1991; **75**: A167.

182 Muzzi DA, Losasso TJ, Dietz NM, Faust RJ, Cucchiara RF, Milde LN. The effect of desflurane and isoflurane on cerebrospinal fluid pressure in humans with supratentorial mass lesions. *Anesthesiology* 1992; **76**: 720–4.

183 Manohar M. Regional brain blood flow and cerebral cortical O_2 consumption during sevoflurane anesthesia in healthy isocapnic swine. *J Cardiovasc Pharmacol* 1986; **8**: 1268–75.

184 Scheller MS, Tateishi A, Drummond JC, Zornow MH. The effects of sevoflurane on cerebral blood flow, cerebral metabolic rate for oxygen, intracranial pressure, and the electroencephalogram are similar to those of isoflurane in the rabbit. *Anesthesiology* 1988; **68**: 548–51.

185 Scheller MS, Nakakimura K, Fleischer JE, Zornow MH. Cerebral effects of sevoflurane in the dog: comparison with isoflurane and enflurane. *Br J Anaesth* 1990; **65**: 388–92.

186 Lu GP, Gibson Jr JA, Frost EAM, Goldiner PL. Cerebral vasodilating effect of sevoflurane versus isoflurane. *Anesthesiology* 1990; **73**: A625.

187 Lu GP, Gibson Jr JA, Frost EAM, Nagashima H, Goldiner PL. Effects of sevoflurane MAC factors on brain microcirculation in the rat. *Anesth Analg* 1990; **70**: S249.

188 Forbes AM, Dolly FG. Acute hypertension during induction of anaesthesia and endotracheal intubation in normotensive man. *Br J Anaesth* 1970; **42**: 618–24.

189 Wohlner EC, Usubiago LJ, Jacoby RM, Hill GE. Cardiovascular effects of extubation. *Anesthesiology* 1979; **51**: S194.

190 Alexander SC, Lassen NA. Cerebral circulatory response to acute brain disease. *Anesthesiology* 1970; **32**: 60–8.

191 Strandgaard S, MacKenzie ET, Sengupta D. Upper limit of autoregulation of cerebral blood flow in the baboon. *Circ Res* 1974; **34**: 435–40.

192 Schutta EH, Kassel NF, Langfitt TW. Brain swelling produced by injury and aggravated by arterial hypertension. *Brain* 1968; **91**: 281–94.

193 Piepgras DG, Morgan MK, Sundt TM, Yanagihara T, Mussman LM. Intracerebral hemorrhage after carotid endarterectomy. *J Neurosurg* 1988; **68**: 532–6.

194 Van Aken H, Cottrell JE, Anger Ch, Puchstein Ch. Treatment of intraoperative hypertensive emergencies in patients with intracranial disease. *Am J Cardiol* 1989; **63**: 43c–7c.

195 Stoelting RK. Circulatory changes during direct laryngoscopy and tracheal intubation. Influence of duration of laryngoscopy with or without prior lidocaine. *Anesthesiology* 1977; **47**: 381–4.

196 Hamill J, Bedford RF, Pobereskin LH, Weaver D, Colahan A. Lidocaine before endotracheal intubation: LTA of IV? *Anesthesiology* 1980; **53**: 26–32.

197 Kreye VAW. Sodium nitroprusside. In: Scriabine A (Ed.), *Pharmacology of antihypertensive drugs*. New York: Raven Press, 1980: 373.

198 Michenfelder JD, Tinker JH. Cyanide toxicity and thiosulfate protection during chronic administration of sodium nitroprusside in the dog. Correlation with a human case. *Anesthesiology* 1977; **47**: 441–8.

199 Stoyka WW, Schutz H. The cerebral response to sodium nitroprusside and trimethaphan controlled hypotension. *Can Anaesth Soc J* 1975; **22**: 275–83.

200 Fitch W, Ferguson GG, Sengupta D, Garibi J, Harper AM. Autoregulation of cerebral blood flow during controlled hypotension in baboons. *J Neurol Neurosurg Psychiatry* 1976; **39**: 1014–22.

201 Larsen R, Teichmann J, Hilfiker O, Busse C, Sonntag H. Nitroprusside-hypotension: cerebral blood flow and central oxygen consumption in neurosurgical patients. *Acta Anaesthesiol Scand* 1982; **26**: 327–30.

202 Crockard HA, Brown FD, Mullan JF. Effects of trimethaphan and sodium nitroprusside on cerebral blood flow in rhesus monkeys. *Acta Neurochir* 1976; **35**: 85–9.

203 Brown FD, Hanlon K, Crockard HA, Mullan S. Effect of sodium nitroprusside on cerebral blood flow in conscious human beings. *Surg Neurol* 1977; **24**: 509–14.

204 Miletich DJ, Gil KSL, Albrecht RF, Zahed B. Intracerebral blood flow distribution during hypotensive anesthesia in the goat. *Anesthesiology* 1980; **53**: 210–14.

205 Turner JM, Powell D, Gibson RM, McDowall DG. Intracranial pressure changes in

129

neurosurgical patients during hypotension induced with sodium nitroprusside or trimethaphan. *Br J Anaesth* 1977; **49**: 419–25.

206 Cottrell JE, Patel KP, Turndorf H, Ransohoff J. Intracranial pressure changes induced by sodium nitroprusside in patients with intracranial mass lesions. *J Neurosurg* 1978; **48**: 329–31.

207 Fitch W, Pichard JD, Tamura A, Graham DI. Effects of hypotension induced with sodium nitroprusside on the cerebral circulation before, and one week after, the subarachnoid injection of blood. *J Neurol Neurosurg Psychiatry* 1988; **51**: 88–93.

208 Marsh ML, Shapiro HM, Smith RW, Marshall LF. Changes in neurologic status and intracranial pressure associated with sodium nitroprusside administration. *Anesthesiology* 1979; **51**: 336–8.

209 Mason DT, Zelis R, Amsterdam EA. Actions of the nitrates on the peripheral circulation and myocardial oxygen consumption. Significance in the relief of angina pectoris. *Chest* 1971; **59**: 296–305.

210 Rogers MC, Hamburger C, Owen K, Epstein MH. Intracranial pressure in the cat during nitroglycerine-induced hypotension. *Anesthesiology* 1979; **51**: 227–9.

211 Cottrell JE, Gupta B, Rappaport H, Turndorf H, Ransohoff J, Flamm ES. Intracranial pressure during nitroglycerine-induced hypotension. *J Neurosurg* 1980; **53**: 309–11.

212 James DJ, Bedford RF. Hydralazine for controlled hypotension during neurosurgical operations. *Anesth Analg* 1982; **61**: 1016–19.

213 Emmelin N, Feldberg W. Systemic effects of adenosine triphosphate. *Br J Pharmacol* 1948; **3**: 273–84.

214 Fukanaga AF, Flacke WE, Bloor BC. Hypotensive effects of adenosine and adenosine triphosphate compared to sodium nitroprusside. *Anesth Analg* 1982; **61**: 273–8.

215 Van Aken H, Puchstein C, Fitch W, Graham DI. Haemodynamic and cerebral effects of ATP-induced hypotension. *Br J Anaesth* 1984; **56**: 1409–16.

216 Van Aken H, Puchstein C, Anger C, Heinecke A, Lawin P. Changes in intracranial pressure and compliance during adenosine triphosphate-induced hypotension in dogs. *Anesth Analg* 1984; **63**: 381–5.

217 Lagerkranser M, Bergstrand G, Gordon E, *et al*. Cerebral blood flow and metabolism during adenosine-induced hypotension in patients undergoing cerebral aneurysm surgery. *Acta Anaesthesiol Scand* 1989; **33**: 15–20.

218 Kolassa N, Beller KD, Sanders KH. Evidence for the interaction of urapidil with 5-HT$_{1A}$ receptors in the brain leading to a decrease in blood pressure. *Am J Cardiol* 1989; **63**: 36c–9c.

219 Puchstein C, Van Aken H, Anger C, Hidding J. Influence of urapidil on intracranial pressure and intracranial compliance in dogs. *Br J Anaesth* 1983; **55**: 443–8.

220 Anger C, Van Aken H, Feldhaus P, *et al*. Permeation of the blood-brain barrier by urapidil and its influence on intracranial pressure in man in the presence of compromised intracranial dynamics. *J Hypertens* 1988; **6**: S63–4.

221 Sicking K, Puchstein C, Van Aken H. Blutdrucksenkung mit Urapidil: Einfluss auf die Hirndurchblutung. *Anesth Intensivmed* 1986; **27**: 147–51.

222 Kick O, Van Aken H, Wouter PF, Wieland W, Van Hemelrijck J. Vital organ blood flow during deliberate hypotension in dogs. *Anesth Analg* 1993; **77**: 737–42.

223 Turlapaty P, Laddu A, Murthy VS, Singh B, Lee R. Esmolol: a titratable short-acting intravenous beta-blocker for acute critical care settings. *Am Heart J* 1987; **114**: 866–85.

224 Blau WS, Kafer ER, Anderson JA. Esmolol is more effective than sodium nitroprusside in reducing blood loss during orthognathic surgery. *Anesth Analg* 1992; **75**: 172–8.

225 Ornstein E, Matteo RS, Weinstein JA, Schwartz A. A controlled trial of esmolol for the induction of deliberate hypotension. *J Clin Anesth* 1988; **1**: 31–5.

226 Ornstein E, Young WL, Ostapkovich N, Matteo RS, Diaz J. Deliberate hypotension in patients with arteriovenous malformations: esmolol compared with isoflurane and sodium nitroprusside. *Anesth Analg* 1991; **72**: 639–44.

227 Edmondson R, Del Valle O, Shah N, *et al*. Esmolol for potentiation of nitroprusside-induced hypotension: impact on the cardiovascular, adrenergic and renin–angiotensin systems in man. *Anesth Analg* 1989; **69**: 202–6.

228 Van Aken H, Puchstein C, Heinecke A. Effect of labetalol on intracranial pressure in dogs with and without intracranial hypertension. *Acta Anaesth Scand* 1982; **126**: 615–19.

229 Durieux M, Mork C, Sperry R, Matthern GE, Longnecker DE. Labetalol preserves blood flows to vital organs during deliberate hypotension induced by isoflurane. *Anesthesiology* 1988; **69**: A899.

230 Modica PA, Tempelhoff R, White PF. The pro- and anticonvulsant effects of anesthetics. Part I and Part II. *Anesth Analg* 1990; **70**: 303–15; 433–44.

231 White PF. Propofol: pharmacokinetics and pharmacodynamics. *Semin Anesth* 1988; **7**: 4–20.

232 De Riu PL, Petruzzi V, Tester C, *et al*. Propofol anticonvulsant activity in experimental epileptic status. *Br J Anaesth* 1992; **69**: 177–81.

233 Simpson KH, Hallsall PJ, Carr CME, Steward KG. Seizure duration after methohexitone or propofol for induction of anaesthesia for electroconvulsive therapy (E.C.T.). *Br J Anaesth* 1987; **59**: 1323–4.

234 Yanny HF, Christmas D. Propofol infusions for status epilepticus. *Anaesthesia* 1988; **43**: 514.

235 Wood PR, Brown GPR, Pugh S. Propofol infusion for the treatment of status epilepticus. *Lancet* 1988; **i**: 480–1.

236 Chilvers CR, Laurie PS. Successful use of propofol in status epilepticus. *Anaesthesia* 1990; **45**: 995–6.

237 Musella L, Wilder BJ, Schmidt RP. Electroencephalographic activation with intravenous methohexital in psychomotor epilepsy. *Neurology* 1971; **21**: 594–602.

238 Barron DW, Dundee JW. Clinical studies of induction agents XVII. Relationship between dosage and side effects of intravenous barbiturates. *Br J Anaesth* 1967; **39**: 24–30.

239 Ryder W. Methohexitone and epilepsy. *Br Dent J* 1969; **126**: 343.

240 Opitz A, Marschall M, Degan R, Koch D. General anesthesia in patients with epilepsy and status epilepticus. In: Degado-Escueta AV, Wasterlain CG, Treiman DM, Porter RJ (Eds), *Status epilepticus: mechanisms of brain damage and treatment*. New York: Raven Press, 1983: 531–5.

241 Brown AS, Horton JM. Status epilepticus treated by intravenous infusions of thiopentone sodium. *BMJ* 1967; **i**: 127–8.

242 Young GB, Blume WT, Bolton CF, Warren KG. Anesthetic barbiturates in refractory status epilepticus. *Can J Neurol Sci* 1980; **7**: 291–3.

243 Gumpert J, Hansotia P, Paul R, Upton A. Methohexitone and the EEG (letter). *Lancet* 1969; **ii**: 110.

244 Ghoneim MM, Yamada T. Etomidate: a clinical and electroencephalographic comparison with thiopental. *Anesth Analg* 1977; **56**: 479–85.

245 Doenicke A, Loffler B, Kugler J, Suttmann H, Gorte B. Plasma concentration and EEG after various regimens of etomidate. *Br J Anaesth* 1982; **54**: 393–9.

246 Morgan M, Lumley J, Whitwam JG. Respiratory effects of etomidate. *Br J Anaesth* 1977; **49**: 233–6.

247 Ebrahim ZY, DeBoer GE, Luders H, Hahn JF, Lesser RP. Effect of etomidate on the electroencephalogram of patients with epilepsy. *Anesth Analg* 1986; **65**; 1004–6.

248 DeCastro J, van de Water A, Wouters L, Xhonneuz R, Reneman R, Kay B. Comparative study of cardiovascular, neurological and metabolic side effects of eight narcotics in dogs. *Acta Anaesthesiol Belg* 1979; **30**: 6–99.

249 Hoffmann P, Schokenhoff B. Etomidate as an anticonvulsive agent. *Anaesthesist* 1984; **33**: 142–4.

250 Schwartz MS, Virden S, Scott DF. Effects of ketamine on the electroencephalograph. *Anaesthesia* 1974; **29**: 135–40.

251 Thompson GE. Ketamine-induced convulsions (letter). *Anesthesiology* 1972; **37**: 662–3.

252 Page P, Morgan M, Loh L. Ketamine anaesthesia in paediatric procedures. *Acta Anaesthesiol Scand* 1972; **16**: 155–60.

253 Ferrer-Allado T, Brechner VL, Dymond A, Cozen H, Crandall P. Ketamine-induced electroconvulsive phenomena in the human limbic and thalamic regions. *Anesthesiology* 1973; **38**: 333–44.

254 Bennett DR, Madsen JA, Jordan WS, Wiser WC. Ketamine anesthesia in brain-damaged epileptics: electroencephalographic and clinical observations. *Neurology* 1973; **23**: 449–60.

255 Fink M, Wienfeld RE, Schwartz MA, Irwin P. Blood levels and electro-encephalographic effects of diazepam and bromazepam. *Clin Pharmacol Ther* 1976; **20**: 184–91.

256 Prior PF, Maclaine GN, Scott DF, Laurance BM. Tonic status epilepticus precipitated by intravenus diazepam in a child with petit mal status. *Epilepsia* 1972; **13**: 467–72.
257 Jawad S, Oxley J, Wilson J, Richens A. A pharmacodynamic evaluation of midazolam as an antiepileptic compound. *J Neurol Neurosurg Psychiatry* 1986; **49**: 1050–4.
258 Smith NT, Dec-Silver H, Sanford TJ, *et al.* EEGs during high dose fentanyl-, sufentanil- or morphine–oxygen anesthesia. *Anesth Analg* 1984; **63**: 386–93.
259 Borgeat A, Biollaz J, Depierraz B, Neff R. Grand mal seizure after extradural morphine analgesia. *Br J Anaesth* 1988; **60**: 733–5.
260 Goetting MG, Thirman MJ. Neurotoxicity of mepéridine. *Ann Emerg Med* 1985; **14**: 1007–9.
261 Scott JC, Sarnquist FH. Seizure-like movements during a fentanyl infusion with absence of seizure activity in a simultaneous EEG recording. *Anesthesiology* 1985; **62**: 812–14.
262 Bowdle TA. Myoclonus following sufentanil without EEG seizure activity. *Anesthesiology* 1987; **67**: 593–5.
263 Freye E, Kuschinsky K. Effects of fentanyl and droperidol on the dopamine metabolism of the rat striatum. *Pharmacology* 1976; **14**: 1–7.
264 Krenn J, Porges P, Steinbereithner K. Case of anaesthesia convulsions under nitrous oxide–halothane anesthesia. *Anaesthesist* 1967; **16**: 83–5.
265 Poulton TJ, Ellingson RJ. Seizures associated with induction of anesthesia with isoflurane. *Anesthesiology* 1984; **61**: 471–6.
266 Smith RA, Winter PM, Smith M, Eger EI II. Convulsions in mice after anesthesia. *Anesthesiology* 1979; **50**: 501–4.
267 Hornbein TF, Eger EI II, Winter PM, Smith G, Wetstone D, Smith KH. The minimum alveolar concentration of nitrous oxide in man. *Anesth Analg* 1982; **61**: 553–6.
268 Yamamura T, Fukuda M, Takeya H, Goto T, Furukawa K. Fast oscillatory EEG activity induced by analgesic concentrations of nitrous oxide in man. *Anesth Analg* 1981; **60**: 283–8.
269 Lebowitz MH, Blitt CD, Dillon JB. Clinical investigation of compound 347 (Ethrane). *Anesth Analg* 1970; **49**: 1–10.
270 Bart AJ, Homi J, Linde HW. Changes in power spectra of electroencephalograms during anesthesia with fluroxene, methoxyflurane and Ethrane. *Anesth Analg* 1971; **50**: 53–63.
271 Niedjadlik K, Galindo A. Electrocorticographic seizure activity during enflurane anesthesia. *Anesth Analg* 1975; **54**: 722–4.
272 Lebowitz MH, Blitt CD, Dillon JB. Enflurane-induced central nervous system excitation and its relation to carbon dioxide tension. *Anesth Analg* 1972; **51**: 355–63.
273 Smith PA, McDonald TR, Jones CS. Convulsions associated with halothane anaesthesia. *Anaesthesia* 1966; **21**: 229–33.
274 Delgado-Escueta AV, Wasterlain CG, Treiman DM, Porter RJ. Management of status epilepticus. *N Engl J Med* 1982; **306**: 1337–40.
275 Clark DL, Hosick EC, Adam N, Castro AD, Rosner BS, Neigh JL. Neural effects of isoflurane (Forane) in man. *Anesthesiology* 1973; **39**: 261–70.
276 Schwartz AE, Tuttle RH, Poppers PJ. Electroencephalographic burst suppression in adults and young patients anesthetized with isoflurane. *Anesth Analg* 1989; **60**: 9–12.
277 Hymes JA. Seizure activity during isoflurane anesthesia. *Anesth Analg* 1985; **64**: 367–8.
278 Kofke WA, Snider MT, Young RSK, Ramer JC. Prolonged low flow isoflurane anesthesia for status epilepticus. *Anesthesiology* 1985; **62**: 653–6.
279 Kofke WA, Snider MT, O'Connell BK, *et al.* Isoflurane stops refractory seizures. *Anesthesiol Rev* 1987; **15**: 58–9.
280 Rampil IJ, Weiskopf RB, Brown JG, *et al.* I-653 and isoflurane produce similar dose-related changes in the electroencephalogram. *Anesthesiology* 1988; **69**: 298–302.
281 Rampil IJ, Lockhart SH, Eger EI II, Yasuda N, Weiskopf RB, Cahalan MK. The electroencephalographic effects of desflurane in humans. *Anesthesiology* 1991; **74**; 434–9.
282 Avramov MN, Shingu K, Omatsu U, Osawa M, Mori K. Effects of different speed of induction with sevoflurane on the EEG in man. *J Anesth* 1987; **1**: 1–7.

5: Fluid management in neurosurgical patients

CONCEZIONE TOMMASINO, MICHAEL M TODD

Neurosurgical patients often receive diuretics (for example, mannitol, frusemide or furosemide) to treat cerebral oedema and to reduce intracranial hypertension. Conversely, they may also require large amounts of intravenous fluids for resuscitation, for blood replacement, as part of therapy for vasospasm, to correct preoperative dehydration, and/or to maintain intraoperative and postoperative haemodynamic stability. These two interventions seem to be in conflict: if diuretics are "good" for patients, is it not reasonable to argue that fluids (and volume expansion) might be "bad"? In general terms, this is the origin of the common belief in fluid restriction and the argument for the prohibition of aggressive administration of fluids. There would be little point in discussing the subject if fluid restriction were benign, its efficacy proven, or if the infusion of large amounts of fluid had been shown conclusively to exacerbate cerebral oedema or intracranial hypertension. This may not be the case, however, and thus there are a variety of cluttered opinions scattered throughout the literature, for example:

- ". . . a negative fluid balance will never diminish brain oedema, but it could endanger the circulation, including the cerebral circulation and the renal function."[1]
- "It is agreed that some cerebral edema follows brain injury, and its prevention or control by the avoidance of overhydration . . . is widely recommended."[2]

This disagreement continues to the present day. It would be beneficial if it could be resolved by the examination of clinical data, but the cerebral effects of fluid restriction and aggressive fluid infusion have not been systematically studied in humans, leaving recourse only to anecdotal reports or to the animal literature.

Few substantial human data exist that concern the impact of fluids on the brain or that could guide rational fluid management in neurosurgical patients. It is possible, however, to examine those factors that influence water movement into the brain and to make some reasonable recommendations.

133

Osmolality, colloid oncotic pressure, crystalloids, and colloids

To start it is important that the reader be familiar with a number of important definitions and distinctions, particularly as they apply to the brain.

Osmotic pressure This is the hydrostatic force acting to equalise the concentration of *water* on both sides of the membrane, which is impermeable to substances dissolved in that water. Water will move along its concentration gradient. This means that if a solution containing 10 mmol/l Na$^+$ and 10 mmol/l Cl$^-$ is placed on one side of a semipermeable membrane with water on the other, water will move "towards" the saline solution. The saline solution has a concentration of 20 mosmol/l, and the force driving water will be about 19·3 mm Hg/mosmol or 386 mm Hg. Note that the driving force is proportional to the *gradient* across the membrane; if two solutions of equal concentration are placed across a membrane, there is no driving force. Similarly, if the membrane is permeable to the solutes (for example, Na$^+$ and Cl$^-$), this will act to reduce the gradient and hence the osmotic forces.

Osmolarity and osmolality Osmolarity describes the molar number of osmotically active particles per litre of solution. In practice, this value is typically calculated by adding up the millimolar concentrations of the various ions in the solution. Osmolality describes the molar number of osmotically active particles per kilogram of solvent. This value is directly measured by determining either the freezing point or the vapour pressure of the solution (each of which is reduced by dissolved solute). Note that osmotic activity of a solution demands that particles be "independent:" as NaCl dissociates into Na$^+$ and Cl$^-$, two osmotically active particles are created. If electrostatic forces act to prevent dissociation of the two charged particles, osmolality will be reduced. For most dilute salt solutions, osmolality is equal to or slightly less than osmolarity. For example, commercial Ringer's lactate solution has a calculated osmolarity of about 275 mosmol/l but a measured osmolality of about 254 mosmol/kg, indicating incomplete dissociation.

Colloid oncotic pressure Osmolarity/osmolality is determined by the total number of dissolved "particles" in a solution, regardless of their size. Colloid oncotic pressure is that portion of that total osmolality which is produced by large molecules, typically plasma proteins. This factor becomes particularly important in biological systems where vascular membranes are often permeable to small ions but not to proteins. In such situations, proteins may be the only osmotically active particles. Normal colloid oncotic pressure is about 20 mm Hg (or equal to about 1 mosmol/kg).

Starling's hypothesis In 1898, Starling published his equations describing the forces driving water across vascular membranes.[3] The two major factors that control this movement are (1) the hydrostatic pressure gradient and (2) osmotic and oncotic gradients. His equation is as follows:

$$FM = k(P_c + \pi_i - P_i - \pi_c)$$

where FM = fluid movement, k = the filtration coefficient of the capillary wall (how leaky it is), P_c = hydrostatic pressure in the capillaries, P_i = hydrostatic pressure in the interstitial (extravascular) space, and π_i and π_c = interstitial and capillary osmotic pressures respectively. This can be restated in a simplified fashion to say that fluid movement is proportional to the hydrostatic pressure gradient minus the osmotic gradient across a vessel wall. The magnitude of the osmotic gradient will depend on the relative permeability of the vessels to solute. In the periphery (muscle, bowel, lung, etc), the capillary endothelium has a pore size of 6·5 nm and is freely permeable to small molecules and ions (Na^+, Cl^-) but not to large molecules, such as proteins (fig 5.1).[4] As a result, π is defined by only colloids and the Starling's equation can be simplified by the following:

Fluid will move into a tissue whenever the hydrostatic gradient increases (either intravascular pressure rises or interstitial pressures fall), or when the osmotic gradient decreases.

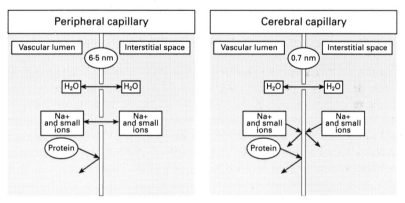

Fig 5.1 Schematic diagram of a peripheral and cerebral capillary. In the periphery, approximate "pore" size is about 6·5 nm, making the vessel wall permeable to both water and small ions (but not to protein). As a result, changes in intravascular colloid oncotic pressure (protein concentration) will alter the transcapillary gradient and hence a change in osmotic driving forces. By contrast, the estimated pore size of about 0·7 nm in the cerebral vascular bed renders the blood–brain barrier impermeable to both small ions and protein (but not to water). Changes in the concentrations of both ions and protein should hence alter driving forces. However, the total driving force that can be achieved even by reducing protein concentration (colloid oncotic pressure) to zero is only equal to that produced by, for example, a change in Na^+ concentration of 1 mmol/l.

135

In normal situations, intravascular protein concentration is higher than interstitial concentrations, acting to draw water back into the vascular space. If colloid oncotic pressure is reduced, for example, by dilution with large amounts of isotonic crystalloids, fluid will start to accumulate in the interstitium, producing oedema. This fact is familiar to all surgeons and anaesthetists who have seen marked peripheral oedema in patients given many litres of crystalloids during surgery or resuscitation. By contrast, in the brain, where the blood–brain barrier is impermeable to both ions and proteins, π is determined by the total osmotic gradient, of which colloid oncotic pressure contributes only a tiny fraction.

Interstitial clearance   In peripheral tissues, there is a net outward movement of fluid (that is, the value of FM is positive). The reason that oedema is not normally present is that this extravasated fluid is cleared by the lymphatics. Although many workers agree that there is some lymphatic drainage of the brain,[5] most interstitial fluid is cleared by either bulk fluid flow into the cerebrospinal fluid (CSF) spaces, or via pinocytosis back into the vasculature.[6 7] This is a slow process, and probably does not act as an important buffer to rapid fluid movement.

Hydrostatic forces and interstitial compliance   In tissue, the net hydrostatic gradient is determined by (1) intravascular pressures and (2) interstitial tissue compliance. Normally, the direction is outward (capillary to interstitium). There is no question that in brain (or in any organ) elevated vascular pressures, such as those produced by high jugular venous pressures or a head down posture, can increase oedema formation.[8 9] An often overlooked factor that influences the pressure gradient is, however, interstitial compliance, that is, the tendency with which tissue resists fluid influx. The loose interstitial space in most peripheral tissues does little to impede the influx of fluid. This explains the ease with which oedema develops around, for example, the face and eyes even with minor hydrostatic stresses (for example, a face down posture). By contrast, the interstitial space of the brain is extremely non-compliant, resisting fluid movement.[7] As a result, minor changes in driving forces (either hydrostatic or osmotic/oncotic) do not produce measurable oedema. A "vicious cycle" can, however, develop; as oedema forms in the brain, the interstitial matrix is disrupted, compliance increases, and additional oedema can form more easily. In addition, the closed cranium and intracranial pressure (ICP) can act to retard fluid influx. This may partly explain the exacerbated oedema formation which can occur after rapid decompression of the intracranial space.[9–13]

Can we take this information and explain the influence of certain fluids on the brain? In contrast to capillaries elsewhere in the body, the endothelial cells in the brain are joined together by continuous tight junctions. There are

136

no intracellular gaps, the cells are not fenestrated, and they do not have channels or chains of vesicles that form transendothelial pathways.[4 14 15] The effective pore size of the blood–brain barrier is only 0·7 nm, making this unique structure normally impermeable to large molecules, and relatively impermeable to many small polar solutes (fig 5.1). By contrast, it is fairly permeable to water. This should serve to make the brain an exquisitely sensitive osmometer. Reduction in serum osmolality (for example, by infusing water) would then be predicted as increasing cerebral oedema (or, conversely, increasing osmolality would reduce water content). This experiment was first done by Weed and McKibben[16] in 1919, who showed a rapid and large increase in brain volume. Since that time, innumerable experiments have shown the exquisite sensitivity of brain water content to changes in serum osmolality.[4 13 17–22] One example is shown in fig 5.2. In this experiment, osmolality in rats was altered by the injection of either water or hypertonic saline. One hour later, brains were removed and water content assessed. The linear relationship between measured arterial osmolality and water content is readily evident. It must be stressed that even small changes in osmolality can produce measurable changes; this is not difficult to accept as a 5 mosmol/kg gradient is equivalent to a force driving water of 100 mm Hg (see above).

What about changes in colloid oncotic pressure? As mentioned, colloidally active molecules contribute to only a tiny fraction of total osmolality and, when the blood–brain barrier is intact, can be responsible for only a small driving force. (Normal plasma colloid oncotic pressure is about 20 mm Hg, whereas that in the brain interstitium is about 0·6 mm Hg.[23] This is equal to the force that could be generated by a change in capillary/tissue osmotic gradient of only 1 mosmol/kg.) It could therefore be predicted that changes in colloid oncotic pressure would have only minimal effect on brain water content. This hypothesis has been tested directly in several experiments. In 1984, Zornow et al[20] subjected normal rabbits to plasmapheresis with various isotonic crystalloid and colloid solutions, intended to reduce colloid osmotic pressure selectively without altering total osmolality. No change in brain water content was seen. More recently, Hindman et al[24] placed rabbits on cardiopulmonary bypass after circuit priming with either a crystalloid or a colloid. Again, no change in brain water content was observed although marked oedema was seen in peripheral tissues (muscle, small bowel, etc) (fig 5.3).

These experiments demonstrate that normal brain water content can be altered by small changes in osmolality, but not by clinically achievable changes in colloid oncotic pressure. What about more clinically relevant conditions, where the blood–brain barrier is abnormal? Again, these have never been examined in humans, but have been studied in a number of animal models. Based on the above comments, it can be predicted that if the blood–brain barrier is made permeable to both small and large molecules (as

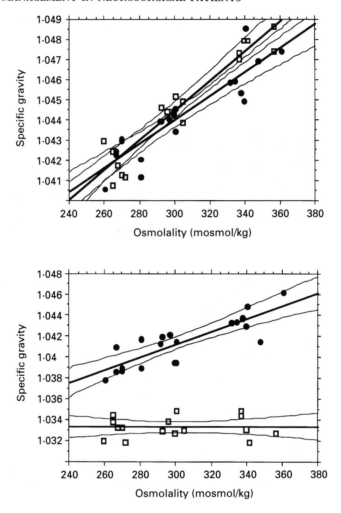

Fig 5.2 Measured brain tissue specific gravity in the rat brain during induced changes in serum osmolality. Specific gravity is determined by immersing small tissue samples in a bromobenzene/kerosene density gradient. As the specific gravity of water is 1·000, lower measurements of specific gravity indicate an *increase* in water content. In the top panel, a linear relationship between osmolality and specific gravity in normal brain tissue is seen. In the bottom panel, two regression lines can be seen: the upper is for an implanted tumour with an intact blood–brain barrier. As in normal brain, changing osmolality produced a linear change in tumour water content. The lower line is from an area of cortical tissue injured by freezing. As the blood–brain barrier is open (as evidenced by the extravasation of a protein tracer—not shown), interstitial ion/protein concentrations change in parallel with changes in blood concentrations. No change in gradient can occur and hence osmotic changes produce no changes in tissue water content. (Figure constructed from data found in Hansen, Warner, Traynelis and Todd. Plasma osmolality and brain water content in a rat glioma model. *Neurosurgery* 1994; **34**: 505–11)

138

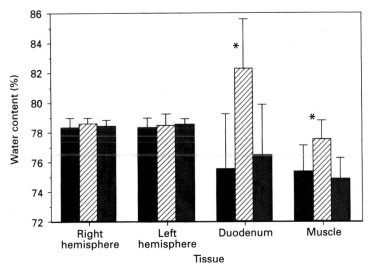

Fig 5.3 Directly measured water contents in the left and right cerebral hemispheres and in two peripheral tissues (duodenum and skeletal muscle). Control animals are denoted by the black bars. The light-hatched bars were samples taken from animals subjected to 1 h of cardiopulmonary bypass using a circuit primed with crystalloid (final colloid oncotic pressure or COP about 5 mm Hg). The dark hatched bars were from animals perfused with a colloid prime (final COP about 20 mm Hg). There were no differences between groups for cerebral tissue. By contrast, there were marked increases in peripheral tissue oedema in animals perfused with crystalloid (*). (Figure constructed from data found in Hindman et al. Differential effect of oncotic pressure on cerebral and extracerebral water content during cardiopulmonary bypass in rabbits. *Anesthesiology* 1990; **73**: 951–7)

is common with several experimental and clinical injuries), it should be impossible to maintain any form of osmotic or oncotic gradient between the blood and brain interstitium. As a result, no changes in water content would be expected with change in either. This has been demonstrated experimentally. Both Kaieda et al[25,26] and Zornow et al[27] studied the acute and delayed impact of changes in osmolality and colloid oncotic pressures in rabbits subjected to a cryogenic cortical injury (which results in a blood–brain barrier that is permeable to protein) and a rise in interstitial colloid oncotic pressure.[23] It was not possible to demonstrate any water content changes in any region as a result of a large reduction in colloid oncotic pressure (produced by isotonic crystalloids). By contrast, changes induced by reductions in total osmolality were seen only in apparently normal brain regions relatively distant from the injury focus. This finding is similar to the several studies showing that acute hyperosmolality or hypo-osmolality (mannitol, urea, hypertonic saline, or free water) reduced water content only in relatively normal brain tissue (that is, where the blood–brain barrier was intact).[22,28–32]

Some exceptions to these findings can be found. In 1954, Bakey et al[17] reported that the rapid infusion of saline could increase ICP. Oedema was not measured. This result can probably be explained either by the large increases in central venous pressure with a resultant increase in cerebral blood volume (CBV)[33] or by an increase in cerebral blood flow (CBF) and CBV resulting from haemodilution. In 1984, Albright et al[34] demonstrated that very high concentrations of hetastarch could reduce oedema even within the boundaries of a cryogenic injury. One possible explanation of this phenomenon is the very high molecular weight of hetastarch, which may have limited its permeability even after damage to the blood–brain barrier. More recently, Hyodo et al[35] showed that haemodilution with large amounts of Ringer's lactate solution increased oedema in animals with focal cerebral ischaemia. There are two possible explanations, both related to the osmolality of the administered solution. First, as noted by Tommasino et al,[21] Ringer's lactate is not strictly isotonic and can lead to decreases in plasma osmolality. As focal ischaemia does not widely disrupt the blood–brain barrier, this effect is more likely to be osmotic in nature.[21] In addition, Hatashita et al[36] have shown that ischaemia results in an increase in tissue osmolality. If fluid therapy reduces plasma osmolality, the blood–brain gradient will increase even further, acting to increase oedema. Again, the important factor is osmolality, not colloid oncotic pressure. Tranmer et al[37] showed that crystalloid infusions could increase ICP, suggesting that this was caused by changing colloid oncotic pressure.[37] Osmolality was not, however, measured and it is probable that the changes were again entirely the result of this factor.[38] Several studies have examined the impact of crystalloids versus colloids in shock/resuscitation models after brain injury. Gunnar et al[39] noted that post-resuscitation ICP was greater in animals resuscitated with saline compared with a hypertonic solution.[39] Both they and Wisner et al,[40] however, noted similar ICP increases with colloids, suggesting that the problem is not that "crystalloids make things worse," but rather that hypertonicity may have some therapeutic value.

Summary: clinical fluid management of neurosurgical patients

As stated, there are essentially few data concerning fluid management in neurosurgical patients. However, the available information can be used to make a series of "reasonable" suggestions.

Fluid restriction
Although fluid restriction is widely practised in patients with mass lesions or cerebral oedema, the only directly applicable data indicate that clinically acceptable restriction has little effect on oedema produced by triethyl-tin

poisoning,[41] by meningitis,[42] or by implanted tumours (unpublished observations), although at least one study has been published in which brain water content was reduced by carrying restriction to extremes (osmolalities of 330–350 mosmol/kg!).[18] Nevertheless, some "logic" behind modest restriction can be found in the work of Shenkin et al.[2] These authors noted that postoperative patients given standard "maintenance" amounts of intravenous fluids (for example, 2000 ml/day of 0·45 physiological saline in 5% dextrose) developed a progressive reduction in serum osmolality, whereas patients given half this volume showed no changes. Although no CNS related parameters were measured, the result suggests that usual maintenance fluids contain excess free water for the typical postoperative craniotomy patient. In this light, fluid restriction can be viewed as "preventing" hypo-osmotically driven oedema. This does not, however, imply that even greater degrees of restriction are beneficial, or that the adminstration of a fluid mixture that does not reduce osmolality is detrimental.

Volume replacement/resuscitation

The available data indicate that volume replacement/expansion will have no effects on cerebral oedema as long as normal serum osmolality is maintained, and as long as cerebral hydrostatic pressures are not markedly increased (for example, resulting from true volume overload and elevated right heart pressures). Whether this is achieved with crystalloid or colloid seems irrelevant, although the osmolality of the selected fluid is crucial. With respect to this issue, it should be noted that Ringer's lactate solution is not strictly iso-osmotic (measured 252–255 mosmol/kg), particularly when administered to patients whose baseline osmolality has been increased by either fluid restriction or the use of hyperosmolar fluids (mannitol, hypertonic saline, etc). The personal recommendation of the authors is that osmolalities be checked repeatedly during resuscitation or surgery, with the goal being to maintain this value either constant or slightly increased. Fluid administration that results in a reduction in osmolality should be avoided. Small volumes of Ringer's lactate (1–3 l) are unlikely to be detrimental and can be safely used, for example, to compensate for the changes in venous capacitance that typically accompany the induction of anaesthesia. If large volumes are needed (resulting from either blood loss or compensation for some other source of volume loss), a change to a more isotonic compound is probably advisable. This could be saline, some other balanced salt solution, or an isotonic colloid (plasma, albumin, hetastarch). (Hetastarch should be used with caution as a result of coagulation factor VIII depletion and possible coagulation difficulties encountered with volumes of more than 1000 ml.[43 44]) However, these recommendations should not be interpreted as "give all the isotonic fluid you like;" volume overload can have detrimental effects on both ICP (via increasing CBV[33]) or via hydrostatically driven oedema formation.[8 45]

In the postoperative period, large fluid requirements should cease. In such cases, the recommendations of Shenkin et al[2] are probably reasonable (about 1000 ml/day), although the authors would again recommend periodic measurements of serum osmolality, particularly if neurological status deteriorates. If cerebral oedema does develop, further restriction is unlikely to be of value and can result in hypovolaemia. Specific treatment with mannitol, frusemide, etc, combined with normovolaemia achieved with fluids that will maintain the increased osmolality, appears to be reasonable. There seems to be little advantage (and some disadvantages) to inducing/permitting hypovolaemia of such a degree that vasopressors are required to maintain acceptable haemodynamic parameters.

Miscellaneous issues

Hypertonic saline

Hypertonic salt solutions have been evaluated for use as resuscitation fluids since the 1960s, particularly as haemodynamic improvement can be achieved with very small volumes of liquid (which can be given very quickly).[46-49] As hyperosmolality is known to reduce brain volume, similar fluids have attracted attention for specific use in patients with head injuries or who are otherwise at risk for increased ICP.[19][50-56] There is no question that such solutions can quickly restore intravascular volume while reducing ICP—something that could be predicted from the above discussion. Unfortunately, what remains unclear is whether this approach is truly unique—or could the identical CNS end point be achieved with any resuscitation method that increased osmolality? In addition, concerns about marked hypertonicity have prevented the widespread use of hypertonic fluids. More recent attention has been directed at hypertonic/hyperoncotic solutions (typically hypertonic hetastarch or dextran solutions).[53][54][57-60] Again, small volumes of such solutions can restore normovolaemia rapidly, without increasing ICP. Although these fluids may increase the speed of resuscitation, it is unclear what they offer in major therapeutic advantages over isotonic fluids combined with more traditional osmotic diuretics.

Diuretics

Both mannitol and frusemide (and occasionally other diuretics) are used to control ICP and brain swelling in neurosurgical patients. The mechanism by which mannitol accomplishes this goal has been discussed (that is, removal of water from areas of brain with a relatively intact blood–brain barrier). Several issues related to mannitol have also been clarified in recent years. It was once believed that mannitol could transiently elevate ICP, and that this might be detrimental.[61] The mechanism of this effect is clearly the result of the vasodilator effects of hyperosmolality, with a resultant increase in

CBV.[62 63] It has now been shown in both dogs and humans, however, that this is a phenomenon that does not seem to occur in the presence of intracranial hypertension, and it does not occur when mannitol is given at moderate rates. There does not, therefore, appear to be any important reasons to avoid mannitol in most neurosurgical patients, other than in those patients with significant cardiovascular disease in whom transient volume expansion might precipitate congestive heart failure. The only other important concern is the excessive and/or repeated use of the drug. Excessive hyperosmolality can be deadly.[64] In addition, mannitol does accumulate progressively in the interstitium with repeated doses.[65] If interstitial osmolality rises excessively, it is possible that the normal brain–blood gradient might be reversed, with a resultant worsened oedema. In addition, if brain osmolality is increased, there is a risk of enhancing oedema by subsequent normalisation of serum osmolality.

The mechanism of frusemide's action remains controversial (although it certainly is related to the drug's ability to block Cl^- transport).[66] Frusemide and similar drugs may also act primarily by reducing cell swelling, rather than by changing extracellular fluid volume. Other non-diuretic drugs related to the loop diuretics may also have directly therapeutic effects.[67 68] One item is clear. Frusemide's maximal effect is delayed compared with mannitol.[69] For this reason, mannitol probably remains the agent of choice for rapid ICP control.

Glucose

In 1977, Myers and Yamaguchi[70] noted a relationship between elevated blood glucose and poor neurological outcome in primates subjected to a cardiac arrest. Subsequent studies have verified this finding, and have shown that glucose administration can worsen outcome from both focal and global ischaemia, presumably as a result of enhanced tissue acidosis.[71 72] Other studies confirmed a relationship between plasma glucose on admission and outcome in patients with stroke, cardiac arrest, and head injury.[73–76] More recent studies suggest that this correlation is not necessarily one of cause and effect (that is, perhaps the high glucose reflects worsened primarily CNS damage), nor has it been possible to demonstrate that the administration of glucose to humans is detrimental.[77–79] Nevertheless, since Sieber et al[80] showed that withholding glucose from adult neurosurgical patients was not associated with hypoglycaemia most writers have suggested that glucose containing fluids not be given to either acutely injured or elective surgical patients. It should be noted that this caveat does not appear to apply to the use of hyperalimentation fluids in such patients, perhaps because these hyperglycaemic fluids are typically started several days after the primary insult. It is also not clear that aggressive control of hyperglycaemia with insulin will improve outcome, although this has not been carefully studied in humans.

Diabetes insipidus

Diabetes insipidus is a common sequela of pituitary and hypothalamic lesions, but it can also occur with other cerebral pathology, such as head trauma or intracranial surgery. Polyuria, progressive dehydration and hypernatraemia occur subsequently. Diabetes insipidus is present when the urine output is excessive, the urine osmolality is inappropriately low relative to serum osmolality (above normal because of water loss), and the urine specific gravity is lower than 1·002. Management of diabetes insipidus requires careful balancing of intake and output, mostly to avoid fluid overload. Each hour the patient should receive maintenance fluids plus three quarters of the previous hour's urine output, or plus the previous hour's urine output minus 50 ml. Saline that is half the concentration of physiological saline and D5W are commonly used as replacement fluids, with frequent controls of glycaemic values. In the presence of urine output higher than 300 ml/h, at least for two hours, it is now standard practice to administer aqueous vasopressin or (desmopressin) (DDAVP).

Syndrome of inappropriate antidiuretic hormone secretion

Various cerebral pathological processes can result in excessive release of antidiuretic hormone (ADH), which causes continued renal excretion of sodium (>20 mmol/l), in spite of hyponatraemia and associated hypo-osmolality. Urine osmolality is therefore high relative to serum osmolality. The mainstay of treatment of the syndrome of inappropriate ADH secretion (SIADH) is fluid restriction, usually to about 1000 ml/24 h of an iso-osmolar solution. If hyponatraemia is severe (<110–115 mmol/l) administration of hypertonic (3–5%) saline and frusemide may be appropriate—but the rapid correction of hyponatraemia has been connected with the occurrence of pontine myelinolysis, and great care is required in correcting it.[81-83]

Haemodilution

One common (but usually inadvertent) accompaniment of fluid infusion is a reduction in haemoglobin/haematocrit. In the face of active blood loss, the use of asanguineous fluids can result in marked acute anaemia. This haemodilution is typically accompanied by an increase in cerebral blood flow, and doctors have long argued about whether the haemodilution is beneficial, benign, or detrimental. The answer probably depends on the disease state and on the degree of haemodilution. In the normal brain, the increase in CBF

144

produced by haemodilution is almost certainly an active compensatory response to a decrease in arterial oxygen content.[84-87] This response is essentially identical to that seen with hypoxia.[84 88 89] This is extremely well tolerated, with little change in O_2 delivery during haemodilution to haematocrits in the low 20s. In the face of brain injury, however, the normal CBF responses to hypoxia and haemodilution are attenuated, and both changes may contribute to secondary tissue damage.[90 91]

The one situation in which haemodilution may be beneficial is in the period immediately during/after a focal cerebral ischaemia event. Several studies have shown that regional O_2 delivery in this situation may be increased (or at least better maintained) in the face of modest haemodilution (haematocrit of about 30%) and animal studies demonstrated some reductions in infarction volumes.[92-98] In spite of this, however, several trials have failed to demonstrate any benefit of haemodilution in human stroke patients, except in patients who are polycythaemic to start with.[99-103] One possible explanation is that haemodilution was started too late to be of value.

What clinical lessons can be learned from this work? It is our opinion that in elective neurosurgical patients and patients with head injuries, haemodilution to haematocrit values below 30–35% is unlikely to be any more "beneficial" than hypoxia. Haemodilution into this range may be better tolerated in patients at risk for focal ischaemia. Nevertheless, active attempts to lower haematocrit are probably not advisable at the present time.

1 Gordon E, Ponten U. In: Winken PJ, Bruyn GW (Eds), *Handbook of clinical neurology*; New York: Elsevier, 1975: 599–626.
2 Shenkin HA, Benzier HO, Bouzarth W, Restricted fluid intake: Rational management of the neurosurgical patient. *J Neurosurg* 1976; **45**: 432–6.
3 Starling EH. In Schaefer E (Ed.), *Textbook of physiology*. London: Caxton, 1898: 285–311.
4 Fenstermacher JD, Johnson JA. Filtration and reflection coefficients of the rabbit blood–brain barrier. *Am J Physiol* 1966; **211**: 341–6.
5 Cserr HF, Harlingberg CJ, Knopf PM. Drainage of brain extracellular fluid into blood and deep cervical lymph and its immunological significance. *Brain Pathol* 1992; **2**: 269–76.
6 Hochwald GM, Wald A, Malhan C. The sink action of cerebrospinal fluid volume flow. *Arch Neurol* 1976; **33**: 339–44.
7 Reulen HJ, Graham R, Spatz M, Klatzo I. Role of pressure gradients and bulk flow in dynamics of vasogenic brain edema. *J Neurosurg* 1977; **46**: 24–35.
8 Cuypers J, Matakas F, Potolicchio SJ. Effect of central venous pressure on brain tissue pressure and brain volume. *J Neurosurg* 1976; **45**: 89–94.
9 Durward QJ, Del Maestro RF, Amacher AL, Farrar JK. The influence of systemic arterial pressure and intracranial pressure on the development of cerebral vasogenic edema. *J Neurosurg* 1983; **59**: 803–9.
10 Cooper PR, Hagler H, Clark WK, Barrett P. Enhancement of experimental cerebral edema after decompressive craniotomy: Implications for the management of severe head injuries. *Neurosurgery* 1979; **4**: 296–300.
11 Hatashita S, Koike J, Sonokawa T, Ishi S. Cerebral edema associated with craniectomy and arterial hypertension. *Stroke* 1985; **16**: 661–8.
12 Cao M, Lisheng H, Shouzheng S. Resolution of brain edema in severe brain injury at controlled high and low intracranial pressures. *J Neurosurg* 1984; **61**: 707–12.
13 Kuncz A, Doczi T, Bodosi M. The effect of skull and dura on brain volume regulation after hypo- and hyperosmolar fluid treatment. *Neurosurgery* 1990; **27**: 509–15.

14 Fenstermacher JD. In: Staub NC, Taylor AE (Eds), *Edema*. New York: Raven Press, 1984: 383–404.
15 Betz AL, Goldstein GW, Katzman R. In: Siegel GJ, Albers RW, Agranoff BW, Malinoff P (Eds), *Basic neurochemistry*. New York: Raven Press, 1989: 591–606.
16 Weed LH, McKibben PS. Pressure changes in the cerebrospinal fluid following intravenous injection of solutions of various concentrations. *Am J Physiol* 1919; **48**: 512–30.
17 Bakay L, Crawford JD, White JC. The effects of intravenous fluids on cerebrospinal fluid pressure. *Surg Gynecol Obstet* 1954; **99**: 48–52.
18 Jelsma LF, McQueen JD. Effect of experimental water restriction on brain water. *J Neurosurg* 1967; **26**: 35–40.
19 Todd MM, Tommasino C, Moore S. Cerebral effects of isovolemic hemodilution with a hypertonic saline solution. *J Neurosurg* 1985; **63**: 944–8.
20 Zornow MH, Todd MM, Moore SS. The acute cerebral effects of changes in plasma osmolality and oncotic pressure. *Anesthesiology* 1987; **67**: 936–41.
21 Tommasino C, Moore S, Todd MM. Cerebral effects of isovolemic hemodilution with crystalloid or colloid solutions in normal rabbits. *Crit Care Med* 1988; **16**: 862–8.
22 Hansen TD, Warner DS, Traynelis V, Todd MM. Plasma osmolality and brain water content in a rat glioma model. *Neurosurgery* 1994; **34**: 505–11.
23 Gazendam J, Go KG, Van Zanten AK. Composition of isolated edema fluid in cold-induced brain edema. *J Neurosurg* 1979; **51**: 70–7.
24 Hindman BJ, Funatsu N, Cheng DCH, Bolles R, Todd MM, Tinker JH. Differential effect of oncotic pressure on cerebral and extracerebral water content during cardiopulmonary bypass in rabbits. *Anesthesiology* 1990; **73**: 951–7.
25 Kaieda R, Todd MM, Cook LN, Warner DS. Acute effects of changing plasma osmolality and colloid oncotic pressure on the formation of brain edema after cryogenic injury. *Neurosurgery* 1989; **24**: 671–8.
26 Kaieda R, Todd MM, Warner DS. Prolonged reduction in colloid oncotic pressure does not increase brain edema following cryogenic injury in rabbits. *Anesthesiology* 1989; **71**: 554–60.
27 Zornow MH, Scheller MN, Todd MM, Moore SS. Acute cerebral effects of isotonic crystalloid and colloid solutions following cryogenic brain injury in the rabbit. *Anesthesiology* 1988; **69**: 185–91.
28 Clasen RA, Cooke PM, Pandolfi S, Carnecki G, Bryar G. Hypertonic urea in experimental cerebral edema. *Arch Neurol* 1965; **12**: 424–34.
29 Pappius HM, Dayes LA. Hypertonic urea. Its effects on the distribution of water and electrolytes in normal and edematous brain tissues. *Arch Neurol* 1965; **13**: 395–402.
30 Wisner D, Schuster L, Quinn C. Hypertonic saline resuscitation of head injury: effects of fluid resuscitation on the brain. *J Trauma* 1990; **30**: 75.
31 Hartwell RC, Sutton LN, Roberts PA, Rosner MJ. Mannitol, intracranial pressure, and vasogenic edema. *Neurosurgery* 1993; **32**: 444–50.
32 Go KG, Lange WED, Sluiter WJ, Woudenberg FV, Ebels EJ, Blaauw EH. The influence of salt-free solutions on cold-induced cerebral oedema. A chemical and morphological study in the rat. *J Neurol Sci* 1973; **18**: 323–31.
33 Todd MM, Weeks JB, Warner DS. The influence of intravascular volume expansion on cerebral blood flow and blood volume in normal rats. *Anesthesiology* 1993; **78**: 945–53.
34 Albright AL, Latchaw RE, Robinson AG. Intrancranial and systemic effects of hetastarch in experimental cerebral edema. *Crit Care Med* 1984; **12**: 496–500.
35 Hyodo A, Heros RC, Tu YK, *et al*. Acute effects of isovolemic hemodilution with crystalloids in a canine model of focal cerebral ischemia. *Stroke* 1989; **20**: 534–40.
36 Hatashita S, Hoff JT, Salamat SM. Ischemic brain edema and the osmotic gradient between blood and brain. *J Cereb Blood Flow Metab* 1988; **8**: 552–9.
37 Tranmer BI, Iacobacci RI, Kindt GW. Effects of crystalloid and colloid infusions on intracranial pressure and computerized electroencephalographic data in dogs with vasogenic brain edema. *Neurosurgery* 1989; **25**: 173–9.
38 Todd MM, Zornow M. Effects of crystalloid and colloid infusions on intracranial pressure (Letter). *Neurosurgery* 1990; **26**: 546–8.
39 Gunnar W, Jonasson O, Merlotti G, Stone J, Barrett J. Head injury and hemorrhagic shock: Studies of the blood brain barrier and intracranial pressure after resuscitation with normal saline solution, 3% saline solution, and dextran-40. *Surgery* 1988; **103**: 398–407.

146

40 Wisner D, Busche F, Sturm J, Gaab M, Meyer H. Traumatic shock and head injury: effects of fluid resuscitation on the brain. *J Surg Res* 1989; **46**: 49.

41 Morse ML, Milstein JM, Haas JE, Taylor E. Effect of hydration on experimentally induced cerebral edema. *Crit Care Med* 1985; **13**: 563–5.

42 Tauber MG, Sande E, Fournier MA, Tureen JH, Sande MA. Fluid administation, brain edema, and cerebrospinal fluid lactate and glucose concentrations in experimental *Escherichia coli* meningitis. *J Infect Dis* 1993; **168**: 473–6.

43 Strauss RG. Review of the effects of hydroxyethyl starch on the blood coagulation system. *Transfusion* 1981; **21**: 299–302.

44 Claes Y, Van Hemelrijck J, Van Gerven M, *et al.* Influence of hydroxyethyl starch on coagulation in patients during the perioperative period. *Anesth Analg* 1992; **75**: 24–30.

45 Mayhan WG, Heistad DD. Role of veins and cerebral venous pressure in disruption of the blood–bain barrier. *Circ Res* 1981; **59**: 216–20.

46 Messmer K, Mokry G, Jesch F. The protective effects of hypertonic solutions in shock. *Br J Surg* 1969; **56**: 626.

47 Monafo WW, Chuntrasakul C, Ayvazian VH. Hypertonic sodium solutions in the treatment of burn shock. *Am J Surg* 1973; **126**: 778–83.

48 De Filippe J, Timoner J, Velasco IT, Lopes OU. Treatment of refractory hypovolemic shock by 7.5% sodium chloride injections. *Lancet* 1980; **ii**: 1002–4.

49 Shackford SR, Sise MJ, Fridlund PH, *et al.* Hypertonic sodium lactate versus lactated ringer's solution for intravenous fluid therapy in operations on the abdominal aorta. *Surgery* 1983; **94**: 41–51.

50 Prough DS, Johnson JC, Poole GV, Stullken EH, Johnston WE, Royster R. Effects on intracranial pressure of resuscitation from hemorrhagic shock with hypertonic saline vs lactated Ringer's solution. *Crit Care Med* 1985; **13**: 407–11.

51 Prough DS, Johnson JC, Stump DA, Stullken EH, Poole GV, Howard G. Effects of hypertonic saline versus lactated Ringer's solution on cerebral oxygen transport during resuscitation from hemorrhagic shock. *J Neurosurg* 1986; **64**: 627–32.

52 Zornow MH, Scheller MS, Shackford SR. Effect of a hypertonic lactated Ringer's solution on intracranial pressure and cerebral water content in a model of traumatic brain injury. *J Trauma* 1989; **29**: 484–8.

53 Whitley JM, Prough DS, Taylor CL, Deal DD, DeWitt DS. Cerebrovascular effects of small volume resuscitation from hemorrhagic shock: Comparison of hypertonic saline and concentrated hydroxyethyl starch in dogs. *J Neurosurg Anesth* 1991; **3**: 47–55.

54 Prough DS, Whitley JM, Olympio MA, Taylor CL, DeWitt DS. Hypertonic/hyperoncotic fluid resuscitation after hemorrhagic shock in dogs. *Anesth Analg* 1991; **73**: 738–44.

55 Schmoker JD, Zhuang J, Shackford SR. Hypertonic fluid resuscitation improves cerebral oxygen delivery and reduces intracranial pressure after hemorrhagic shock. *J Trauma* 1991; **31**: 1607–13.

56 Shackford SR, Zhuang J, Schmoker J. Intravenous fluid tonicity. Effect on intracranial pressure, cerebral blood flow, and cerebral oxygen delivery in focal brain injury. *J Neurosurg* 1992; **76**: 91–8.

57 Armistead CW, Vinvent JL, Preiser JC, De Backer D, Minh TL. Hypertonic saline solution–hetastarch for fluid resuscitation in experimental septic shock. *Anesth Analg* 1989; **69**: 714–20.

58 Prough DS, Whitley JM, Taylor CL, Deal DD, DeWitt DS. Small-volume resuscitation from hemorrhagic shock in dogs: Effects on systemic hemodynamics and systemic blood flow. *Crit Care Med* 1991; **19**: 364–72.

59 Kreimeier U, Bruckner UB, Niemczyk S, Messmer K. Hyperosmotic saline dextran for resuscitation from traumatic-hemorrhagic hypotension: effect on regional blood flow. *Circ Shock* 1990; **32**: 83–99.

60 Schurer L, Dautermann C, Hartl R, *et al.* Treatment of hemorrhagic hypotension with hypertonic/hyperoncotic solutions: effects on regional cerebral blood flow and brain surface oxygen tension. *Eur Surg Res* 1992; **24**: 1–12.

61 Cottrell JE, Robustelli A, Post K, Turndorf H. Furosemide- and mannitol-induced changes in intracranial pressure and serum osmolality and electrolytes. *Anesthesiology* 1977; **47**: 28–30.

62 Ravussin P, Archer DP, Meyer E, Abou Madi M, Yamamoto L, Trop D. The effects of

147

rapid infusions of saline and mannitol on cerebral blood volume and intracranial pressure in dogs. *Can Anaesth Soc J* 1985; **32**: 506–15.

63 Ravussin P, Archer DP, Tyler JL, *et al*. Effects of rapid mannitol infusion on cerebral blood volume. A positron emission tomographic study in dogs and man. *J Neurosurg* 1986; **64**: 104–13.

64 Star RA. Hyperosmolar states. *Am J Med Sci* 1990; **300**: 402–12.

65 Kaufman AM, Cardoso ER. Aggravation of vasogenic cerebral edema by multiple-dose mannitol. *J Neurosurg* 1992; **77**: 584–9.

66 Garay RP, Hannaert PA, Nazaret C, Cragoe EJ. The significance of the relative effects of loop diuretics and anti-brain edema agents on the Na^+, K^+, Cl^- cotransport system and the $Cl^-/NaCO_3^-$ anion exchanger. *Arch Pharmacol* 1986; **334**: 202–9.

67 Kimelberg HK, Rose JW, Barron KD, Waniewski RA, Cragoe EJ. Astrocytic swelling in traumatic–hypoxic brain injury. Beneficial effects of an inhibitor of anion exchange transport and glutamate uptake in glial cells. *Mol Chem Neuropathol* 1989; **11**: 1–31.

68 Kimelberg HK, Barron KD, Bourke RS, Nelson LR, Cragoe EJ. Brain anti-cytoxic edema agents. *Progr Clin Biol Res* 1990; **361**: 363–85.

69 Wilkinson HA, Rosenfeld S. Furosemide and mannitol in the treatment of acute experimental intracranial hypertension. *Neurosurgery* 1983; **12**: 405–10.

70 Myers RE, Yamaguchi SI. Nervous system effects of cardiac arrest in monkeys. *Arch Neurol* 1977; **34**: 65–74.

71 Siesjo BK. Pathophysiology and treatment of focal cerebral ischemia. Part I: Pathophysiology. *J Neurosurg* 1992; **77**: 169–84.

72 Siesjo BK. Pathophysiology and treatment of focal cerebral ischemia. Part II. Mechanism of damage and treatment. *J Neurosurg* 1992; **77**: 337–54.

73 Pulsinelli WA, Levy DE, Sigsbee B, Scherer P, Plum F. Increased damage after ischemic stroke in patients with hyperglycemia with or without established diabetes mellitus. *Am J Med* 1983; **74**: 540–3.

74 Longstreth WT, Inui TS. High blood glucose level on hospital admission and poor neurological recovery after cardiac arrest. *Ann Neurol* 1984; **15**: 59–63.

75 Young B, Ott L, Dempsey R, Haack D, Tibbs P. Relationship between admission hyperglycemia and neurologic outcome of severely brain-injured patients. *Ann Surg* 1989; **210**: 466–73.

76 Lam AM, Winn HR, Cullen BF, Sundling N. Hyperglycemia and neurological outcome in patients with head injury. *J Neurosurg* 1991; **75**: 545–51.

77 Robertson CS, Goodman JC, Narayan RK, Contant CF, Grossman RG. The effect of glucose administration on carbohydrate metabolism after head injury. *J Neurosurg* 1991; **74**: 43–50.

78 Longstreth WT, Copass MK, Dennis LK, Rauchmatthews ME, Stark MS, Cobb LA. Intravenous glucose after out-of-hospital cardiopulmonary arrest – a community-based randomized trial. *Neurology* 1993; **43**: 2534–41.

79 Sieber FE, Toung TJ, Diringer MN, Wang H, Long DM. Preoperative risks predict neurological outcome of carotid endarterectomy related stroke. *Neurosurgery* 1992; **30**: 847–54.

80 Sieber F, Smith DS, Kupferberg J, *et al*. Effects of intraoperative glucose on protein catabolism and plasma glucose levels in patients with supratentorial tumors. *Anesthesiology* 1986; **64**: 453–9.

81 Norenberg MD, Leslie KO, Robertson AS. Association between rise in serum sodium and central pontine myelinolysis. *Ann Neurol* 1982; **11**: 128–35.

82 Sterns RH, Riggs JE, Schochet SS. Osmotic demyelination syndrome following correction of hyponatremia. *N Engl J Med* 1986; **314**: 1535–42.

83 Kroll M, Juhler M, Lindholm J. Hyponatraemia in acute brain disease. *J Intern Med* 1992; **232**: 291–7.

84 Jones MD, Traystman RJ, Simmons MA, Molteni RA. Effects of changes in arterial O_2 content on cerebral blood flow in the lamb. *Am J Physiol* 1981; **240**: H209–15.

85 Brown MM, Wade JPH, Marshall J. Fundamental importance of arterial oxygen content in the regulation of cerebral blood flow in man. *Brain* 1985; **108**: 81–93.

86 Hudak ML, Koehler RC, Rosenberg AA, Traystman RJ, Jones MD. Effect of hematocrit on cerebral blood flow. *Am J Physiol* 1986; **251**: H63–70.

87 Harrison MJG. Influence of haematocrit in the cerebral circulation. *Cerebrovasc Brain Metab Rev* 1989; **1**: 55–67.
88 Korosue K, Heros RC. Mechanism of cerebral blood flow augmentation by hemodilution in rabbits. *Stroke* 1992; **23**: 1487–93.
89 Todd MM, Wu B, Maktabi M, Hindman B, Warner DS. Cerebral blood flow and oxygen delivery during hypoxemia and hemodilution: role of oxygen content. *Am J Physiol* 1994; **267**: H2025–31.
90 Lewelt W, Jenkins LW, Miller JD. Effects of experimental fluid–percussion injury of the brain on cerebrovascular reactivity to hypoxia and to hypercapnia. *J Neurosurg* 1982; **56**: 332–8.
91 Todd MM, Wu B, Warner DS. The hemispheric cerebrovascular response to hemodilution is attenuated by a focal cryogenic brain injury. *J Neurotrauma* 1994; **11**: 149–60.
92 Wood JH, Kee DB. Hemorheology of the cerebral circulation in stroke. *Stroke* 1985; **16**: 765–72.
93 Kee DB, Wood JH. In: Wood JH (Ed.), *Cerebral blood flow: physiologic and clincial aspects.* New York: McGraw Hill, 1987: 173–85.
94 Tu KY, Heros RC, Karacostas D, *et al.* Isovolemic hemodilution in experimental focal cerebral ischemia. Part 2: Effects on regional cerebral blood flow and size of infarction. *J Neurosurg* 1988; **69**: 82–91.
95 Cole DJ, Drummond JC, Shapiro HM, Hertzog RE, Brauer FS. The effect of hypervolemic hemodilution with and without hypertension on cerebral blood flow following middle cerebral artery occlusion in rats anesthetized with isoflurane. *Anesthesiology* 1989; **71**: 580–5.
96 Hartmann A, Rommel T, Dettmers C, Tsuda Y, Lagreze H, Broich K. Hemodilution in cerebral infarcts. *Arzneimittel Forschung* 1991; **41**: 348–51.
97 Yamauchi H, Fukuyama H, Ogawa M, Ouchi Y, Kimura J. Hemodilution improves cerebral hemodynamics in internal carotid artery occlusion. *Stroke* 1993; **24**: 1885–90.
98 Cole DJ, Schell RM, Drummond JC, Reynolds L. Focal cerebral ischemia in rats – effect of hypervolemic hemodilution with diaspirin cross-linked hemoglobin versus albumin on brain injury and edema. *Anesthesiology* 1993; **78**: 335–42.
99 Scandinavian Stroke Study Group. Multicentre trial of hemodilution in acute ischemic stroke: Results in the total patient population. *Stroke* 1987; **18**: 691–9.
100 Scandinavian Stroke Study Group. Multicenter trial of hemodilution in acute ischemic stroke. Results of subgroup analyses. *Stroke* 1988; **19**: 464–71.
101 Italian Acute Stroke Study Group. Haemodilution in acute stroke: results of the Italian Haemodilution Trial. *Lancet* 1988; **i**: 318–21.
102 Grotta JC. Hypervolemic hemodilution treatment of acute stroke: Results of a randomized multicenter trial using pentastarch. *Stroke* 1989; **20**: 317–23.
103 Mast H, Marx P. Neurological deterioration under isovolemic hemodilution with hydroxyethyl starch in acute cerebral ischemia. *Stroke* 1991; **22**: 680–3.

6: Intraoperative and postoperative monitoring of the CNS for neurosurgery

CHRISTIAN WERNER, EBERHARD KOCHS

During anaesthesia and critical care, cerebral hypoxia and/or ischaemia commonly develops as a function of systemic hypotension, intracranial hypertension, cerebral vasospasm, cerebral embolism, temporary or permanent vascular occlusion, retractor pressure, or respiratory failure.[1] Measuring secondary insults in head injured patients, Jones et al[2] have shown a close relationship of variables such as hypoxia, increased intracranial pressure (IOP), arterial hypotension or seizures, and neurological outcome. The data reported by Jones et al[2] suggest that monitoring of the central nervous system, including measurements of neuronal function, cerebral blood flow (CBF), and cerebral oxygenation, could lead to pharmacological and surgical treatment according to the individual status of the patient. This will reduce neuronal injury and neurological deficit associated with cerebral ischaemia which is not diagnosed clinically in anaesthetised and sedated patients.

Neurophysiological monitoring: electroencephalography

EEG generation

Brain electrical activity which can be recorded from the skull is characterised by a complex pattern of voltage fluctuations. The amplitude of action potentials from intracellular sites measures 80–100 mV. In contrast, the amplitudes of extracellular field potentials are only about 100 μV. Action potentials cannot be demonstrated in surface EEG recordings. This indicates that the generators of the EEG are not directly linked to intracellular action potentials but to synaptic activity which induces membrane potentials locally restricted to connected neurons. The immediate relationship between EEG waveforms and postsynaptic membrane potentials of cortical neurons could be demonstrated in simultaneous recordings of the EEG and of intracellular potential fluctuations (fig 6.1). In apical dendrites, summation of excitatory postsynaptic potentials (EPSPs) results in the generation of electric dipoles which induce direct current components (fig 6.2). As less than 35% of the

150

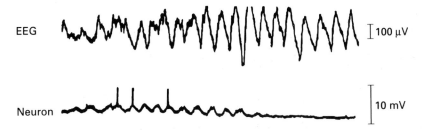

EEG

Neuron

$\left]\right. 100\,\mu V$

$\left]\right. 10\,mV$

Fig 6.1 Bottom tracing: intracellular recording of the membrane potential with rhythmic fluctuations and superimposed action potentials. Upper tracing: in the simultaneous recorded EEG the rhythmic fluctuations are seen; however, there is no correlation to the action potentials. (Modified according to Creutzfeld[3a])

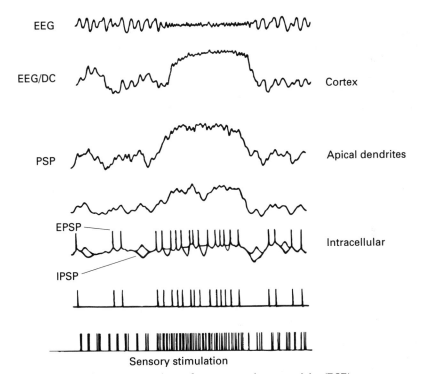

EEG

EEG/DC   Cortex

PSP   Apical dendrites

EPSP   Intracellular

IPSP

Sensory stimulation

Fig 6.2 Schematic representation of postsynaptic potentials (PSP) as generator sources for the EEG. The input induced by sensory stimulation is transmitted via specific and non-specific thalamic afferent pathways to the cortex. The PSPs are summed up in the area of apical dendrites and the cell body of large pyramidal cells of layer V in the cerebral cortex. The summation of excitatory postsynaptic potentials (EPSP) and inhibitory postsynaptic potentials (IPSP) results in a shift of the cortical slow waves (DC shift). As a result of filtering this DC shift may not be seen in the EEG

151

cortex is located on the surface of the hemispheres, direct recording of the total brain electrical activity is limited. The cortex is, however, connected to subcortical areas via projection pathways which may modulate cortical EEG activity. Functional abnormalities in subcortical brain structures may thus induce characteristic changes in the surface EEG.

Methods

Electrodes

For intraoperative recording of spontaneous and evoked EEG, standard disc or needle electrodes made of gold, silver, platin, or tin may be used. Disc electrodes are applied with conductive paste or glue to establish appropriate contact with the skin. As an alternative, electrodes may be fixed with collodion which secures a permanent fixation. As a result of a smaller contact area, needle electrodes produce higher impedances in comparison with disc electrodes. Using modern amplifiers with input impedances of more than 10 MΩ it is not usually necessary to reduce the electrode impedance below 1–2 kΩ. Careful application to achieve impedances that do not vary between electrodes is more important. Impedances greater than 20 kΩ may indicate damaged electrodes which should be removed.

For assessment of cerebral ischaemic events the anatomical distribution of the supplying arteries has to be considered. An anterior–posterior montage is suitable for assessment of drug effects. Following an international standardisation agreement (International Federation of Societies for Electroencephalography and Clinical Neurophysiology) electrodes should be placed according to the International 10–20 system (fig 6.3). For a most comprehensive evaluation of brain electrical activity 16 or 32 channel recordings are used. However, two or four channel recordings are usually appropriate for intraoperative monitoring purposes.

Amplifier

For intraoperative monitoring differential amplifiers are widely used. This type of amplifier rejects common signals ("common mode rejection") to two electrodes or connecting lines such noise from the power line (60 Hz or 50 Hz) or ECG. Different impedances in the pairs of electrodes or poor grounding of the patient causes the quality of the biosignal to deteriorate. Modern amplifiers are designed to achieve input impedances of greater than 10 MΩ which reduces the influence of small differences in electrode impedances.

Filter

For intraoperative monitoring, frequencies below 0·5 Hz and above 30 Hz are discriminated using specific filter arrangements. A filter setting that excludes frequencies below 2 Hz should not be accepted because anaesthetic

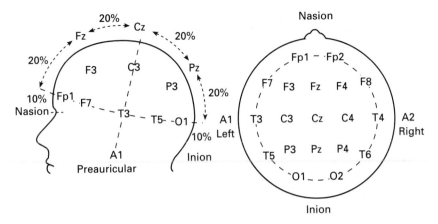

Fig 6.3 The 10–20 system makes use of prominent landmarks of the skull. Using the inion (point of maximum height of the occipital protuberance), the nasion (bridge of the nose), and the external auditory meatus, an array of exact locations can be devised across the scalp. Along the line between the nasion and the inion five points are marked in 10% or 20% intervals: frontopolar (Fp), frontal (F), central (C), parietal (P), and occipital (O). The lateral positions are defined according to coronary planes with 10% and 20% distances from the midline and parallel to a line between the external auditory meatuses. Points on the right hemispheres are assigned even numbers and points above the left hemispheres odd numbers

induced EEG changes may result in increases in slow wave activity below 2 Hz.

EEG display

The amplified and filtered EEG waves are displayed as a graph of voltage (amplitude) over time. The EEG is characterised in terms of voltage, frequencies, degree of organisation, rhythms and patterns, symmetry or asymmetry, and reactivity to sensory stimulation. In addition, activity in selected frequency bands may be evaluated separately. Conventional EEG frequency bands are divided into: δ (0·5–4 Hz), θ (4–8 Hz), α (8–13 Hz), and β (>13 Hz). Conventional multichannel EEG recordings may be performed in the operating room. For the control of a multichannel EEG, however, an experienced neurophysiologist must continuously monitor the strip recordings. In addition, small changes over time may be difficult to detect using paper strips. Currently, intraoperative EEG monitoring is performed using processed EEG which preferentially displays time compressed trends in single EEG parameters. For assessment of intraoperative EEG patterns, the generation and appearance of possible artefacts must be taken into account.

EEG analysis may be performed according to two fundamentally different techniques. In the "time domain" the EEG signal is evaluated over time,

153

whereas in the "frequency domain" the signal is transformed into the frequency range. Zero crossing analysis and aperiodic analysis are two examples for the "time domain" technique; this simply measures the time intervals for waves with either positive or negative polarity. Following this, the frequency is calculated as the number of polarity changes divided by two (fig 6.4). Aperiodic analysis uses two different algorithms. The time between two successive minima with an interposed maximum is calculated by the slow wave algorithm. The fast wave algorithm calculates the time between two successive minima irrespective of the polarity.

In a different approach to EEG analysis the signals are transformed into the "frequency domain." In a first step, the signals are digitised in assigning the different voltages to discrete numbers. By subjecting the digitised signals to Fast Fourier Transformation (FFT), the data are converted to the "frequency domain" (fig 6.5). One assumption of FFT is that the signal is stationary and periodic which may not hold true for short EEG segments or for short lasting EEG changes (that is, burst suppression activity). An epoch length between two and eight seconds allows an almost continuous calculation and display of EEG parameters. Following FFT, power spectrum analysis may be used to calculate the distribution of power (an amplitude measure) at each frequency point. Based on these analyses, several monitoring parameters such as median frequency, spectral edge frequency, peak power frequency, or the power ratio of selected frequency bands, etc may be calculated and displayed as a trend parameter over time (fig 6.6).

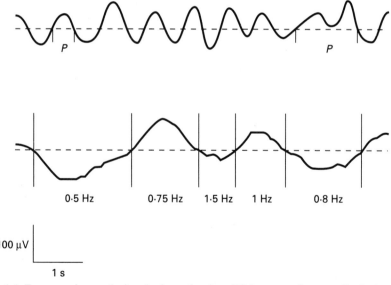

Fig 6.4 Zero crossing analysis calculates the time (P) between changes of polarity of the signal. The frequency is calculated as $F = 1/P$.

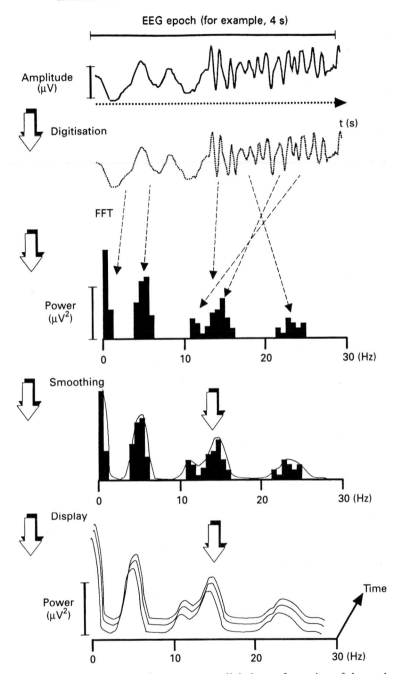

Fig 6.5 Power spectrum analysis represents a digital transformation of the analogue signal followed by Fast Fourier Transformation (FFT) for calculation of the power at each frequency component

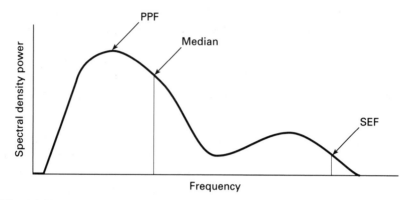

Fig 6.6 From the spectral density power several univariate parameters can be calculated: peak power frequency (PPF), median frequency (frequency that cuts the area under the curve by half), and spectral edge frequency (SEF; frequency below which 95% of the power is found)

Calculated EEG parameters can be displayed in several ways. The power spectrum may be displayed as a graph of individual epochs over time (fig 6.6). Small spectral power changes may, however, be obscured by previous epochs of higher amplitudes. By rotating the time axis, this problem of hidden line plots may be partly overcome. More detailed analysis is possible with selected frequency bands plotted over time. The spectral edge frequency has originally been defined as the upper limit of the power spectrum. In more recent applications the spectral edge frequency has been used to describe the frequency below which 95% or 90% of the spectral power is found. The median frequency is defined as the frequency which divides the area under the spectral power curve by half. Other univariate descriptors are the peak power frequency, the mean frequency, or several ratios of selected frequency bands.

Effects of anaesthetics

Inhalational anaesthetics

Nitrous oxide (>40%) results in loss of α activity and induction of faster waves followed by 4–8/s rhythms. Volatile anaesthetics when given in subanaesthetic concentrations produce fast wave activity which is changed to slower waves with the onset of unconsciousness. At about 0·4 MAC (minimum alveolar concentration) a shift from occipital to frontal high amplitude slow wave activity will be observed. At the same time, cerebral oxygen demand is decreased.

Halothane—A dominant frequency in the range of 11–16 Hz is seen at 1 MAC of halothane. Increasing halothane concentrations produce EEG slowing to 1 Hz activity (4 MAC). Seizure activity or burst suppression patterns will not occur with clinically relevant halothane concentrations.

Enflurane—Enflurane produces high amplitude 7–14 Hz activity at an anaesthetic level of 1 MAC. Further increases in enflurane concentrations may produce seizure activity. Hypocapnia may facilitate sharp wave activity at lower concentrations.

Isoflurane—With loss of consciousness isoflurane produces a mixture of slow wave activity superimposed with faster waves. At 1 MAC the EEG is dominated by 4–8 Hz activity. Increasing isoflurane concentrations produce progressive EEG slowing until burst suppression occurs. The addition of nitrous oxide (60%) produces EEG silence at 1·3–1·5 MAC of isoflurane.

Sevoflurane—Sevoflurane produces similar EEG changes to those seen with isoflurane.

Desflurane—Desflurane produces prominent θ and β activity at 1 MAC. Similar to isoflurane, desflurane may produce suppression of the EEG. No epileptiform activity has been observed so far.

Intravenous anaesthetics
Barbiturates—During induction of anaesthesia, barbiturates produce EEG activation which is followed by slowing and increases in amplitude. Progressive increases in concentration may result in burst suppression and electrical silence. At this stage maximal reduction in cerebral metabolism is achieved.

Etomidate may produce uncoordinated movements of the extremities. No epileptiform activity has, however, been observed in scalp recordings following etomidate. Similar to the action of barbiturates, burst suppression and electrical silence may be produced with etomidate.

Propofol also produces EEG slowing with increases in amplitude. Propofol may be titrated until burst suppression patterns occur. Controversy exists on the generation of epileptiform activity. Although some studies suggest anticonvulsive properties of propofol,[3] others have demonstrated generalised convulsions with propofol.[4]

Benzodiazepines—Benzodiazepines produce EEG activation with irregular faster waves of low amplitude. Increases in benzodiazepine plasma concentrations may result in EEG slowing and increases in amplitude. Unlike the effects of hypnotics, however, no burst suppression is produced.

Ketamine—Ketamine produces synchronised high amplitude θ activity superimposed with low amplitude high frequency activity (20–40 Hz).

157

Opioids

Administration of opioids results in a progressive EEG slowing with prominent activity of high amplitude δ and θ waves ($>50~\mu V$). Fentanyl when given in doses below 3 $\mu g/kg$ produces only minimal EEG changes. Maximal EEG alterations may be seen at doses up to 100 $\mu g/kg$ with development of a plateau in the EEG in response to the drug. Experimental studies have shown that supraclinical doses of fentanyl may produce epileptic activity.[5]

Intraoperative EEG monitoring

Carotid endarterectomy

For EEG monitoring during carotid endarterectomy, the electrode montage must represent brain areas supplied by the carotid artery. Cerebral ischaemia may occur following carotid artery occlusion or with insertion of a temporary shunt. In these circumstances, improvement of cerebral perfusion may help to avoid serious neurological sequelae. As hypoxic/ischaemic EEG changes may not be different from anaesthetic induced EEG alterations, the anaesthetic technique (for example, $<1\cdot0\%$ isoflurane in nitrous oxide) should avoid rapid changes in anaesthetic or opioid plasma concentrations.[6][7] Blood pressure may be maintained with vasopressor or hypotensive drugs. The EEG has to be carefully monitored during the critical phases of the surgical procedure: internal carotid cross clamping and shunt insertion. In response to ischaemia the EEG changes may vary considerably. Most frequently, a reduction in amplitude of fast wave activity and a shift to high amplitude, slow wave activity may be seen in the ipsilateral hemisphere. Following the onset of ischaemia, initial EEG changes may be noted within 60 s.[8] With persisting cerebral ischaemia, brain electrical silence may eventually occur.

Seizure surgery

A variety of clinical seizures may represent epileptogenic disorders. In spite of the progress in drug treatment of seizure activity, some patients with epilepsy are refractory to medical therapy. In these patients, resection of the cortical area with the epileptogenic focus may be indicated. The EEG may serve as a marker for the underlying hyperexcitable area of the cortex.[9] The surgical procedure may be performed either in conscious patients under local anaesthesia of the scalp and cranium or in anaesthetised patients. For local anaesthesia, excellent cooperation of the patient is necessary. General anaesthesia improves patient comfort but traditional cortical stimulation and mapping techniques may no longer be used. The anaesthetic technique has to be planned carefully to provide adequate patient management plus optimal conditions for surgery with minimal effects on neurophysiological monitoring. In anaesthetised patients, the EEG activity may be considerably altered.

The anaesthetic technique has to take into account the anticonvulsant effects that occur with a variety of anaesthetics. A major goal is to achieve a light steady state of anaesthesia with minimal effects on the EEG and seizure activity.

Epileptiform activity without motor manifestations has been observed after administration of methohexitone (methohexital) and etomidate.[10] Induction of anaesthesia may be performed with an ultrashort acting barbiturate and small doses of an opioid. If no electrocorticography is planned, anaesthesia may be maintained using a combination of low dose isoflurane or halothane with nitrous oxide in oxygen. All volatile and intravenous anaesthetics may confound identification of the seizure foci. Enflurane and methohexitone have, however, been reported to activate epiletogenic foci, thus facilitating their localisation.[11] If intraoperative stimulation and electrocorticography are planned, small doses of methohexitone (10–20 mg) in combination with a nitrous oxide–opioid technique may be favourable. Hyperventilation can induce or potentiate seizure activity and should be avoided unless this is required for surgical exposure.[12]

Neurophysiological monitoring: evoked responses

In the operating room somatosensory (SEPs), auditory (AEPs), visual evoked responses (VEPs), and motor evoked potentials (MEPs) may be used for intraoperative monitoring. In contrast to the EEG, which represents the spontaneous activity of the cortex, evoked responses (EPs) reflect changes in electrical activity of the central and peripheral nervous system induced by exogenous stimuli. The amplitude of sensory evoked responses recorded at the scalp is small ($0\cdot5$–$5~\mu V$) when compared with the EEG. The responses to the individual stimuli are averaged so that the randomly generated EEG will be eliminated. For each stimulus modality and specific component the required number of stimuli depends on the relative size of the response in question.[13] SEP and VEP components may be assessed with as few as 64–128 stimuli whereas smaller EP amplitudes such as early AEPs (BAEPs) may require the averaging of more than 1000 responses. EP waveforms are quantified according to their latencies following stimulus onset and their amplitudes.

Somatosensory evoked responses

The most frequently used stimulus for SEP recordings is an electrical pulse applied to the skin near a large peripheral nerve (for example, median nerve, ulnar nerve, tibial nerve). SEPs may also be recorded using mechanical or tactile stimulation techniques. With electrical stimuli, the stimulation intensity has to be adjusted to above motor threshold level to elicit large SEP components. SEPs recorded from the scalp compromise early components generated in peripheral nerves and in the brain stem, as well as short, middle, and long latency components with origins in subcortical and cortical areas. For monitoring purposes during clinical anaesthesia, subcortical (latency 13–15 ms) and early cortical components (latency 18–50 ms) following median or posterior tibial nerve stimulation are usually evaluated.

Technical considerations

The bandpass used for SEP recordings is critical for waveform analysis. For intraoperative monitoring filtering at 10 Hz or higher may be used to minimise baseline shifts and low frequency artefacts. The low pass filter is usually set at 1 kHz or higher. The minimum sampling rate must be at least twice the highest frequency present in the sampled data (Nyquist's theorem) to avoid spurious low frequency components that are not present in the original signals.

SEP components are identified by their respective polarity (P = positive, N = negative) and the peak latency of the individual SEP amplitude following the trigger pulse (fig 6.7). Short latency SEPs (<20 ms) are generated in the peripheral nerves, spinal cord, and subcortical and primary cortical structures. Intermediate (20–100 ms) and long (>100 ms) latency SEPs are generated in the cerebral cortex. They are sensitive to anaesthetic agents and changes in physiological variables such as cerebral blood flow, arterial oxygen tension (Pao_2), haematocrit, and body temperature. Long latency SEPs are very sensitive to the effects of anaesthetics but are also subject to changes in vigilance, attention, and the individual emotional state. A frontal scalp reference is most often used for intraoperative SEP monitoring because it appears to be less noisy than non-cephalic references.

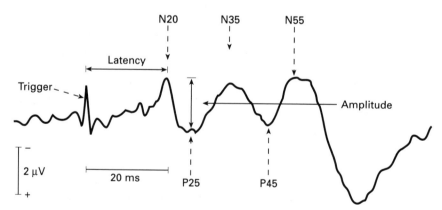

Fig 6.7 SEP recordings following median nerve stimulation at the contralateral somatosensory projection area with frontal reference. The individual SEP components are identified by their respective polarity (P = positive; N = negative) and their peak latency following the trigger impulse

Hypothermia decreases conduction velocity and delays synaptic trans-mission. For 1°C the nerve conduction velocity decreases about 2·5 m/s, affecting latencies of SEP components. A linear relationship between latency and tympanic temperature has been calculated for the temperature range of 25–35°C.[14] The difference between the major cervical SEP N13 and the first negative thalamocortical peak N20 recorded over the scalp represents the central conduction time (CCT; normal value: 5·8 + 0·5 ms). The CCT reflects the time interval for the evoked response to travel through the intracranial portion of the somatosensory pathway. The central conduction time may vary as a logarithmic function or exponentially with decreasing temperature.

In anaesthetised patients, arterial carbon dioxide tensions in a range of 2·66–6·65 kPa (20–50 mm Hg) exert small or no changes in subcortical and cortical SEP components.[15] Cortical SEPs are depressed at a mean arterial blood pressure below 40 mm Hg. Sequential recovery of SEPs upon resto-ration of a compromised blood flow or mean arterial blood pressure is dependent on the length of hypotension.

Effects of anaesthetics

Inhalational anaesthetics—Inhalational agents reduce SEP amplitudes and increase latencies to a different degree. Increasing concentrations of up to 50% nitrous oxide cause graded reductions in SEP amplitudes without changes in latencies. Volatile anaesthetics also depress cortical SEPs and, quantitatively different from the effects of nitrous oxide, increase latencies in a dose dependent manner. Enflurane in comparison with halothane and isoflurane produces the greatest, and halothane the least, depressing effect on early cortical SEPs. However, high dose enflurane may increase SEP amplitudes. This effect has been attributed to an enflurane induced synchronisation of cortical neurons and excitation.[16] Isoflurane results in more pronounced SEP depression than halothane when given in equipotent doses. In contrast to 2% halothane, administration of equipotent concentra-tions of isoflurane in 66% nitrous oxide may result in complete loss of cortical SEPs. Recent data suggest that sevoflurane given with increasing concentra-tions up to 1·5 MAC has similar effects on median nerve SEPs as isoflurane. Reproducible SEP recordings may be obtained with all volatile anaesthetics within the range of 0·5–1 MAC.

Intravenous anaesthetics—Spinal and subcortical SEPs are not affected by intravenous anaesthetics. With the exception of etomidate, most intravenous anaesthetics decrease amplitudes of early cortical SEPs in a dose related manner with abolishment of later cortical SEPs. In contrast to the depressing effects of barbiturates, etomidate administration results in a large increase of the early SEP component N20P25. Propofol infused for induction (2–2·5 mg/ kg) and for maintenance of anaesthesia (9 mg/kg per h) does not suppress subcortical and early cortical SEPs.[17] SEP latencies are prolonged with all intravenous anaesthetics. Variable findings suggesting either no change or a moderate increase in early cortical SEP amplitudes have been reported for ketamine.[18][19]

Opioids—Administration of opioids (morphine, fentanyl, alfentanil, sufentanil) results in moderate decreases of cortical SEPs with minimal changes in latencies. Changes in upper or lower extremity SEPs induced by opioids are smaller compared with the effects of intravenous or inhalational anaesthetics. An opioid based anaesthetic technique allows adequate SEP signal acquisition in most instances.[20]

Surgical procedures

SEP monitoring has reached a stage of widespread application in neurosurgery, orthopaedic surgery, vascular surgery, and interventional neuroradiology.

Spinal cord monitoring—A major problem during spinal cord monitoring is a poor baseline recording in patients with intramedullary tumours or vascular lesions caused by preoperative neurological deficits. Patients scheduled for scoliosis surgery, vascular surgery, or interventional neuroradiology rarely present with pre-existing neurological deficits so that normal potentials may be recorded. In these cases intraoperative neurological complications may be recognised by decreases in amplitude and increases in latency. However, false negative as well as false positive waveform changes may occur.[21]

Carotid endarterectomy—SEP monitoring during carotid endarterectomy has been suggested as superior to EEG monitoring[22] because SEPs are generated in brain stem structures as well as in the cortex. Following contralateral median nerve stimulation, SEPs are evoked in the ipsilateral postcentral region. Early shunt insertion following loss of SEPs has been reported to prevent neurological deficits. Once the SEPs have been depressed as a result of cross clamping of the carotid artery, the recovery of SEPs may be used to ensure proper functioning of the shunt. Neurological deficits may, however, occur in the presence of stable SEPs throughout the surgical procedure.[23] The failure of SEPs to predict all strokes may be related to the regional specificity of this monitoring modality or to the different types of ischaemia (that is, focal versus incomplete hemispherical). In a study comparing EEG with SEP during carotid endarterectomy, however, the SEP was more sensitive to neuronal injury compared with the EEG.[24]

Aneurysm surgery—Accidental or intentional vessel occlusion during aneurysm surgery may result in severe SEP changes. If SEP changes occur, transient or permanent neurological deficits may develop. Unchanged SEPs do not, however, necessarily indicate preserved neurological function because the vascular territory at risk does not always include sensory pathways. If the surgical procedure involves the vascular region for the sensory pathways, SEP deterioration appears to be a reliable indicator of ischaemia.

Auditory evoked responses

AEPs reflect the response of the central nervous system to auditory stimulation at different areas of the brain. Similar to evoked responses of other modalities, AEPs consist of a series of positive and negative waves following activation of relay structures in the auditory pathway. The different components of early AEPs (BAEPs: I–VI) are thought to originate in specific sites of the brain stem.[25] Early cortical AEPs (MLAEPs: middle latency waves: No, Po, Na, Pa, Nb) are thought to originate from the medial geniculate and primary auditory cortex.[26] Late cortical waves (P1, N1, P2, N2, P3) are generated in the cortex and association areas.[27]

Technical considerations

BAEPs and MLAEPs are evoked by electronic square waves (clicks, duration: 100–500 μs) with a stimulation rate around 10 Hz. For assessment of late cortical AEP (>80 ms) components, slow and irregular repetition frequencies have to be chosen (>1–2/s) so as to minimise habituation and cumulative interactions between AEP subcomponents. The stimulus intensity is preferentially set to an individual threshold or above the average threshold for a specific population. AEPs are best recorded at the vertex (Cz) versus linked mastoids. The reference electrode may be placed at the frontal head. Hypothermia may induce an increase in latency ($+0.2$ ms/°C) and a reduction in AEP amplitude. AEPs with latencies of more than 30 ms are affected by the state of vigilance. Early MLAEPs may increase in amplitude with raised levels of alertness and arousal.[28] The late component N2 may increase in amplitude with decreases in vigilance.

Effects of anaesthetics

BAEPs are rather resistant to the effects of intravenous anaesthetics and opioids. Volatile anaesthetics prolong BAEP latencies in a graded manner with increasing concentrations.[13] The effects of anaesthetics on MLAEPs are more pronounced compared with BAEPs. Recent studies have shown that halothane, enflurane, isoflurane, etomidate, althesin, thiopentone, propofol, or the infusion of saline, in addition to a constant mixture of 70% nitrous oxide and 30% oxygen, decrease MLAEP amplitudes and increase latencies of the components Pa and Nb.[13] These findings indicate that the primary sensory processing in the brain is blocked at the level of the primary sensory cortex whereas receptor specific anaesthetics (for example, benzodiazepines, opioids, ketamine) do not suppress MLAEPs.[29] Using 0·3% end tidal halothane in 70% nitrous oxide in oxygen, MLAEPs increase in amplitude with surgical stimulation.[30] A close correlation between intraoperative preservation of MLAEPs and implicit memory has been established.[29] General anaesthetics seem to provide more effective suppression of auditory sensory processing and unconscious perceptions during general anaesthesia than receptor specific agents.

Surgical procedures

The physiological basis for monitoring AEPs during intracranial surgical procedures is the sensitivity of AEPs to sensorineural and conductive hearing deficits.[31] BAEP monitoring may be used to assess brain stem function during interventions at the base of the skull or in head injured patients. BAEPs appear to be less sensitive to global hypoxia or raised intracranial pressure when compared with SEPs or EEG. The integrity of cranial nerve VIII may be monitored using BAEPs during resection of acoustic neuroma and other tumours of the cerebellopontine angle, or during microvascular decompression which has substantial risk for hearing loss.[32] Bilateral alterations in BAEPs are indicative of a compromised brain stem function.

Visual evoked responses

Visual evoked cortical responses (VEPs) are produced by flash stimuli applied using a pair of goggles containing light emitting electrodes. No subcortical VEPs have been identified so far. Following stimulation of the retina, VEPs may be recorded for assessment of the integrity of the visual pathway. VEPs are best recorded at the occipital cortex (O1, O2). VEP recording may be used during surgical procedures, such as resection of pituitary tumours or craniopharyngiomas, or near the optic tract to monitor damage of the visual system. VEPs are affected by disorders of the lens or optic neuritis; they are very sensitive to the effects of anaesthetics and increases in latencies and decreases in amplitude were found with inhalational anaesthetics.[33 34] VEPs are also sensitive to increases in ICP and hypothermia.[35]

Monitoring of intracranial pressure

Intracranial pressure (measured in mm Hg) is an important variable in the perioperative management of patients with head injury, intracranial tumour, spontaneous intracranial haemorrhage, cerebral vascular occlusive disease, meningitis, encephalitis, and encephalopathy. Changes in intracranial pressure are determined by alterations of the components of intracranial volume such as parenchyma (oedema), blood (hypercapnia, dysregulation, venous hypertension, venous outflow obstruction), and cerebrospinal fluid (CSF) (hydrocephalus). Langfitt *et al*[36 37] have identified the relationship between changes in intracranial volume and intracranial pressure. This relationship has been defined as cerebral elastance ($\Delta P/\Delta V$). With the additional invasive measurement of mean arterial blood pressure (MAP) (measured in mm Hg), cerebral perfusion pressure (CPP) (measured in mm Hg) can be calculated according to the following formula:

$$CPP = MAP - ICP$$

Monitoring of ICP (and CPP) has several useful clinical implications but the decision to measure ICP should be confirmed by the following clinical situation and radiological imaging studies:[38]

1 Elevated ICP associated with a midline shift can indicate intracranial mass lesions.
2 ICP trends facilitate early diagnosis and treatment of a developing mass lesion.
3 Intracranial elastance can be determined by fluid injections and withdrawal.
4 CSF drainage following ventriculostomy can temporarily decrease ICP pressure and allows for CSF sampling.
5 Therapeutic interventions to treat intracranial hypertension (hyperventilation, diuretics, hypnotics) can be titrated according to the dynamic ICP response.[39]

The non-uniformity of the intracranial compartment with irregularly shaped CSF spaces, and bony, dural, and arachnoid barriers may produce an inhomogeneous pressure pattern within the calvarium. Thus, increased ICP may exist in the supratentorial but not in the infratentorial compartment. Likewise, regional supratentorial hypertension may occur next to supratentorial normotensive areas. This indicates that intracranial hypertension may be missed by ICP monitoring in patients with local or regional abnormalities distant to the ICP probe.

A variety of techniques for chronic ICP monitoring has been developed, and the decision to use one specific technique should be based on the experience of the surgeon, and on the clinical indications. ICP monitoring techniques may be classified as supratentorial, infratentorial, and lumbar. The supratentorial approach is by far the most commonly indicated, and may be subclassified as epidural, subdural–subarachnoid, intraventricular, or parenchymal (fig 6.8). All of the clinically available monitors have recognised advantages and disadvantages because they vary in their accuracy, the ease of insertion, and relative risks (table 6.1). Nevertheless, there is no doubt that ICP monitoring serves as a warning system, indicating changes in ICP associated with changes in intracranial volume or displacement of cerebral structures. During intracranial surgery, monitoring of ICP and arterial blood pressure permits precise titration of pharmacological agents for induction and maintenance of anaesthesia. ICP monitoring allows observation of the consequences of venous engorgement during positioning or application of the bone flap during cranial closure.[40] Postoperative measurements of ICP include early detection and immediate treatment of brain oedema and intracranial haemorrhage.

Monitoring of cerebral haemodynamics

Transcranial Doppler ultrasonography

Transcranial Doppler ultrasonography measures blood flow velocity (cm/s) in major basal cerebral arteries both non-invasively and continuously. The anterior, middle, and posterior cerebral arteries can be insonated via the thin layers of the temporal bone above the zygomatic arch. The infratentorial vasculature (vertebral arteries, basilar artery) can be insonated by the transoccipital approach through the foramen magnum. Several methodological limitations apply when using transcranial Doppler ultrasonography as a monitor of cerebral blood flow (CBF). Doppler measurements are sensitive to changes in the angle between the ultrasonic beam and the vessel.[41] It is therefore essential to keep the insonation depth and the insonation angle

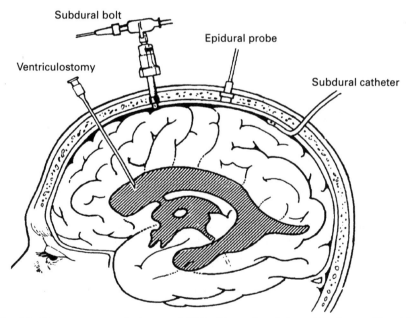

Fig 6.8 Measurement techniques of ICP. (Reproduced from Bendo *et al*[39a] with permission)

Table 6.1 Advantages and disadvantages of measurement techniques of ICP

Device	Advantage	Disadvantage
Supratentorial		
Epidural	Dura intact Low infection rate	Potential risk of haemorrhage Accuracy questionable Recalibration with changes in head position
Subdural–subarachnoid bolt	No brain invasion Low infection rate No ventricular cannulation	Port blockade by swollen brain Artefact from tube movement Fluid filled column may be blocked by air and debris Recalibration with changes in head position
Fibreoptic	Sudural, intraparenchymal, or intraventricular placement Minimal artefact and drift High resolution of waveform	Once inserted, calibration check is impossible Fibre breakage Infection
Ventricular	Gold standard of accuracy Allows drainage of CSF for: ICP control, CSF sampling Intrathecal antibiotics	Difficult cannulation Fluid filled column may be blocked by air and debris Artefact from tube movement Infection
Infratentorial		
Subdural		Difficult percutaneous access Presence of fragile neural and vascular structures Pseudomeningocele formation
Lumbar		
Subarachnoid		Brain herniation Infection

constant during the investigation period. Maintenance of the probe position during surgical procedures and intensive care, however, still creates significant practical problems. As the diameter of the insonated vessel segment remains unknown, absolute CBF values cannot be inferred from transcranial Doppler ultrasonography data.

Cerebral blood flow and cerebral perfusion pressure
   The flow spectra of transcranial Doppler ultrasonography closely reflect changes in CBF regardless of the status of CBF autoregulation or cerebral metabolism. Studies in humans have shown that blood flow velocity changes within the middle cerebral artery correlate with regional CBF in the corresponding perfusion territory.[42 43] This is consistent with studies in dogs where transcranial Doppler ultrasonography was a semiquantitative monitor of changes in CBF when intravenous and volatile anaesthetics or opioids were given.[44-46]
   In human volunteers, Newell *et al*[47] found a close correlation between

167

changes in transcranial Doppler ultrasonic spectra and internal carotid flow during induction of arterial hypotension. This is in support of studies in laboratory animals and humans with and without intracranial pathology, where transcranial Doppler ultrasonography indicated changes in CBF associated with decreases in CPP.[48–52] The diastolic flow velocity pattern appears to be the most sensitive Doppler parameter of CBF. Data from animals subjected to progressive decreases in CPP show that decreases in CBF and EEG activity resulted in concomitant decreases of the diastolic frequency spectrum.[48 53 54] This is consistent with a close relationship between the diastolic flow velocity pattern and neuronal function.

Thus, transcranial Doppler monitoring allows discrimination of changes in CBF induced by anaesthetics and sedatives from those associated with changes in CPP (for example, head injury, arteriovenous malformations, systemic hypotension). With persisting diastolic zero flow or further decreases in CPP, cerebral circulatory arrest occurs. Transcranial Doppler ultrasonic spectra of brain dead subjects show five typical blood flow velocity patterns (figs 6.9 and 6.10):

1 Systolic flow without diastolic flow
2 Systolic flow with combined diastolic forward and reversed flow
 • oscillating flow (biphasic flow) with reversed diastolic flow
 • systolic peaks without diastolic flow
 • no detectable flow.[55 56]

Cerebral embolism
Transcranial Doppler ultrasonography detects cerebral embolic events

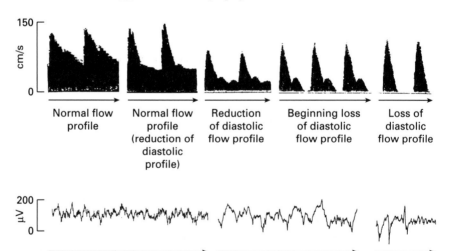

Fig 6.9 Changes of the transcranial Doppler ultrasonic frequency spectra and the EEG pattern during progressive decreases in CPP. (Reproduced from Werner[54a] with permission)

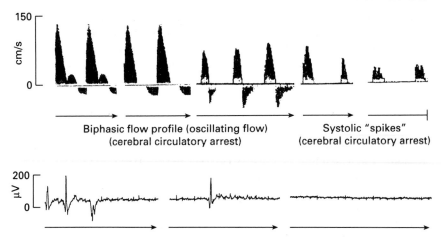

Fig 6.10 Transcranial Doppler ultrasonic frequency spectra and EEG pattern with impeding and persisting cerebral circulatory arrest. (Reproduced from Werner[54a] with permission)

during cardiac or neurovascular surgery.[57–59] These emboli appear as short duration, high intensity signals in the Doppler spectrum. The Doppler emboli signals vary according to stroke subtype.[58] Results from in vitro studies suggest a positive correlation between the size of an embolus and the amplitude of the transcranial Doppler signal for materials such as atheroma, thrombus, platelets, or fat.[60 61] Additionally, algorithms detecting the power increase occurring with emboli provide a high sensitivity and specificity to discriminate artefact from true embolic events.[62] In support of the embolic hypothesis of perioperative stroke, prospective transcranial Doppler monitoring and postoperative neurological examination in patients undergoing cardiopulmonary bypass found a close correlation between the occurrence of intraoperative embolism and postoperative neurological deficit.[63]

Carotid endarterectomy and cerebral vasospasm

Several studies have evaluated the changes of the blood flow velocity pattern on transcranial Doppler ultrasonography during various ischaemic challenges. In conscious patients undergoing balloon occlusion tests of the internal carotid artery or carotid endarterectomy, decreases in average blood flow velocity (>65%) indicated ischaemic CBF and low stump pressures parallel to clinical symptoms of cerebral ischaemia.[64 65] Investigations in patients undergoing carotid endarterectomy indicate that the sensitivity and specificity to detect intraoperative cerebral ischaemia are increased with the combination of transcranial Doppler ultrasonography and EEG monitoring.[66 67]

Abnormal increases in flow velocity occur with both cerebral vasospasm

169

and hyperaemia. Transcranial Doppler ultrasonic monitoring can discriminate between these non-hyperaemic and hyperaemic pathophysiologies. In patients with cerebral vasospasm, the Doppler waveform showed a diastolic notch which is consistent with increased cerebrovascular resistance. This diastolic notch did not develop with post-traumatic hyperaemia.[68] The value of pathological increases in CBF as a parameter for cerebral ischaemia is, however, unclear. Grosset et al[69] have shown, in 121 patients with subarachnoid haemorrhage, that increases in transcranial Doppler ultrasonic spectra correlate with delayed ischaemic deficits. In contrast, other studies indicate that increases in CBF are not predictive of the development of delayed ischaemic deficits.[70–72] This is consistent with a study in head injured patients where CO_2 reactivity in the early days following trauma did not correlate with outcome.[73] Thus, the mechanisms of delayed ischaemic deficits following subarachnoid haemorrhage and head injury appear to be multifactorial. As a consequence, transcranial Doppler frequency spectra should be combined with variables such as clinical grade and CPP to guide therapeutic interventions.

Laser Doppler flowmetry

Laser Doppler flowmetry measures relative changes in cerebral and spinal cord blood flow (arbitrary units or mV).[74–76] Several methodological and technical limitations apply, however, with the use of laser Doppler flowmetry as a cerebral perfusion monitor. Laser Doppler flowmetry is an invasive technique and requires craniotomy and exposure of the brain or spinal cord to place the probe on the surface of neuronal tissue. This may produce microtrauma, CSF fistulae, and infection. Changes in the probe position and fibre movement artefacts produce deviations from true organ blood flow. It is therefore important to maintain the laser Doppler probe in a constant position and fix the device in a self retaining retractor or micromanipulator to minimise movements. This allows comparisons of cerebral or spinal cord blood flow over time.

Clinical studies have demonstrated the use of laser Doppler flowmetry as a continuous CBF measurement technique for the perioperative period and during neurocritical care.[77–82] In patients undergoing craniotomy for resection of arteriovenous malformations, tumour, and occlusion of aneurysms, laser Doppler flowmetry reflected changes in CBF during manipulations of Pa_{CO_2} and MAP.[80–82] The application of laser Doppler flowmetry to measure CO_2 reactivity may guide early therapeutic intervention with decreases in the cerebrovascular response to CO_2, or the level of hyperventilation necessary to improve CBF. Laser Doppler flowmetry can be used to assess CBF autoregulation[83] which may be impaired or abolished with the use of anaesthetics, in patients with intracranial mass lesions or following head injury. The status of CBF autoregulation, however, varies between patients and insult. Manipulations to increase CPP may be of advantage[84] but may also be detrimental to the brain depending on the autoregulatory status.[85] The application of laser Doppler flowmetry to measure changes in CBF during changes in arterial blood pressure permits adjustment of CPP to maintain adequate CBF levels. There is potential use of laser Doppler flowmetry monitoring in the clinical evaluation of cerebral ischaemia.[77 78] During neurosurgery, brain retractor pressure may produce brain contusion and infarction which may be diagnosed intraoperatively using laser Doppler techniques.[86] Dirnnagl et al[87] have correlated changes in CBF with changes in laser Doppler flow in a rat model of cerebral ischaemia. Although the authors have shown a close correlation between relative changes in CBF and laser Doppler flow, they did not define or identify specific laser Doppler flow patterns that indicate cerebral ischaemia. Although the ischaemic threshold level of laser Doppler signals is still unclear, this technique may significantly improve the quality of treatment in patients with intracranial pathology, particularly when combined with measurements of ICP, brain electrical activity, or jugular bulb venous oxygen saturation (Sjo_2).

Thermal measurement systems

Thermal measurement systems monitor changes in CBF using heated thermistors placed on the cortical surface. The heat is conducted into the surrounding tissue and dissipated at a rate related to tissue perfusion. Wei et al[88] have validated the responses of thermal measurement systems to rapid changes in mean arterial blood pressure in rats. Using microthermistor probes, the results of Wei et al[88] indicate that the thermal measurement system can quantitate changes in CBF. These results are consistent with experiments by Voorhees et al[89] who found a linear relationship between nitroprusside induced changes in CBF measured with microspheres and CBF data from thermal clearance measurements. In patients undergoing craniotomy for cerebral aneurysm clipping after subarachnoid haemorrhage, Abe et al[90 91] have employed thermal gradient CBF measurements to monitor the effects of nicardipine and prostaglandin on CBF and CO_2 reactivity. The results from these clinical studies show that thermal measurement systems assess dynamic CBF during neurosurgical procedures.

Near infrared techniques

Near infrared spectroscopy measures changes in oxyhaemoglobin, deoxyhaemoglobin, and cytochrome aa_3 redox status both non-invasively and continuously. It is possible that near infrared spectroscopy measures changes in CBF. Following injection of indocyanine green into the right atrium, the transmission of the bolus through the cerebral circulation can be detected, and the resulting high resolution time–activity curve depicts the influx and decay of this non-diffusible tracer signal. With simultaneous recordings over an arterial vessel, the cerebral mean cortical transit time can be generated.[92] Alternatively, the induction of sudden increases in arterial oxygen saturation (Sao_2) produces increases in oxyhaemoglobin concentrations, thus simulating the arterial tracer. Organ blood flow may be derived by consideration of the haemoglobin concentration in whole blood and the integral of the change in Sao_2 over time. In support of this, studies in critically ill pre-term infants have shown that the estimation of CBF using the near infrared spectroscopy principle was closely correlated with measurements of CBF with xenon-133.[93] Although there is limited experience with this technique, the available data suggest that non-invasive near infrared spectroscopy may be a potential bedside monitor of cerebral perfusion.

Monitoring of cerebral oxygenation and metabolism

Jugular bulb venous oxygen saturation (Sjo_2)

Measurements of jugular bulb venous oxygen saturation have been employed as a monitoring technique to estimate changes in CBF and cerebral oxygen consumption ($CMRo_2$) in patients at risk of developing perioperative cerebral ischaemia or hypoxia.[94] The description of the relationship between CBF and $CMRo_2$ is based on the calculation of the arterial–jugular venous oxygen content difference ($ajDo_2$) according to the Fick principle:

$$ajDo_2 = CMRo_2/CBF.$$

With constant Sao_2, arterial oxygen tension (Pao_2), and haemoglobin concentration, the ratio of CBF to $CMRo_2$ is proportional to Sjo_2.[95] In healthy subjects, CBF and $CMRo_2$ are coupled as indicated by $ajDo_2$ values of 5–9 ml % and Sjo_2 values of 55–75%. Increases in Sjo_2 to values over 75% indicate relative or absolute hyperaemia, whereas decreases of Sjo_2 to values of less than 50% indicate relative hypoperfusion.[95] With Sjo_2 values of less than 40%, increases in cerebral venous lactate concentrations indicate global cerebral ischaemia (fig 6.11). Changes in arterial blood gases (Pao_2, $Paco_2$, and pH), body temperature, haemoglobin concentration, ICP, and the administration of drugs will, however, modulate the relationship between CBF and Sjo_2.

Sjo_2 can be measured continuously using a fibreoptic catheter or intermittently by drawing blood samples through the catheter. In patients with focal or diffuse intracranial pathology, the catheter should be placed on the side with the dominant venous drainage. This side may be identified by manual compression of each internal jugular vein and observation of concomitant changes in ICP.[96] Following cannulation of the internal jugular vein at the level of the thyroid cartilage in a retrograde fashion, a catheter is inserted through the introducer with the tip positioned at the level of the base of the

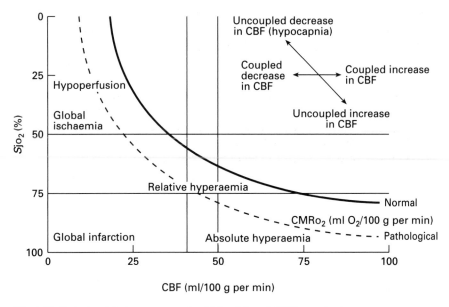

Fig 6.11 Relationship between cerebral blood flow (CBF), cerebral oxygen consumption or cerebral metabolic rate ($CMRO_2$), and jugular bulb venous oxygen saturation (Sjo_2) in head injured patients. High, normal, or reduced levels of CBF are indicated by high, normal, or low Sjo_2 values. Sjo_2 values of less than 40% indicate global cerebral ischaemia with increases in cerebral venous lactate concentrations. Global infarction is associated with cessation of cerebral metabolism which in turn increases Sjo_2 to constant high values. (Reproduced from Dearden[95] with permission)

skull. A lateral radiograph should be taken to confirm the position of the catheter tip within the jugular bulb (photograph). Catheters should not be placed in patients suffering from cervical spine injury or coagulopathies.[97]

Jugular bulb venous oxygen saturation and cerebral ischaemia

With constant Sao_2 and haemoglobin concentration, changes in Sjo_2 reflect dynamic CBF. Robertson *et al*[98] have shown, in head injured patients, that changes in CBF can be reliably estimated based on the calculation of ajDo_2 and the arteriovenous difference of lactate content. Several studies indicate that desaturation of jugular venous blood ($Sjo_2 < 40\%$) is associated with development of EEG abnormalities, neurological deterioration, unconsciousness, and depletion of cerebral energy stores, indicating cerebral ischaemia.[99-101] This is consistent with data from head injured patients showing desaturation of jugular venous blood as a function of intracranial hypertension, hypotension, hypocapnia, and hypoxia.[102] In patients undergoing carotid endarterectomy, neurological dysfunction was associated with lateral sinus oxygen saturation below 50% whereas no neurological complication occurred in patients with lateral sinus oxygen saturation over 60%.[103]

These results confirm that monitoring of Sjo_2 indicates critical cerebral perfusion (and $CMRo_2$) associated with vascular engorgement or decreases in CPP. In patients with intracranial hypertension, prolonged hyperventilation may be associated with a worse outcome.[104] Cruz[105] has suggested that the level of hyperventilation necessary to reduce acute increases in ICP should be geared according to the optimum O_2 extraction ratio (as derived from the arterial–venous oxygen content difference or ajDo_2 and arterial O_2 content) of the patients. Brain tumours, arteriovenous malformations, head injury, or stroke may be associated with impaired or abolished CBF autoregulation.[84 106] In these patients, monitoring Sjo_2 can identify the level of CPP necessary to maintain CBF and $CMRo_2$ above the individual ischaemic threshold.

Near infrared techniques

Regional cerebrovascular oxygen saturation can be measured non-invasively using near infrared transmission spectroscopy. Clinical studies have demonstrated a close correlation between cerebrovascular oxygen desaturation to values of less than 55% and the earliest burst of θ–δ background slowing in the EEG or with systemic hypoxia.[107 108] This is consistent with correlation studies between near infrared spectroscopy and Sjo_2 measurements suggesting that near infrared spectroscopy is sensitive to hypoxic challenges.[109] A significant proportion of near infrared light is, however, absorbed by extracerebral tissue. Thus, changes in flow or oxygenation in these tissues will have clinically relevant impact on near infrared data.[108] Measurements of the concentrations of oxyhaemoglobin, deoxyhaemoglobin, and cytochrome aa_3 using near infrared spectroscopy may reflect the cerebral oxygen supply and the intracellular (mitochondrial) oxygen availability. Further validation studies to prove the accuracy of near infrared spectroscopy are, however, required before clinical application is recommended.

Cerebral and spinal tissue oxygen tension

Neuronal ischaemia and hypoxia are considered to be the major mecha-nisms of secondary brain and spinal cord injury. Measurements of local tissue oxygen tension have been recently introduced as a continuous, although invasive, technique of CNS monitoring. Using polarographic needle probes, Maas et al[110] have measured Po_2 in CSF and neuronal tissue in both cats and humans during changes in CPP and during hypoxic challenges. Both CSF Po_2 and brain tissue Po_2 reflected changes in cerebral oxygenation caused by abnormal cerebral oxygen supply and CBF. This is consistent with clinical data indicating alterations of brain tissue Po_2 in pathological human brain cortex.[111] The results from these invasive studies suggest an improvement in the monitoring of ischaemic/hypoxic events. The critical threshold of cerebral spinal and brain surface oxygen tension still, however, needs to be identified.

Cerebral microdialysis

The analysis of dialysate derived from cerebral microdialysis indicates trends in the concentration of substances in the extracellular fluid that are related to hypoxic or ischaemic neuronal injury. Illievich et al[112] have shown in rabbits that changes in glutamate and glycine concentrations can be measured during repeated transient global ischaemia. Persson et al[113] have shown that microdialysis can be used in critically ill patients to monitor changes in ischaemia related substances. Landolt et al[114] have used microdialysis for on line pH determination by continuously sampling extracellular fluids in ischaemic rat brain. This technique promises to increase the understanding of the pathophysiology of neurological damage. Microdialysis is, however, an invasive measure and the local irritation next to the site of insertion of the microdialysis probe may no longer represent the brain as a whole.

Conclusion

Brain electrical monitoring is sensitive to changes in neuronal function caused by ischaemic or traumatic neuronal injury. The sensitivity and specificity to detect these functional changes vary with the type of insult and the choice of background anaesthetic. Measurements of depth of anaesthesia (using arousal patterns of the EEG or incomplete suppression of evoked potential signals), as well as specific EEG patterns for pharmacodynamic quantification of drug effects, promise to achieve the optimum relationship between anaesthetic dose and anaesthetic effect.

Monitoring of ICP indicates changes in intracranial volume or displacement of cerebral structures. This modality allows observation of the consequences of drug administration, hyperventilation, venous engorgement during positioning, or application of the bone flap during cranial closure. Postoperative measurements of ICP include early detection and immediate treatment of brain oedema and intracranial haemorrhage.

Transcranial Doppler ultrasonography is a semiquantitative, non-invasive, and continuous measure of changes in CBF induced by anaesthetics and opioids. Monitoring of the diastolic blood flow velocity pattern is a sensitive parameter of critical CBF and ischaemic neuronal dysfunction caused by decreases in CPP.

Laser Doppler flowmetry and thermal measurement systems are invasive but continuous techniques used to assess changes in microcirculatory CBF within brain lesions. Monitoring of Sj_{O_2} reflects the balance between cerebral oxygen delivery and cerebral oxygen demand. This allows for determination of the cerebral hypoperfusion associated with increases in oxygen extraction.

Near infrared spectroscopy promises to be a technique with potential for non-invasive measurements of cerebral oxygen saturation, mitochondrial oxygen availability, and CBF. The combination of monitoring of cerebral function (EEG, evoked potentials) and ICP with monitoring of cerebral haemodynamics, Sjo_2, and cerebral venous lactate concentration allows determination of the critical threshold level of CPP below which increasing oxygen extraction leads to cerebral hypoperfusion. This will optimise diagnosis and treatment of cerebral hypoperfusion and ischaemia.

1 Gentleman D, Jennett B. Audit of transfer of unconscious patients to a neurosurgical unit. *Lancet* 1990; **335**: 330–4.

2 Jones PA, Andrews PJD, Midgley S, *et al.* Measuring the burden of secondary insults in head-injured patients during intensive care. *J Neurosurg Anesth* 1994; **6**: 4–14.

3 Dwyer R, McCaughey W, Lavery J, McCarthy G, Dundee JW. Comparison of propofol and methohexitone as anesthetic agents for electroconvulsive therapy. *Anaesthesia* 1988; **43**: 459–62.

3a Creutzfeldt O, Houchin J. Neuronal basis of EEG waves. In: Rèmon A (Ed.), *Electroencephalography and clinical neurophysiology*, Vol 2C. Amsterdam: Elsevier, 1974: 5–55.

4 Hodkinson BP, Frith RW, Mee WE. Propofol and the electroencephalogram. *Lancet* 1987; **ii**: 1518.

5 Carlsson C, Smith DS, Keykah MM, Englebach I, Harp JR. The effects of high-dose fentanyl on cerebral circulation and metabolism in rats. *Anesthesiology* 1982; **57**: 375–80.

6 Cucchiara RF, Theye RA, Michenfelder JD. The effects of isoflurane on canine cerebral metabolism and blood flow. *Anesthesiology* 1974; **40**: 571–4.

7 Messick JM Jr, Casement B, Sharbrough FW, Milde LN, Michenfelder JD, Sundt TM. Correlation of regional cerebral blood flow (rCBF) with EEG changes during isoflurane anesthesia for carotid endarterectomy: Critical rCBF. *Anesthesiology* 1987; **66**: 344–9.

8 Muzzi DA, Wilson PR, Daube JR, Sharbrough FW. Electrophysiologic neurologic monitoring. In: Cucchiara RF, Michenfelder JD (Eds), *Clinical neuroanesthesia*. New York: Churchill Livingstone, 1990: 117–70.

9 Steinkeler JA, Sharbrough FW. Seizure surgery. In: Cucchiara RF, Michenfelder JD (Eds), *Clinical neuroanesthesia*. New York: Churchill Livingstone, 1990: 309–24.

10 Opitz A, Marschall M, Degan R, Koch D. General anesthesia in patients with epilepsy and status epilepticus. *Adv Neurol* 1983; **34**: 531–5.

11 Ito BM, Sato S, Kufta CV, Tran D. Effect of isoflurane and enflurane on the electrocorticogram of epileptic patients. *Neurology* 1988; **38**: 924–8.

12 Kofke A, Tempelhoff R, Dasheff RM. Anesthesia for epileptic patients and for epilepsy surgery. In: Cottrell JE, Smith DS (Eds), *Anesthesia and neurosurgery*. St Louis: Mosby, 1994: 495–524.

13 Thornton C. Evoked potentials in anaesthesia. *Eur J Anaesth* 1991; **8**: 89–107.

14 Russ W, Sticher J, Scheld H, Hempelmann G. Effects of hypothermia on somatosensory evoked responses in man. *Br J Anaesth* 1987; **59**: 1484–91.

15 Kalkman CJ, Boezeman EH, Ribberink AA, Oosting J, Deen L, Bovill JG. The influence of changes in arterial carbon dioxide tension on the electroencephalogram and posterior tibial nerve somatosensory cortical evoked potentials during alfentanil/nitrous oxide anesthesia. *Anesthesiology* 1991; **75**: 68–74.

16 Lebowitz MH, Blitt CD, Dillon JB. Enflurane-induced central nervous system excitation and its relation to carbon dioxide tension. *Anesth Analg* 1972; **51**: 355–63.

17 Scheepstra GL, De Lange JJ, Booji LHD, Ros HH. Median nerve evoked potentials during propofol anaesthesia. *Br J Anaesth* 1989; **62**: 92–4.

18 Schubert A, Licina MG, Kineberry PJ. The effect of ketamine on human somatosensory evoked potentials and its modification by nitrous oxide. *Anesthesiology* 1989; **72**: 33–9.

19 Kochs E, Blanc I, Werner C, Schulte am Esch J. Electroencephalogram and somatosensory evoked potentials following low-dose ketamine (0·5 mg/kg). *Anaesthesist* 1988; **37**: 625–30.

20 Schulte am Esch J, Kochs E (Eds). *Central nervous system monitoring in anesthesia and intensive care*. Berlin: Springer, 1994.

21 Schmid UD, Hess CW, Ludin HP. Somatosensory evoked potentials following median nerve and segmental stimulation do not confirm cervical radiculopathy with sensory deficit. *J Neurol Neurosurg Psychiatry* 1988; **51**: 182–7.

22 Dinkel M, Lörler H, Langer H, Schweiger H, Rügheimer E. Evoked potential monitoring for vascular surgery. In: Schulte am Esch J, Kochs E (Eds), *Central nervous system monitoring in anesthesia and intensive care*. Berlin: Springer, 1994: 230–47.

23 Schweiger H, Kamp HD, Dinkel M. Somatosensory evoked potentials during carotid artery surgery: experience in 400 operations. *Surgery* 1991; **109**: 602–9.

24 Lam AM, Manninen PH, Ferguson GG, Nantau W. Monitoring of electrophysiologic function during carotid endarterectomy: a comparison of somatosensory evoked potentials and conventional electroencephalogram. *Anesthesiology* 1991; **75**: 15–21.

25 Lev A, Sohmer H. Sources of averaged neural responses recorded in animal and human subjects during cochlear audiometry (electrocochleogram). *Archiv für Klinische und Experimentelle Ohren Nasen und Kopfheilkunde* 1972; **201**: 79–90.

26 Woods DL, Clayworth CC, Knight RT, Simpson GV, Naeser MA. Generators of middle- and long-latency auditory evoked potentials: implications from studies of patients with bitemporal lesions. *Electroencephalogr Clin Neurophysiol* 1987; **68**: 132–48.

27 Lovrich D, Novick B, Vaughan HG. Topographic analysis of auditory event-related potentials associated with acoustic and semantic processing. *Electroencephalogr Clin Neurophysiol* 1988; **71**: 40–54.

28 Woldorff M, Hansen JC, Hillyard SA. Evidence for effects of selective attention in the mid-latency range of the human auditory event-related potential. *Electroencephalogr Clin Neurophysiol* 1987; **40** (suppl): 146–54.

29 Schwender D, Klasing S, Madler C, Pöppel E, Peter K. Auditory evoked potentials to monitor intraoperative awareness. In: Schulte am Esch J, Kochs E (Eds), *Central nervous system monitoring in anesthesia and intensive care*. Berlin: Springer, 1994: 215–29.

30 Thornton C, Konieczko K, Jones JG, Jordan C, Dore CJ, Heneghan CPH. Effect of surgical stimulation on the auditory evoked response. *Br J Anaesth* 1988; **62**: 61–5.

31 Galambos R, Hecox K. Clinical applications of the brainstem auditory potentials. *Prog Clin Neurophysiol* 1972; **2**: 1–19.

32 Watanabe E, Schramm J, Strauss C. Neurophysiologic monitoring in posterior fossa surgery. II. BAEP-waves I and V and preservation of hearing. *Acta Neurochir (Wien)* 1989; **98**: 118–28.

33 Uhl RR, Squire KC, Bruce DL, Starr A. Effect of halothane anesthesia on the human cortical visual evoked response. *Anesthesiology* 1980; **53**: 273–6.

34 Sebel PS, Flynn PJ, Ingram DA. Effect of nitrous oxide on visual, auditory and somatosensory evoked potentials. *Br J Anaesth* 1984; **56**: 1403–7.

35 Russ W, Kling D, Loesevitz A, Hempelmann G. Effect of hypothermia on visual evoked potentials (VEP) in humans. *Anesthesiology* 1984; **61**: 207–10.

36 Langfitt TW, Weinstein JD, Kassell NF. Transmission of increased intracranial pressure. I. Within the craniospinal axis. *J Neurosurg* 1964; **21**: 989–97.

37 Langfitt TW, Weinstein JD, Kassell NF. Cerebral vasomotor paralysis produced by intracranial hypertension. *Neurology* 1965; **15**: 622–41.

38 Schweitzer JS, Bergsneider, Becker DP. Intracranial pressure monitoring. In: Cottrell JE, Smith DS (Eds), *Anesthesia and neurosurgery*, 3rd edn. Chicago: Mosby–Year Book Inc., 1994: 117–35.

39 Feldman Z, Narayan RK. Intracranial pressure monitoring: techniques and pitfalls. In: Cooper PR (Ed.), *Head injury*, 3rd edn. Baltimore, MA: Williams & Wilkins, 1993: 247–74.

39a Bendo AA, Hartung J, Kass IS, Cottrell JE. Neurophysiology and neuroanesthesia. In: Barash PG, Cullen BF, Stoelting RK (Eds), *Clinical anesthesia*, 2nd edn. Philadelphia: JP Lippincott Co, 1992:871–918.

40 Shapiro HM, Wyte SR, Harris AB, *et al.* Acute intraoperative intracranial hypertension in neurosurgical patients: mechanical and pharmacologic factors. *Anesthesiology* 1972; **37**: 399–405.

41 Aaslid R. *Transcranial Doppler sonography*. New York: Springer Verlag, 1986.
42 Bishop CCR, Powell S, Rutt D, Browse NL. Transcranial Doppler measurement of middle cerebral artery blood flow velocity: a validation study. *Stroke* 1986; **17**: 913–15.
43 Dahl A, Russell D, Nyberg-Hansen R, Rootwelt K. A comparison of regional cerebral blood flow and middle cerebral artery blood flow velocities: simultaneous measurements in healthy subjects. *J Cereb Blood Flow Metab* 1992; **12**: 1049–54.
44 Werner C, Hoffmann WE, Baughman VL, Albrecht RF, Schulte am Esch J. Effects of sufentanil on cerebral blood flow, cerebral blood flow velocity and metabolism in dogs. *Anesth Analg* 1991; **72**: 177–81.
45 Werner C, Hoffman WE, Kochs E, Albrecht RD, Schulte am Esch J. The effects of propofol on cerebral blood flow in correlation to cerebral blood flow velocity in dogs. *J Neurosurg Anesth* 1992; **4**: 41–6.
46 Kochs E, Hoffmann WE, Werner C, Albrecht RF, Schulte am Esch J. Cerebral blood flow velocity in relation to cerebral blood flow, cerebral metabolite rate for oxygen, and EEG during isoflurane anesthesia in dogs. *Anesth Analg* 1993; **76**: 1222–6.
47 Newell DW, Aaslid R, Lam A, Mayberg TS, Winn HR. Comparison of flow and velocity during dynamic autoregulation testing in humans. *Stroke* 1994; **25**: 793–7.
48 Barzó P, Dóczi T, Csete K, Buza Z, Bodosi M. Measurements of regional cerebral blood flow and blood flow velocity in experimental intracranial hypertension: Infusion via the cisterna magna in rabbits. *Neurosurgery* 1991; **28**: 821–5.
49 Nelson RJ, Perry S, Hames TK, Pickard JD. Transcranial Doppler ultrasound studies of cerebral autoregulation and subarachnoid hemorrhage in the rabbit. *J Neurosurg* 1990; **73**: 601–10.
50 Aaslid R, Lindegaard K-F, Sorteberg W, Nornes H. Cerebral autoregulation dynamics in humans. *Stroke* 1989; **20**: 45–52.
51 Aaslid R, Newell DW, Stooss R, Sorteberg W, Lindegaard K-F. Assessment of cerebral autoregulation dynamics from simultaneous arterial and venous transcranial Doppler recordings. *Stroke* 1991; **22**: 1148–54.
52 Chan K-H, Miller JD, Dearden NM, Andrews PJD, Midgley S. The effect of changes in cerebral perfusion pressure upon middle cerebral artery blood flow velocity and jugular bulb venous oxygen saturation after severe brain injury. *J Neurosurg* 1992; **77**: 55–61.
53 Werner C, Hoffmann WE, Kochs E, Albrecht RF, Schulte am Esch J. Transcranial Doppler sonography indicates critical brain perfusion during hemorrhagic hypotension in dogs. *Anesth Analg* 1992; **74**: S347.
54 Tranquart F, Berson M, Bodard S, Roncin A, Pourcelot L. Evaluation of cerebral blood flow in rabbits with transcranial Doppler sonography: first results. *Ultrasound Med Biol* 1991; **17**: 815–18.
54a Werner C. Transcranial Doppler sonography: monitoring of cerebral perfusion. In: Schulte am Esch J, Kochs E (Eds), *Central nervous system monitoring in anesthesia and intensive care*. Berlin: Springer-Verlag, 1994: 315–25.
55 Hassler W, Steinmetz H, Gawlowski J. Transcranial Doppler ultrasound in raised intracranial pressure and in intracranial circulatory arrest. *J Neurosurg* 1988; **68**: 745–51.
56 Hassler W, Steinmetz H, Pirschel J. Transcranial Doppler study of intracranial circulatory arrest. *J Neurosurg* 1989; **71**: 195–201.
57 Georgiadis D, Grosset DG, Kelman A, Faichney A, Lees KR. Prevalence and characteristics of intracranial microemboli signals in patients with different types of prosthetic cardiac valves. *Stroke* 1994; **25**: 587–92.
58 Grosset DG, Georgiadis D, Abdullah I, Bone I, Lees KR. Doppler emboli signals vary according to stroke subtype. *Stroke* 1994; **25**: 382–4.
59 Spencer MP, Thomas GI, Nicholls SC, Sauvage LR. Detection of middle cerebral artery emboli during carotid endarterectomy using transcranial Doppler ultrasonography. *Stroke* 1990; **21**: 415–23.
60 Bunegin L, Wahl D, Albin MS. Detection and volume estimation of embolic air in the middle cerebral artery using transcranial Doppler sonography. *Stroke* 1994; **25**: 593–600.
61 Markus H, Brown MM. Differentiation between different pathological cerebral embolic materials using transcranial Doppler in an in vitro model. *Stroke* 1993; **24**: 1–5.
62 Markus H, Loh A, Brown MM. Computerized detection of cerebral emboli and discrimination from artifact using Doppler ultrasound. *Stroke* 1993; **24**: 1667–72.

63 Pugsley W, Klinger L, Paschalis C, Treasure T, Harrison M, Newman S. The impact of microemboli during cardiopulmonary bypass on neuropsychological function. *Stroke* 1994; **25**: 1393–9.

64 Giller CA, Mathews D, Walker B. Prediction of tolerance to carotid artery occlusion using transcranial Doppler ultrasound. *J Neurosurg* 1994; **81**: 15–19.

65 Jørgensen LG, Schroeder TV. Transcranial Doppler for detection of cerebral ischemia during carotid endarterectomy. *Eur J Vasc Surg* 1992; **6**: 142–7.

66 Jansen C, Vriens EM, Eikelboom BC, Vermeulen FEE, van Gijn J, Ackerstaff RGA. Carotid endarterectomy with transcranial Doppler and electroencephalographic monitoring. *Stroke* 1993; **24**: 665–9.

67 Halsey JH, McDowell HA, Gelmon S, Morawetz RB. Blood flow velocity in the middle cerebral artery and regional cerebral blood flow during carotid endarterectomy. *Stroke* 1989; **20**: 53–8.

68 Chan K-H, Dearden NM, Miller JD, Midgley S, Piper IR. Transcranial waveform differences in hyperemic and nonhyperemic patients after severe head injury. *Surg Neurol* 1992; **38**: 433–6.

69 Grosset DG, Straiton J, McDonald I, Cockburn M, Bullock R. Use of Transcranial Doppler sonography to predict development of a delayed ischemic deficit after subarachnoid hemorrhage. *J Neurosurg* 1993; **78**: 183–7.

70 Laumer R, Steinmeier R, Gönner F, Vogtmann T, Priem R, Fahlbusch R. Cerebral hemodynamics in subarachnoid hemorrhage evaluated by transcranial Doppler sonography. Part 1. Reliability of flow velocities in clinical management. *Neurosurgery* 1993; **33**: 1–9.

71 Davis SM, Andrews JT, Lichtenstein M, Rossiter SC, Kaye AH, Hopper J. Correlations between cerebral arterial velocities, blood flow, and delayed ischemia after subarachnoid hemorrhage. *Stroke* 1992; **23**: 492–7.

72 Sander D, Klingelhöfer J. Cerebral vasospasm following posttraumatic subarachnoid hemorrhage evaluated by transcranial Doppler ultrasonography. *J Neurol Sci* 1993; **119**: 1–7.

73 Steiger H-K, Aaslid R, Stooss R, Seiler RW. Transcranial Doppler monitoring in head injury: relations between type of injury, flow velocities, vasoreactivity, and outcome. *Neurosurgery* 1994; **34**: 79–86.

74 Haberl RL, Heizer ML, Ellis EF. Laser Doppler assessment of brain microcirculation: effect of local alterations. *Am J Physiol* 1989; **256**: H1255–60.

75 Haberl RL, Heizer ML, Marmarou A, Ellis EF. Laser Doppler assessment of brain microcirculation: effect of systemic alterations. *Am J Physiol* 1989; **256**: H1247–54.

76 Lindsberg PJ, O'Neill JT, Paakkari IA, Hallenbeck JM, Feuerstein G. Validation of laser–Doppler flowmetry in measurement of spinal cord blood flow. *Am J Physiol* 1989; **257**: H674–80.

77 Bolognese P, Miller JI, Heger IM, Milhorat TH. Laser–Doppler flowmetry in neurosurgery. *J Neurosurg Anesth* 1993; **5**: 151–8.

78 Meyerson BA, Gunasekera L, Linderoth B, Gazelius B. Bedside monitoring of regional cortical blood flow in comatose patients using laser Doppler flowmetry. *Neurosurgery* 1991; **29**: 750–5.

79 Haberl RL, Villringer A, Dirnagl U. Applicability of Laser–Doppler flowmetry for cerebral blood flow monitoring in neurological intensive care. *Acta Neurochir* 1993; **59**(suppl): 64–8.

80 Rosenblum BR, Bonner RF, Oldfield EH. Intraoperative measurement of cortical blood flow adjacent to cerebral AVM using Laser Doppler velocimetry. *J Neurosurg* 1987; **66**: 396–9.

81 Fasano VA, Urciuoli R, Bolognese P, Mostert M. Intraoperative use of laser Doppler in the study of cerebral microvascular circulation. *Acta Neurochir (Wien)* 1988; **95**: 40–8.

82 Arbit E, DiResta GR, Bedford RF, Shah NK, Galicich JH. Intraoperative measurement of cerebral and tumor blood flow with laser–Doppler flowmetry. *Neurosurgery* 1989; **24**: 166–70.

83 Florence G, Seylaz J. Rapid autoregulation of cerebral blood flow: A laser–Doppler flowmetry study. *J Cereb Blood Flow Metab* 1992; **12**: 674–80.

84 Rosner MJ. Cerebral perfusion pressure: link between intracranial pressure and systemic circulation. In Wood JH (Ed.), *Cerebral blood flow*. New York: McGraw-Hill, 1987: 425–48.

179

85 Bouma GJ, Muizelaar JP, Bandoh K, Marmarou A. Blood pressure and intracranial pressure–volume dynamics in severe head injury: relationship with cerebral blood flow. *J Neurosurg* 1992; **77**: 15–19.

86 Andrews RJ, Bringas JR. A review of brain retraction and recommendations for minimizing intraoperative brain injury. *Neurosurgery* 1993; **33**: 1052–64.

87 Dirnagl U, Kaplan B, Jacewicz M, Pulsinelli W. Continuous measurement of cerebral cortical blood flow by laser–Doppler flowmetry in a rat stroke model. *J Cereb Blood Flow Metab* 1989; **9**: 589–96.

88 Wei D, Shea M, Saidel GM, Jones SC. Validation of continuous thermal measurement of cerebral blood flow by arterial pressure change. *J Cereb Blood Flow Metab* 1993; **13**: 693–701.

89 Voorhees WD, DeFord JA, Bleyer MW, Marchosky JA, Moran CJ. Continuous monitoring of cerebral perfusion by thermal clearance. *Neurol Res* 1993; **15**: 75–82.

90 Abe K, Demizu A, Yoshia I. Effect of prostaglandin E_1 induced hypotension on carbon dioxide reactivity and local cerebral blood flow after subarachnoid hemorrhage. *Br J Anaesth* 1992; **68**: 268–71.

91 Abe K, Iwanaga H, Shimada Y, Yoshiya I. The effect of nicardipine on blood flow velocity, local cerebral blood flow, and carbon dioxide reactivity during cerebral aneurysm surgery. *Anesth Analg* 1993; **76**: 1227–33.

92 McCormick PW, Stewart M, Goetting MG, Dujovny M, Lewis G, Ausman JI. Noninvasive cerebral optical spectroscopy for monitoring cerebral oxygen delivery and hemodynamics. *Crit Care Med* 1991; **19**: 89–97.

93 Bucher H-U, Edwards AD, Lipp AE, Duc G. Comparison between near infrared spectroscopy and [133]Xenon clearance for estimation of cerebral blood flow in critically ill preterm infants. *Pediatr Res* 1993; **33**: 56–60.

94 Matta BF, Lam AM, Mayberg TS, Shapira Y, Winn RH. A critique of the intraoperative use of jugular venous bulb catheters during neurosurgical procedures. *Anesth Analg* 1994; **79**: 745–50.

95 Dearden NM. Jugular bulb venous oxygen saturation in the management of severe head injury. *Curr Opinion Anaesth* 1991; **4**: 279–86.

96 Stocchetti N, Paparella A, Bridelli F, Bacchi M, Piazza P, Zuccoli P. Cerebral venous oxygen saturation studied using bilateral samples in the jugular veins. *Neurosurgery* 1994; **34**: 38–44.

97 Andrews PJD, Dearden NM, Miller JD. Jugular bulb cannulation: description of a cannulation technique and validation of a new continuous monitor. *Br J Anaesth* 1991; **67**: 553–8.

98 Robertson C, Narayan RK, Gokaslan ZL, *et al.* Cerebral arteriovenous oxygen difference as an estimate of cerebral blood flow in comatose patients. *J Neurosurg* 1989; **70**: 222–30.

99 Meyer JS, Gotoh F, Ebihara S, Tomita M. Effects of anoxia on cerebral metabolism and electrolytes in man. *Neurology* 1965; **115**: 892–901.

100 Lennox WG, Gibbs FA, Gibbs EL. Relationship of unconsciousness to cerebral blood flow and to anoxemia. *Arch Neurol Psychol* 1935; **34**: 1001–13.

101 Cruz J. On-line monitoring of global cerebral hypoxia in acute brain injury: Relationship to intracranial hypertension. *J Neurosurg* 1993; **79**: 228–33.

102 Sheinberg M, Kanter MJ, Robertson CS, Contant CF, Narayan RK, Grossman RG. Continuous monitoring of jugular venous oxygen saturation in head-injured patients. *J Neurosurg* 1992; **76**: 212–17.

103 Lyons C, Clark LC, McDowell H. Cerebral venous oxygen content during carotid thrombintimectomy. *Ann Surg* 1964; **160**: 561–7.

104 Muizelaar JP, Marmarou A, Ward JD, *et al.* Adverse effects of prolonged hyperventilation in patients with severe head injury: a randomized clinical trial. *J Neurosurg* 1991; **75**: 731–9.

105 Cruz J. Combined continuous monitoring of systemic and cerebral oxygenation in acute brain injury: Preliminary observations. *Crit Care Med* 1993; **21**: 1225–32.

106 Paulson OB, Strandgaard S, Edvinsson L. Cerebral autoregulation. *Cerebrovasc Brain Metab Rev* 1990; **2**: 161–91.

107 McCormick PW, Stewart M, Goetting MG, Balakrishnan G. Regional cerebrovascular oxygen saturation measured by optical spectroscopy in humans. *Stroke* 1991; **22**: 596–602.

108 Germon TJ, Kane NM, Manara AR, Nelson RJ. Near-infrared spectroscopy in adults:

effects of extracranial ischaemia and intracranial hypoxia on estimation of cerebral oxygenation. *Br J Anaesth* 1994; **73**: 503–6.

109 Pollard V, DeMelo E, Deyo DJ, Stoddard H, Hoffmann DJ, Prough DS. Generation and validation of an algorithm for brain oxygen monitoring. *Anesth Analg* 1994; **78**: S343.

110 Maas AIR, Fleckenstein W, de Jong DA, van Santbrink H. Monitoring cerebral oxygenation: experimental studies and preliminary clinical results of continuous monitoring of cerebrospinal fluid and brain tissue oxygen tension. *Acta Neurochir* 1993; **59**: 50–7.

111 Meixensberger J, Dings J, Roosen K. Studies of tissue PO_2 in normal and pathological human brain cortex. *Acta Neurochir* 1993; **59**: 58–63.

112 Illievich UM, Zornow MH, Choi KT, Strnat MAP, Scheller MS. Effects of hypothermia or anesthetics on hippocampal glutamate and glycine concentrations after repeated transient global cerebral ischemia. *Anesthesiology* 1994; **80**: 177–86.

113 Persson L, Hillered L. Chemical monitoring of neurosurgical intensive care patients using intracerebral microdialysis. *J Neurosurg* 1992; **76**: 72–80.

114 Landolt H, Langemann H, Gratzl O. On-line monitoring of cerebral pH by microdialysis. *Neurosurgery* 1993; **32**: 1000–4.

7: Intraoperative and postoperative positioning of the neurosurgical patient

P RAVUSSIN, OHG WILDER-SMITH

The position of a neurosurgical patient has important repercussions on intracranial haemodynamics and homoeostasis. In the postoperative phase, patient position can be freely determined by therapeutic considerations. Such intraoperative therapeutic considerations are, however, frequently in conflict with the positioning necessary for neurosurgery. Although optimisation of the intracranial environment is obviously important for surgical outcome, equally good positioning for surgical access plays a role because of the resultant shorter operating times, the less invasive site access, and reduction of traumatic brain retraction. It is thus clear that the resolution of such opposing interests must be based on a good understanding of the basic physiological principles involved so as to achieve the best possible compromise for the patient.

Theoretical considerations

The position of a neurosurgical patient can be changed either by sitting him or her up or by rotating or flexing/extending the head on the neck. Both types of position change can have marked effects on the intracranial environment. Before describing these effects in detail, it should be emphasised that the results of position change are strongly influenced by the state of intracranial and extracranial circulation, and homoeostasis, *before* the position change. This means, for example, that sitting a hypovolaemic patient up will have effects other than those seen in someone who is normovolaemic. As another example, rotating the head of a young patient without vascular disease will have a very different result from that for a geriatric patient with advanced atherosclerosis and severe carotid stenosis. These differences must be kept in mind when interpreting or comparing the literature in this field. Another problem with the published studies is that most have studied severely head injured patients, so the results are not necessarily directly applicable to other neurosurgical patients.

All the alterations in intracranial environment resulting from change of position can be ascribed to the effects on two main intracranial systems: the circulation of blood and the circulation of cerebrospinal fluid (CSF). These changes result, in turn, from many interacting factors, both intracranial and extracranial; the changes produce the following four major effects:

1 Cerebrospinal fluid transfer
2 Changes in venous drainage
3 Alterations in cerebral arterial perfusion pressure
4 Alterations in cerebral blood flow (CBF).

Cerebrospinal fluid transfer

When a patient is raised to the upright position, there is normally a transfer of CSF from the cerebral to the spinal compartment as a result of gravity,[1] thus reducing intracranial pressure (ICP). Obviously this transfer is only possible in the presence of unimpeded CSF circulation, so that patients with conditions such as transforaminal herniation, cervico-occipital malformations, or adhesions in the CSF channels will not undergo such transfer. Compensatory transfer of CSF from the cerebral to the spinal compartment is physiological with fluctuations in ICP. Thus much less or even no CSF is available for transfer in patients who have intracranial hypertension in the sitting position, which potentially reduces the impact of this manoeuvre on ICP. On the other hand, many patients with intracranial hypertension will undergo significant reductions of pressure with only small reductions of intracerebral CSF volume as a result of the significantly decreased compliance of their intracranial contents.

Venous drainage changes

The venous bed provides the largest single contribution to intracranial compliance,[2] and represents the final outflow pressure for both the CSF and the cerebrovascular systems.[3] Any improvement of venous drainage accompanying the raising of the head is directly communicated to the intracranial space by the valveless internal jugular veins, aided by the external jugular veins and the vertebral venous plexus,[4] resulting in decreased intracerebral venous pressure and blood volume.[5] Again the intra–extracranial volume shift is a physiological buffering mechanism, which may already be largely exhausted in patients with intracranial hypertension. As for CSF, however, the decreased cerebral compliance in such patients will cause small volume changes to be accompanied by larger pressure alterations.

The effect of venous drainage on ICP is almost immediately demonstrated by the rise of ICP with jugular venous compression, which lasts as long as the compression.[6] Compression of the right jugular vein in the conscious or anaesthetised child raises superior longitudinal venous sinus pressure by 5 mm Hg and bilateral compression by 10 mm Hg, independent of the position.[7] Hyperextension of the head, for example, significantly diminishes internal jugular vein diameter,[8] providing an easily forgotten cause of raised ICP. In spite of the effect on ICP just described, jugular compression in the absence of intracranial pathology alter neither CBF nor oxygen consumption.[9]

The application of a positive end expiratory pressure (PEEP) during ventilation will affect venous drainage by raising intrathoracic pressures. The ultimate impact of PEEP on ICP will depend not only on pulmonary (and thoracic) compliance but also on intracerebral pressure–volume relationships, as well as the patient's position.[10] The impact of PEEP on ICP is maximal in the presence of reduced intracerebral and normal pulmonary compliance.[10] It has been shown that elevating the head by 30° can limit the rise in ICP as a result of PEEP ventilation.[11]

Cerebral arterial perfusion pressure and blood flow

Raising the thorax above the haemodynamic neutral position will have effects on cardiac output by altering both the preload and afterload of the heart. Anaesthetised patients are particularly prone to relative hypovolaemia as a result of their impaired vasomotor tonus. Hence, in anaesthetised patients, the sitting position is frequently associated with reduced venous return to the right heart (reduced preload), making possible substantial falls in blood pressure and cardiac output. In addition, the head is well above the heart in the sitting position, not only increasing the afterload for flow in this direction, but also decreasing perfusion pressure caused by hydrostatic column effects. Thus the sitting position will be associated with reductions in both cerebral arterial perfusion pressure and CBF, which are generally considered deleterious in neurosurgical patients.

Even a normal subject who is rapidly sat up will undergo momentary reduction of CBF of up to 80% before systemic and cerebral autoregulation returns it to normal.[12] It must be kept in mind that these autoregulatory mechanisms, both systemic and cerebral, are strongly depressed by anaesthesia as well as by some intracranial pathologies. The intolerance to the sitting position in anaesthesia of patients with vertebrobasilar vascular insufficiency is notorious. The ultimate effects of these reductions in CBF and perfusion pressure depend sensitively upon the actual state of intracranial homoeostasis, particularly of the autoregulatory mechanisms.

Perfusion of the brain can also be impaired by the effects of head positioning on the arterial vessels entering the skull, namely the two internal carotid arteries and the two vertebral arteries fusing to form the basilar trunk. These two systems are normally anastomosed via the circle of Willis to permit collateral circulation if one or more of these arteries become blocked off. On rotating the head to one side by 60°, there is a major reduction in the contralateral vertebral artery flow, with a complete stop occurring at about 80°.[12] If both vertebral arteries are intact this poses no problem. If the patient, however, has a congenitally single vertebral artery, or if one is obstructed, serious reductions in vertebrobasilar flow may result. In the healthy subject, the internal carotid arteries are mobile and flow does not alter with head movement. Should the carotids be adherent to adjacent soft tissues, or in a case of bony abnormalities of, for example, the cervical ribs, head movement may be associated with marked reductions in carotid flow. Again, the impact of these reductions depends not only on how intact the circle of Willis is,[12] but also on the state of intracranial autoregulatory mechanisms.

Practical aspects

The optimal position for neurosurgical patients has continued to be the subject of controversy since Kenning and coauthors described marked diminution of ICP with the semisitting (45°) or sitting (90°) position in neurological patients who had actual or potential intracranial hypertension.[3] Since this time, various groups have advocated either a semisitting position (mostly 30°) for patients with raised ICP,[3 13 14] a flat position (0°) for such patients,[5] or individual titration of the position, taking into account monitoring results for ICP, cerebral perfusion pressure (CPP), and CBF.[15–18]

What factors must be taken into account in deciding the benefit of modification of head position in the neurosurgical patient? All therapy for the neurosurgical patient must aim to maintain adequate supplies of nutrients to the brain cells. To ensure this, not only global but also regional CBF must be maintained. This is the ultimate goal of therapy in neurosurgical patients, and its attainment clearly depends on the quality and detail of information on brain blood supply which monitoring provides.[19]

In the normal brain, CBF is normally held constant by autoregulation between CPP of about 50 and 120 mm Hg, whereas, in the severely traumatised brain, no autoregulation at all may be present, leading to a linear relationship between flow and perfusion pressure. Using the formula:

$$CPP = MAP - ICP$$

it is clear that although increases in ICP will decrease CPP, decreases in mean arterial pressure (MAP) will equally reduce CPP. Thus any assessment of the *global* effects of posture must include, as a minimum, changes of *both* ICP and arterial pressure. As Gaab's group has pointed out,[20] care must be taken with the assumption that peripheral arterial pressures referenced to the skull accurately reflect actual intracranial or even internal carotid arterial pressures.

Another important factor to be taken into account is the finding by

185

Rosner's group[15] that CPPs of, on average, less than 70–80 mm Hg can be associated with reflex, vasodilatory increases of ICP via "plateau" or "B" waves (the so called vasodilatory cascade). In some patients this inferior limit may be as high as 90–100 mm Hg. Put differently, in many patients increased CPP has a vasconstricting effect, reducing cerebral blood volume and thus ICP (the "vasoconstrictive cascade"), a finding that has been confirmed by other groups.[21–23] Indeed, it is increasingly clear that neurosurgical patients, particularly if head injured, are particularly sensitive to falls in CPP (figs 7.1 and 7.2), with the ultimate relationship between perfusion pressure and ICP depending on whether or not autoregulation is intact. In a recent study, Bouma and coauthors[21] demonstrated that, with intact autoregulation, ICP in severely head injured patients rose steeply with falls in blood pressure, although remaining stable with blood pressure increases. In the absence of intact autoregulation, ICP varied directly with blood pressure. Thus falls in blood pressure and CPP should be avoided in head injured patients, even with high basal values.[21]

The effects of position change on *global* CBF can either be measured directly, for example, using the Kety–Schmidt N_2O technique,[24] or estimated using transcranial Doppler flow velocity measurement[25 26] or other indirect methods such as arteriojugular venous oxygen extraction.[27 28] Chan and coauthors[19 23] have demonstrated that, if the cerebral metabolic rate remains unchanged, a stable CBF, as measured by transcranial Doppler, is accompanied by a stable Sjo_2, and that these two parameters remain stable at CPPs above 70 mm Hg (figs 7.1 and 7.2).

Although these methods of assessing global intracranial change are now

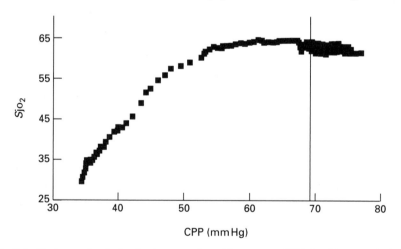

Fig 7.1 Methoxamine bolus for hypotension: Sjo_2 versus CPP. In this severely head injured patient, there is a critical CPP at 69 mm Hg, under which Sjo_2 starts to decline. (With kind permission of Andrews PJD, Wang FC, Miller JD, unpublished data)

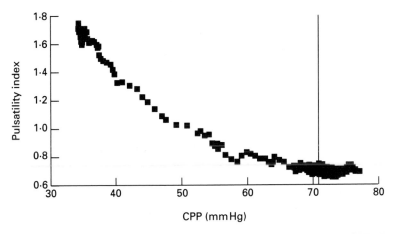

Fig 7.2 Methoxamine bolus for hypotension: pulsatility index versus CPP. In the same patient, the critical CPP under which the pulsatility index starts to rise is set at 71 mm Hg. (With kind permission of Andrews PJD, Wang FC, Miller JD, unpublished data)

well established, methods of assessing regional changes, for example, by transcranial laser Doppler[25] or near infrared transcranial and transcutaneous spectroscopy,[29] are still in their infancy and awaiting full validation. The effects on regional CBF of body position changes have not been systematically studied to date.[30]

What effect, then, do changes in body and head position actually have in clinical practice? Table 7.1 summarises the results of the most important recent studies on this subject. Most of the studies found relatively large interindividual variability in their results, making prediction of the effects of position change in the individual case difficult. In general, moderate head elevation (up to about 30°) decreases ICP, with the effects on CPP being variable. Patients with low initial perfusion pressures are particularly vulnerable to further decreases in CPP. Further increases in head up position not only further decrease CPP but are associated with the tendency to raised ICP. The only study to measure CBF[13] found little effect on flows of 30° head elevation, with the cerebral metabolic rate for oxygen (CMR_{O_2}) and the arteriovenous lactate extraction also being little affected. The study of Yoshida et al[16] also studied the effects of head tilt ("chin on chest") and head extension ("sniffing position"). Both manoeuvres had clear effects in addition to body position, with head tilt increasing ICP and decreasing CPP, whereas head extension decreased ICP and increased CPP.

Other problems specific to the sitting position

As already discussed, sitting a patient up can result in marked haemodynamic changes, caused mainly by relative hypovolaemia and reduced venous

Table 7.1 Studies of the effects of the sitting position on intracranial environment

Study	Positions tested	ICP	CPP	CBF	Others
Feldman[13]	0°, 30°	↓ (all)	⇔	⇔	$CMRo_2$: ⇔; av$D$lac: ⇔
Kenning[3]	0°, 45°, 90°	↓ (all)	NT	NT	NT
Durward[14]	0°, 15°, 30°, 60°	↓ (15°, 30°); ↑ (60°)	⇔ (15°, 30°), ↓ (60°)	NT	NT
Rosner[5]	0°, 10°, 20°, 30°, 40°, 50°	↓ (10° = 1 mm Hg)	↓ (10° = 2–3 mm Hg)	NT	NT
Ropper[18]	0°, 60°	Variable (mainly ↓)	NT	NT	Intracranial compliance: variable
Yoshida[16]	0°, 15°, 30°, 45°	↓ (all)	Variable	NT	Chin: ICP ↑ CPP ↓ ; sniff: ICP ↓ CPP ↑
Davenport[17]	0°, 20°, 40°, 60°	↓ (0, 20°); ↑ (40°, 60°)	↓ (>20°)	NT	Note hepatic coma patients

ICP = intracranial pressure; CPP = cerebral perfusion pressure; CBF = cerebral blood flow; $CMRo_2$ = cerebral metabolic rate for oxygen; av$D$lac = arteriovenous difference for lactate; ↓ = reduced; ↑ = increased; ⇔ = unchanged; NT = not tested; chin = chin on chest position; sniff = sniffing position.

188

return to the heart in patients with cardiovascular tonus and reflexes depressed by anaesthesia. These changes can usually be reduced by attention to adequate volume loading of the patient before position change, although sometimes tonus may need to be supported pharmacologically. The sitting position can also be made less haemodynamically aggressive by measures such as flexing the knees and hips, thus raising the legs, appropriate padding to avoid obstruction of venous return, and bandaging of the extremities or the use of a **G** suit, again to improve venous return. Obviously, the patient should only be sat as upright as absolutely necessary.

Postoperative tetraplegia is another risk associated with the sitting position and extreme flexion of the head on the chest.[31] One reason for this is the aforementioned problem of hypotension and reduced perfusion pressure impinging on a watershed region of truncal and spinal perfusion, particularly in the context of impaired autoregulation. Another factor is the possibility of stretching and even tearing of the cervicomedullary vessels as a result of extreme flexion of the neck. A minimum gap of 3–4 cm between chin and chest should be insisted upon during positioning to prevent this complication, as well as careful attention to the preservation of an adequate perfusion pressure throughout the operation.

Another problem specific to the sitting position is the possibility of venous gas embolisation. This is the result of subatmospheric pressures in the venous system of the head once it is above the level of the heart (at a thoracic angle of about 25°). Thus, if veins, particularly those unable to collapse (for example, if fixed to bone), are opened by the surgeon, air will be sucked into them, causing gas embolism. These emboli descend to the heart where even relatively small volumes of air can have significant haemodynamic consequences. If air emboli reach the arterial circulation the results are even more serious, because they then cause infarctions in vital organs such as the brain or heart. The presence of 0·05 ml air in a coronary artery is enough to cause irreversible damage to the myocardium. The complication of systemic embolisation usually occurs because the foramen ovale is anatomically or functionally patent (present in about 25–35% of the population). As arterial air embolism is such a potentially serious complication, all patients scheduled for surgery in the upright position must be screened for an anatomically or functionally patent foramen by echocardiography. If the foramen ovale is patent, surgery should *not* be performed in the sitting position. This attitude is necessary because the suggested anaesthetic prophylaxes against air embolism (raised central venous pressure, PEEP) are not only problematic but most probably ineffective. Clearly it is unrealistic, even in the most stable haemodynamic conditions, to expect 100% avoidance of air embolism.

Thus anaesthetic management of air embolism must be directed towards its detection and treatment, which require close cooperation with the neurosurgeon, who should immediately inform the anaesthetist of any suspected air embolism. The most effective monitoring for air embolism is via Doppler ultrasonography of the heart, echocardiography, and/or by monitoring of the end expiratory carbon dioxide or nitrogen concentration. Once air embolism has occurred it must be treated immediately by aspiration through a large bore central venous catheter with many openings. Such a catheter *should* be placed prophylactically before starting the operation, and its tip radiologically verified as being in the right atrium, 2 cm distal to the junction of the superior vena cava and right auricular cavity, for all interventions in the sitting position.[32] Aspiration continues until no further air is aspirated. To prevent further air emboli, the operative field should be flooded with water, if possible, and the jugular veins compressed until the venous leak is identified and controlled. Should embolisation continue or haemodynamic instability ensue, consideration should be given to lying the patient flat or even slightly head down.

Conclusions

The main therapeutic goal in neurosurgical patients is the maintenance of blood supplies in the brain. Clearly, therapy directed only—or even primarily—at the ICP is inadequate to this end. Such therapy must be based, as a minimum, on knowledge of CPPs and, preferably, blood flows, with additional information such as cerebral metabolic rates, arteriojugular venous oxygen extraction, and *regional* (as opposed to global) cerebral behaviour being most valuable. At present, the maintenance of a CPP of above at least 70 mm Hg must be considered a minimum goal (see figs 7.1 and 7.2).

With regard to the effects of body position on the intracranial environment, the studies discussed demonstrate a large intraindividual variability in responses, particularly of CPPs or blood flows. Hypovolaemic patients, or those with low initial CPPs, are particularly vulnerable to undesirable effects. Thus individual titration of body position in neurosurgical patients is recommended according to the results of monitoring CBF (for example, transcranial Doppler), CPP, ICP, and cerebral metabolism (for example, jugular bulb oximetry). In general, head up positions of up to 20–30° may result in useful reductions of ICP without major reductions in CPP or blood flow, *provided* hypovolaemia is avoided, by either fluid loading or catecholamine support, and perfusion pressure maintained above 70 mm Hg. The head should be extended on the neck ("sniffing position"). Sitting the patient up further, flexing the head on the neck ("chin on chest"), or extreme rotation of the head on the neck is likely to lower CPP while possibly increasing ICP; these positions should be avoided.

1 Magnaes B. Body position and cerebrospinal fluid pressure. Part 1: Clinical studies of the effect of rapid postural changes. *J Neurosurg* 1976; **44**: 687–97.
2 Marmarou A, Shulman K, LaMorgese J. Compartmental analysis of compliance and outflow resistance of the cerebrospinal fluid system. *J Neurosurg* 1975; **43**: 523–34.

3 Kenning JA, Toutant SM, Saunders RL. Upright patient positioning in the management of intracranial hypertension. *Surg Neurol* 1981; **15**: 148–52.

4 Patterson JL. Circulation through the brain. In: Ruch TC, Patton HD (Eds), *Physiology and biophysics*. Philadelphia: Saunders, 1965: 1242–50.

5 Rosner MJ, Coley IB. Cerebral perfusion pressure, intracranial pressure, and head elevation. *J Neurosurg* 1986; **65**: 636–41.

6 Potts DG, Deonarine V. Effect of positional changes and jugular vein compression on the pressure gradient across the arachnoid villi and granulations of the dog. *Neurosurgery* 1973; **38**: 722–8.

7 Grady MS, Bedford RF, Park TS. Changes in superior sagittal sinus pressure in children with head elevation, jugular venous compression, and PEEP. *J Neurosurg* 1986; **65**: 199–202.

8 Armstrong PJ, Sutherland R, Scott DHT. The effect of position and different manoeuvres on internal jugular vein size. *Acta Anaesthesiol Scand* 1994; **38**: 229–31.

9 Tuoung TJK, Miyabe M, McShane AJ, Rogers MC, Traystman RJ. Effect of PEEP and jugular venous compression on canine blood flow and oxygen consumption in the head elevated position. *Anesthesiology* 1988; **68**: 53–8.

10 Burchiel KJ, Steege TD, Wyler AR. Intracranial pressure changes in brain injured patients requiring PEEP ventilation. *Neurosurgery* 1981; **8**: 443–9.

11 Lodrini S, Montolivo M, Pluchino F, Borroni V. Positive end-expiratory pressure in supine and sitting positions: its effects on intrathoracic and intracranial pressures. *Neurosurgery* 1989; **24**: 873–7.

12 Toole JF. Effects of change of head, limb and body position on cephalic circulation. *N Engl J Med* 1968; **279**; 307–11.

13 Feldman Z, Kanter MJ, Robertson CS, et al. Effect of head elevation on intracranial pressure, cerebral perfusion pressure, and cerebral blood flow in head-injured patients. *J Neurosurg* 1992; **76**: 207–11.

14 Durward QJ, Amacher AL, Del Maestro RF, Sibbald WJ. Cerebral and· cardiovascular responses to changes in head elevation in patients with intracranial hypertension. *J Neurosurg* 1983; **59**: 938–44.

15 Rosner MJ, Daughton S. Cerebral perfusion pressure management in head injury. *J Trauma* 1990; **30**: 933–41.

16 Yoshida A, Shima T, Okada Y, Yamada Y, Kurino H. Effects of postural changes on epidural pressure and cerebral perfusion pressure in patients with serious intracranial lesions. In: Avezaat CJJ, van Eijndhoven JHM, Maas AIR, Tans JTJ (Eds), *Intracranial pressure VIII*. Heidelberg: Springer, 1993: 433–6.

17 Davenport A, Will EJ, Davison AM. Effect of posture on intracranial pressure and cerebral perfusion pressure in patients with fulminant hepatic and renal failure after acetaminophen self-poisoning. *Crit Care Med* 1990; **18**: 286–9.

18 Ropper AH, O'Rourke D, Kennedy SK. Head position, intracranial pressure, and compliance. *Neurology* 1982; **32**: 1288–91.

19 Chan KHM Miller JD, Dearden NM, Andrews PJD, Midgley S. The effect of changes in cerebral perfusion pressure upon middle cerebral artery blood flow velocity and jugular venous oxygen saturation after severe brain injury. *J Neurosurg* 1992; **77**; 55–61.

20 Woischneck D, Gaab MR, Rickels E, Heissler HE, Trost A. Correct measurement of cerebral perfusion pressure. In: Hoff JT, Betz AL (Eds), *Intracranial pressure VII*. Heidelberg: Springer, 1989: 850–2.

21 Bouma GJ, Muizellar JP, Bandoh K, Marmarou A. Blood pressure and intracranial pressure–volume dynamics in severe head injury: relationship with cerebral blood flow. *J Neurosurg* 1992; **77**: 15–19.

22 Shrader H, Lofgren J, Zwetnow NM. Influence of blood pressure on tolerance to an intracranial expanding mass. *Acta Neurol Scand* 1985; **71**: 114–26.

23 Chan KH, Dearden NM, Miller JD, Andrew PJD, Midgley S. Multimodality monitoring as a guide to treatment of intracranial hypertension after severe head injury. *Neurosurgery* 1993; **32**: 547–53.

24 Kety SS, Schmidt CF. The determination of cerebral blood flow in man by the use of nitrous oxide in low concentrations. *Am J Physiol* 1945; **143**: 55–66.

25 Pickard JD, Czosnyka M. Management of raised intracranial pressure. *J Neurol Neurosurg Psychiatry* 1993; **56**: 845–58.

26 Aaslid R, Markwalder TM, Nomes H. Non-invasive transcranial Doppler ultrasound recording of flow velocity in basal cerebral arteries. *J Neurosurg* 1982; 57; 769–74.
27 Robertson CS, Narayan RK, Gokaslan ZL, *et al*. Cerebral arteriovenous oxygen difference as an estimate of cerebral blood flow in comatose patients. *J Neurosurg* 1989; 70: 222–30.
28 Miller JD. Head injury. *J Neurol Neurosurg Psychiatry* 1993; 56: 440–7.
29 Wyatt JS, Cope M, Delpy DT, Wray S, Reynolds EOR. Quantification of cerebral oxygenation and haemodynamics in sick newborn infants by near infrared spectroscopy. *Lancet* 1986; ii; 1063–6.
30 McCormick PW, Stewart M, Goetting MG, Dujovny M, Lewis G, Ausman J. Noninvasive cerebral optical spectroscopy for monitoring cerebral oxygen delivery and hemodynamics. *Crit Care Med* 1991; 19: 89–97.
31 Wilder BL. Hypothesis: The etiology of midcervical quadriplegia after operation with the patient in the sitting position. *Neurosurgery* 1982; 4; 530–1.
32 Bunegin L, Albin MS, Helsel PE, Hoffman A, Hung TK. Positioning the right atrial catheter: a model for reappraisal. *Anesthesiology* 1981; 55: 343–8.

8: Anaesthetic management of cerebral aneurysms and arteriovenous malformations

J ADAM LAW, ADRIAN W GELB

Cerebral aneurysms

Subarachnoid haemorrhage is responsible for 10% of all strokes and rupture of a cerebral aneurysm is the most common cause of subarachnoid haemorrhage. The prevalence of unruptured cerebral aneurysms in the general population is estimated to be 4000 per 100 000,[1] although the annual incidence of subarachnoid haemorrhage from ruptured aneurysms is fortunately much less at 11 per 100 000.[2] The incidence varies somewhat according to country and racial group.[3] The peak age for rupture is 40–60 years with the ratio of women:men being 3:2.[4]

Morbidity and mortality from subarachnoid haemorrhage are high. Of the annual 30 000 new cases in North America, 12 000 will die or become severely disabled before receiving any treatment. Of the remaining 18 000, half experience good functional recovery whereas the other 9000 die or become disabled, 3000 from vasospasm, 3000 from rebleeding, 1000 from medical complications, and 2000 from surgical complications.[5]

Clinical presentation

Cerebral aneurysms most frequently present with subarachnoid haemorrhage but they may also be discovered before rupturing either as an incidental finding or as a consequence of causing increased intracranial pressure. Up to 50% of people will experience a small "warning" bleed, with symptoms ranging from malaise to severe headache with nuchal rigidity. As such it is easily misdiagnosed, accounting for the large percentage dying or becoming severely disabled before presentation.

At the time of aneurysm rupture, intracranial pressure (ICP) increases markedly and may equal systemic blood pressure. If bleeding continues, death from brain stem herniation rapidly ensues. If bleeding stops, the passage of blood through the subarachnoid space may reduce ICP but results in meningeal irritation. This, and the elevated ICP, cause the typical

193

Table 8.1   Modified Hunt and Hess classification of subarachnoid haemorrhage

Grade	Criteria	Perioperative mortality rate (%)
0	Unruptured aneurysm	0–5
I	Asymptomatic or minimal headache and slight nuchal rigidity	0–5
II	Moderate to severe headache, nuchal rigidity, no neurological deficit other than cranial nerve palsy	2–10
III	Drowsiness, confusion, or mild focal deficit	10–15
IV	Stupor, moderate to severe hemiparesis, possibly early decerebrate rigidity, vegetative disturbance	60–70
V	Deep coma, decerebrate rigidity, moribund appearance	70–100

symptoms of subarachnoid haemorrhage: loss of consciousness, severe global headache, nuchal rigidity, photophobia, and fever.

Intracranial pressure may remain somewhat elevated for weeks following subarachnoid haemorrhage and may be associated with reduced cerebral blood flow (CBF), loss of CBF–carbon dioxide reactivity and autoregulation, with these effects being more pronounced in higher grade patients.[6][7]

The severity of subarachnoid haemorrhage can be graded according to one of several available classifications. That of Botterell *et al*, described in 1956[8] was modified by Hunt and Hess in 1968[9] with another subsequent revision which added a grade 0, asymptomatic category (table 8.1). The classification has important prognostic significance in terms of perioperative mortality rates, with most agreeing that grades 0 and 1 patients should have a perioperative mortality rate of less than 5% whereas grade 5 patients will generally not survive. Another classification system, based on the Glasgow coma scale, has been proposed by the World Federation of Neurologic Surgeons (WFNS) (table 8.2).[10]

Table 8.2   WFNS grading scale

WFNS grade	GCS score	Motor deficit
I	15	Absent
II	13–14	Absent
III	13–14	Present
IV	7–12	Present or absent
V	3–6	Present or absent

WFNS, World Federation of Neurologic Surgeons.
GCS, Glasgow coma scale.

Laboratory studies to confirm a clinical suspicion of subarachnoid haemorrhage include lumbar puncture, computed tomography, and angiography. Lumbar puncture with the typical xanthochromic appearance of the centrifuged supernatant cerebrospinal fluid (CSF) can confirm subarachnoid haemorrhage. Computed tomography may provide information about the location of the bleeding and can identify aneurysms greater than 1 cm in diameter. It also yields prognostic information because there is a relationship between the amount of blood in the subarachnoid space and the risk of developing vasospasm. Angiography of the cerebral and vertebral vessels is then performed to confirm the exact cause of the bleeding and the location of the aneurysm.

Preoperative considerations

The preoperative goals are twofold: to recognise and treat systemic effects occurring as a consequence of the subarachnoid haemorrhage which could jeopardise the brain's recovery, and to prevent or treat two of the more dreaded complications—vasospasm and rebleeding.

Systemic effects of subarachnoid haemorrhage

Hypertension—Hypertension is common with acute subarachnoid haemorrhage, possibly reflecting a state of autonomic hyperactivity. It is of significance because it can increase the transmural pressure across the wall of the aneurysm, thus increasing the possibility of rebleeding. The transmural pressure is the difference between the pressure in the aneurysm and the local ICP. The pressure in the aneurysm has been shown to be equal to systemic mean arterial pressure (MAP).[11] Thus any cause of hypertension increases the risk of rupture. On the other hand, these patients are also at risk for cerebral ischaemia. Recalling that cerebral perfusion pressure (CPP) is the difference between MAP and ICP, in a patient with acutely increased ICP as a result of subarachnoid haemorrhage, too low a blood pressure could compromise CPP. This problem may be compounded by the presence of vasospasm or an impairment of cerebral autoregulation. As an empirical compromise, many neurosurgeons favour keeping the systolic blood pressure between 120 and 150 mm Hg before the operation.

Electrocardiogram changes—The automatic hyperactivity at the time of subarachnoid haemorrhage may also account for the frequent occurrence of electrocardiogram (ECG) abnormalities.[12] ECG changes are present in 50–80% of patients and include ST, T, and P wave changes, the presence of U waves, ST interval prolongation, and various dysrhythmias.[13 14] Usually these ECG changes are not indicative of underlying myocardial disease, although some pathological studies have demonstrated microscopic focal changes in the myocardium.

195

Patients with these ECG changes do not experience any increased morbidity or mortality from cardiac causes. ECG studies have failed to show a correlation between myocardial dysfunction and ECG changes in the subarachnoid haemorrhage patient, showing instead a correlation between myocardial dysfunction and the severity of the subarachnoid haemorrhage.[15]

Intravascular blood volume changes—Other haemodynamic changes associated with subarachnoid haemorrhage include plasma volume contraction[16] and contraction of the red cell mass, which may also be the result of the generalised vasoconstriction accompanying the autonomic hyperactivity. These changes appear to be most marked in patients who subsequently develop symptomatic vasospasm, and may be considered as a marker. Other causes of the decreased circulating blood volume include supine diuresis, phlebotomy, and diuresis induced by angiographic dye. Intravascular volume re-expansion should occur before induction of anaesthesia to avoid an exaggerated hypotensive response to anaesthetic agents. Central venous pressure or pulmonary artery occlusion pressure monitoring may be indicated.

Electrolyte abnormalities—Electrolyte disturbances are common. Hyponatraemia often paradoxically accompanies the hypovolaemia which is seen in these patients, and may be related to the release of atrial natriuretic factors as a result of distension of the cerebral ventricles.[17] Hyponatraemia is also associated with vasospasm.[18] Hypokalaemia and hypocalcaemia have also been described.[19]

Vasospasm

Vasospasm and rebleeding are the most serious complications following subarachnoid haemorrhage. Neurological deterioration without evidence of rebleeding suggests a diagnosis of vasospasm which may be confirmed by angiography or suggested by transcranial Doppler ultrasonography.[20] Cerebral arterial spasm occurs angiographically in 60–70% of patients following subarachnoid haemorrhage. Only half of these become clinically symptomatic,[21] however, prompting some to use terms such as "delayed ischaemic deficits" (DID) to describe the symptomatic phenomenon. Symptoms, when they occur, usually begin 5–7 days after the subarachnoid haemorrhage and rarely after two weeks. Symptoms start over a period of hours and begin with features of a global reduction in CBF, such as drowsiness and confusion, leading to stupor. Signs of focal ischaemia (motor and speech) follow.

The aetiology of vasospasm is uncertain but appears to be related to the presence of blood in the subarachnoid space.[22] Other clinical correlates are the grade of the subarachnoid haemorrhage, with a higher occurrence of vasospasm in poor grade patients, and the location of the aneurysm, with site of subarachnoid blood corresponding to the location of vasospasm.

The pathophysiology of the spasm appears multifactorial and is probably the result of a combination of both vascular smooth muscle spasm and thickening of the vessel wall. Mediators in this process continue to be proposed with recent interest focusing on free radicals such as oxyhaemoglobin,[23] although other possible substances include serotonin, histamine, catecholamines, prostaglandins, angiotensin, and lipid peroxidase.[24] Mechanical distortion or disruption of vessel architecture may also be a factor.

A number of modalities have been described to prevent and treat vasospasm. Approaches are aimed at prevention or a reversal of the arterial narrowing, prevention of cerebral ischaemia, or protecting the brain from the effects of ischaemia and involve the following:

1 Prevention:
   (a) Ca^{2+} channel blockers
   (b) evacuation of subarachnoid blood
   (c) hypervolaemic hypertensive haemodilution.
2 Treatment:
   (a) hypervolaemic hypertensive haemodilution
   (b) angioplasty
   (c) Ca^{2+} channel blockers.

There has been much interest in early surgery as well as thrombolytic drugs such as tissue plasminogen activator (tPA) to remove the blood, thus preventing vasospasm and both of these have resulted in some success.[25-27]

Prevention or reversal of cerebral ischaemia is predicated based on measures that increase CBF. As flow is related to perfusion pressure, viscosity, and density, haemodynamic manipulations involving induced hypertension and hypervolaemia have been successful in reversing cerebral ischaemia caused by vasospasm. Crystalloids or colloids are used to maintain central venous pressure or pulmonary artery occlusion pressure in the region of 12–14 mm Hg. Recent studies have shown no benefit from raising filling pressures beyond this level,[28] and to do so increases the morbidity. Complications include pulmonary oedema, dilutional hyponatraemia, and myocardial infarction. Vasopressors may also be needed to raise the blood pressure, the most frequently used being dopamine, dobutamine, and phenylephrine. Vasopressin may be used to limit diuresis to less than 200 ml/ h, and atropine may be needed to maintain heart rate. With a clipped aneurysm, target blood pressure is in the 160–200 mm Hg range, whereas, with an unclipped aneurysm, systolic blood pressure should be limited to 120–150 mm Hg to reduce the risk of rebleeding.[29 30] Treatment should be continued until the vasospasm resolves or the presence of cerebral infarction

197

is confirmed. Transluminal angioplasty is a mechanical means that has also been successfully used to dilate narrowed vessels and improve flow.[31]

Many drugs have been studied in the attempt to produce better prevention and treatment of vasospasm. Nimodipine, a calcium channel blocking drug, has been the most successful to date, with studies showing a significant (40–70%) reduction in the morbidity rate.[32] It should be noted that many studies using nimodipine have failed to demonstrate reversal of the angiographic vasospasm, suggesting alternative mechanisms of effect, perhaps by a direct cytoprotective effect on the ischaemic neuron, or by acting on the microvasculature.[33] Many other calcium channel antagonists are currently under investigation.

Rebleeding

The risk of rebleeding is maximal on the first day after subarachnoid haemorrhage and carries with it a mortality rate of 80%. Thereafter, the risk of rebleeding diminishes with time (table 8.3). Unlike the initial bleed, when blood can spread freely through the subarachnoid space, clots and adhesions restrict the spread of blood causing a high rate of intracerebral haematoma formation.

Approaches to decreasing the risk of rebleeding include early surgery, meticulous blood pressure control, and the use of antifibrinolytic agents. After subarachnoid haemorrhage, some degree of hypertension is common. Although usually responsive to sedation, antihypertensive agents may be needed together with very careful titration of blood pressure, because cerebral ischaemia can occur. A systolic blood pressure of 120–150 mm Hg is the range with the lowest mortality and incidence of rebleeding.[34]

Antifibrinolytic agents such as aminocaproic acid and tranexamic acid have been used to decrease fibrinolytic activity in the CSF. Inhibition of this activity should lead to stabilisation of the clot in the aneurysm and a lower incidence of rebleeding. Although studies have confirmed this, the results have been tempered by an increased occurrence of ischaemic complications such as vasospasm so that mortality at three months is similar with or without use of these agents.[35] An additional complication of the use of antifibrinolytics is a higher occurrence of hydrocephalus.

Table 8.3 Risk of haemorrhage from ruptured aneurysms

Time period	Percentage risk
24 hours	50
14 days	30
90 days	5
6 months	3
1 year	3
> 1 year	3

The definitive prevention of rebleeding is surgical clipping of the aneurysm. The International Cooperative Study on Timing of Aneurysm Surgery found a rebleeding rate of 6% for patients undergoing surgery within three days, compared with 22% for those operated on from days 15 to 20.[36] Currently, early clipping is probably the best modality for the prevention of rebleeding.

Timing of surgery

Early surgery (within 2–5 days) has certain advantages as does delaying the surgery until 10–14 days after the subarachnoid haemorrhage as the following shows:

Early:
- less risk of rebleeding
- early evacuation of subarachnoid clot; reduced risk of vasospasm
- reduced risk of aneurysm rupture during hypervolaemic hypertensive treatment of vasospasm
- shorter hospital stay.

Delayed:
- improved operating conditions as a result of resolution of brain oedema and inflammation
- less risk of intraoperative aneurysm rupture as a result of clot stabilisation
- more time for medical evaluation of the patient
- easier (elective) scheduling for the operating room.

The International Cooperative Study on the Timing of Aneurysm Surgery,[36] although not a controlled study, suggested that low grade neurologically intact patients did well at all times, that is, with surgery being done within three days or after day 11, but that they had a lower mortality with later surgery. Patients who were operated on between days 7 and 10 fared worst, this being the period of maximal risk for vasospasm. When the subset of North American patients was examined, results were better with early surgery. It should be noted that, at the time of completion of this study (1980–3), the use of the calcium channel blocker nimodipine was not widespread, nor was hypervolaemic hypertensive therapy practised as aggressively. Use of these modalities may now tip the balance further in favour of early surgery.

Hydrocephalus

Hydrocephalus occurs in 15% of patients after subarachnoid haemorrhage[37] and is caused by the interference with CSF reabsorption by blood in the subarachnoid space. It is usually treated after the aneurysm is secured because reducing the ICP will increase the gradient across the wall of the aneurysm, predisposing to another rupture.

Surgical considerations

A number of different surgical techniques exist for the treatment of cerebral aneurysms. Most involve placing a spring loaded clip across the neck of the aneurysm exposed during craniotomy. This follows meticulous dissection, in an attempt to preserve the parent vessel and as many of the involved branches as possible. Other less satisfactory methods include the occlusion of the feeding parent vessel, trapping of the aneurysm by proximal and distal vessel occlusion, hunterian proximal ligation of the carotid or vertebral arteries, and wrapping of the aneurysm with gauze, muscle, or synthetic material.

More recently, interest has developed in the use of endovascular techniques. Percutaneous endovascular balloon embolisation has been used, but carries with it a significant risk of aneurysm rupture.[38] Of recent interest is the use of intra-aneurysmal electrothrombosis using platinum coils. These are placed within the lumen of the aneurysm, following which an electric current is passed through them. Reports of the success of this technique, which can obliterate from 70% to 100% of the aneurysm, have been encouraging.[39] So far, these techniques are used mainly in patients in whom the aneurysm is not amenable to surgical clipping.

Anaesthetic management

Goals

The goals of anaesthetic management are to facilitate operating conditions for the surgeon while minimising the risk of intraoperative rupture of the aneurysm, and avoiding other conditions that could worsen the neurological deficit. These aims are met by careful control of the aneurysm's transmural pressure, control of ICP, and maintenance of cerebral oxygen delivery.

Preoperative assessment

Before surgery, the patient should be carefully evaluated with special attention paid to the following. A neurological examination should be performed with the level of consciousness and presence of focal neurological deficits being noted, because these may indicate the presence of vasospasm or increased ICP. It will also give some indication of the neurological status that can be anticipated at the end of the procedure. The lower level of blood pressure at which a neurological deterioration occurs should be noted, if available. Computed tomography (CT) scans should be reviewed for location of the aneurysm, amount of blood in the subarachnoid space, and evidence of increased ICP.

The respiratory system should be examined for evidence of aspiration pneumonia, atelectasis, or pulmonary oedema.

Cardiac manifestations of subarachnoid hemorrhage have already been discussed. If significant ECG changes are present, a decision must be made on appropriate invasive monitoring. In addition, the patient's intravascular volume must be assessed, and appropriate blood products reserved.

Preoperative sedation is rarely needed in these patients and is preferably not used. Sedation could interfere with neurological assessment both pre-operatively and postoperatively. Opioids or barbiturates used as sedatives could result in hypercapnia, causing an increase in ICP. Alert patients usually respond to a reassuring visit from the anaesthetist. If needed, a small dose of a benzodiazepine can be administered.

Other drugs that the patient has been on preoperatively should be assessed individually. Nimodipine should be continued perioperatively, as should steroids and anticonvulsants.

Monitoring
Routine monitors are as follows:

- ECG
- Pulse oximetry and capnography
- Intra-arterial blood pressure monitoring
- Central venous pressure monitoring
- Urine output
- ± Pulmonary artery pressure monitoring
- Temperature
- ± ICP monitoring
- ± EEG monitoring
- ± Brain stem auditory and/or somatosensory evoked potentials.

This must include ECG and blood pressure monitoring. Non-invasive blood pressure monitoring, with an automatic cuff cycling at one minute intervals, is looked upon as adequate by some for induction in good grade patients, and has the advantage of having no potential for a blood pressure increase as a result of pain of insertion of an arterial line. Others, however, argue that it is critical to have beat to beat monitoring during the critical phase of induction (laryngoscopy and intubation), and therefore advocate placement of intra-arterial blood pressure monitoring under local anaesthesia preinduction. One alternative is to place the arterial line postinduction but preintubation.[40]

All other monitors and procedures can be done postinduction. This includes placement of central venous access. Whether to rely on central venous pressure measurement or to place a pulmonary artery catheter is at the discretion of the anaesthetist; however, factors suggesting pulmonary artery catheter placement would include a history of cardiac disease, a high grade subarachnoid haemorrhage, or known need for postoperative hyper-volaemic therapy. At least one study suggests a poor correlation between central venous pressure and pulmonary wedge pressure, mandating the need for pulmonary artery catheter monitoring during hypervolaemic therapy.[28]

Other monitors to be inserted postinduction include temperature probes and a urinary catheter.

Further monitors which are sometimes used include auditory brain stem and/or somatosensory evoked potentials, electroencephalogram (EEG) monitoring, and ICP monitors.

Finally, insertion of a lumbar subarachnoid drain may be considered. Operating conditions are improved by having a slack brain which can result from drainage of CSF. A polyethylene catheter may be inserted through a Tuohy needle, or a spinal needle may be used, with the malleable end of the 18 gauge needle being bent back parallel to the back postinsertion. Care must be taken during insertion that minimal CSF is lost, because a sudden decrease in the ICP will increase transmural pressure, thereby increasing the risk of aneurysm rupture.

Induction

The actual agents used for induction are less important than attention to detail and smoothness of the procedure. Any hypertensive peak puts the patient at further significant risk of haemorrhage. The goal during induction is the maintenance of a normal or slightly reduced transmural pressure. This will reduce the likelihood of rupture without increasing the risk of cerebral ischaemia. The aim is for a smooth induction with good attenuation of the sympathetic response to laryngoscopy and intubation, and minimal straining, bucking, or coughing on the endotracheal tube postintubation.

The patient should be preoxygenated with 100% oxygen by mask. An opioid (fentanyl 3–7 μg/kg, sufentanil 0·3–0·7 μg/kg, or alfentanil 25–50 μg/kg) is then administered. Induction of anaesthesia then follows. Sodium thiopentone (thiopental) 3–7 mg/kg is commonly used for this purpose, in a dose titrated to effect. Equally effective are propofol, methohexitone (methohexital), and midazolam. Most will cause a transient 10–15% lowering of blood pressure, which will help to decompress the aneurysm at a time when the ICP is also reduced and will also help offset the sympathetic response to laryngoscopy and intubation.

Immediately before intubation, lignocaine (lidocaine) or an additional bolus of induction agent may be given in an effort to prevent the pressor response to laryngoscopy and intubation. Other agents used for this purpose include α and/or β blockers, for example, labetalol and esmolol. Vasodilating drugs, if used, can cause significant increases in ICP. Anaesthesia may also be deepened by instituting an inhaled anaesthetic such as isoflurane by positive pressure ventilation via a mask before intubation. The vasodilator effect can be attenuated by concomitant hyperventilation.

None of the neuromuscular blocking agents crosses the blood–brain barrier or has any direct effect on the neurovasculature. Any changes in intracranial dynamics usually reflect the systemic effect of the agent. Suxamethonium (succinylcholine) is the neuromuscular blocking agent of choice when rapid onset and maximal relaxation are required. Hyperkalaemia has not been a problem in the authors' experience[41] and increases in ICP can be attenuated by the use of a defasciculating dose of a non-depolarising neuromuscular blocking agent.[42] Non-depolarising agents are very frequently used for intubation.

Maintenance

Maintenance of anaesthesia can be with one of many combinations of agents. The authors routinely use nitrous oxide (N_2O), oxygen, and an opioid such as fentanyl, together with isoflurane. Alternatively a higher dose opioid technique can be used, to which droperidol or a benzodiazepine, or a propofol infusion, is added. Hyperventilation to a $Paco_2$ of 28–30 mm Hg may be instituted in the presence of an increased ICP; it can, however, otherwise be kept at about 35 mm Hg. It is not known if hyperventilation is useful in a patient with angiographic cerebral vasospasm: on the one hand, hyperventilation may further constrict the vasospastic vessels thus predisposing to cerebral ischaemia, although, on the other, by causing vasoconstriction of normal cerebral vessels more blood could actually be forced through the non-autoregulating vasospastic vessels.

The pressor response to head pinning should be attenuated, either by additional doses of propofol, thiopentone, or an opioid, or by injection of local anaesthetic at the pin insertion site. After final positioning, the lungs should be reauscultated to confirm endotracheal tube position. All bony prominences should be well padded as these procedures may be long, and there should be provision made for maintaining the patient's temperature, for example, with use of a heating blanket.

Intraoperative considerations

Brain relaxation—Both mannitol and frusemide (furosemide) are used for brain shrinkage. The use of one or the other or a combination depends more on surgical preference than on scientific evidence, as is the case with the doses used. A typical mannitol dose is 0·25–1·0 g/kg. In the experience of the authors it works effectively if given over 20–25 minutes, which then avoids precipitous changes in intravascular volume and ICP. It begins to take effect within 4–5 minutes, with a maximal effect in 45 minutes (range 20–120 minutes). Frusemide 0·1–1 mg/kg decreases total body water content, CSF production, and intracranial astroglial swelling. Clinical efficacy of these medications should be judged by the degree of brain relaxation *not* by urine production.

If a lumbar drain has been placed, it can be opened carefully once the dura is opened. Drainage of CSF should not exceed 5 ml/min to avoid a Cushing's response, that is, hypertension and bradycardia. Drainage of CSF is a very effective way of decreasing the intracranial volume; 50–150 ml are withdrawn, as required. The drain is closed once dural closure starts.

Fluid and electrolyte management—Before clipping the aneurysm, fluid administration is usually limited to that needed for maintenance. After the aneurysm has been clipped, the aim is to achieve a central venous pressure in the high normal range to prevent symptomatic vasospasm. Crystalloid (Ringer's lactate or physiological saline) is usually used as the maintenance fluid and glucose containing fluids should be avoided as a result of concerns that glucose may worsen cerebral ischaemia. Colloid solutions may also be needed. Blood should be transfused as required. The optimal haematocrit to maintain cerebral oxygen delivery is thought to be in the range 30–35%.

Electrolytes should be checked intraoperatively at periodic intervals. Some concern has existed about the propensity of mannitol to cause disturbances in electrolytes, but doses under 2 g/kg probably have no effect in this regard.[43]

Controlled hypotension—Hypotension is used intraoperatively to decrease intra-aneurysmal pressure and thereby wall tension. This makes the aneurysm softer and more pliable during surgical manipulation and, in addition, if rupture occurs, blood loss may be decreased and the haemorrhage more easily controlled. Hypotension is used in two forms: systemic hypotension, in which systemic arterial blood pressure is reduced, and local hypotension, in which the aneurysm's proximal feeding artery is temporarily occluded with clips.

Systemic hypotension was the technique of choice until recently when a transition to temporary clips started to occur. This reflects the availability of clips that can be repeatedly applied without injuring the vessel and also perhaps the absence of convincing evidence that systemic hypotension indeed reduces the incidence of rupture or the associated blood loss.[44] Avoiding systemic hypotension also reduces the risk of injury to other parts of the brain or body.

The safe lower limit for systemic hypotension has not been definitively established. As autoregulation is normally maintained to a mean blood pressure of 50 mm Hg, this pressure is frequently regarded as the safe lower limit. Others have also argued that in good grade patients the brain will tolerate a 10–20% decrease in CBF without a detrimental effect and have therefore allowed mean blood pressure to decrease to as low as 40 mm Hg. In poor grade patients, autoregulation is lost and, in chronic hypertension, the limits of autoregulation are shifted to the right. In these patients hypotension should be more carefully used and a more conservative lower limit also used. Relative contraindications to systemic hypotension include severe uncontrolled hypertension, valvular heart disease, ischaemic disease of the brain, heart, or kidney, and significant pulmonary, renal, or hepatic insufficiency.

Before the induction of systemic hypertension, anaemia and hypovolaemia should be corrected. Blood pressure control is much more labile in the presence of hypovolaemia and hypovolaemic hypotension is associated with more tissue dysfunction than normovolaemic drug induced hypotension. The adequacy of pulmonary gas exchange during hypotension should be confirmed by arterial blood gas analysis.

The most commonly used agents are sodium nitroprusside and isoflurane. Nitroprusside has the advantages of rapid onset and offset but has the disadvantage of reflex tachycardia, difficulty of control, and possible cyanide toxicity. Isoflurane has a slightly slower onset and offset of action, but is easier to control and, if already part of the anaesthetic, avoids the use of another drug.[45] Glyceryl trinitrate (nitroglycerin) also has been used but seems less potent and may not induce deep levels of hypotension. Trimetaphan is still used by some and has less propensity to disrupt autoregulation. Urapidil is an antihypertensive agent used in Europe during neuroanaesthesia. Its mechanisms of action include peripheral α blockade as well as interaction with brain serotonin (5-hydroxytryptamine) 5-HT$_{1a}$ receptors. It does not affect CBF or ICP[46] and does not cause either significant sympathetic activation or rebound hypertension. It is often used in combination with isoflurane.

Local hypotension may be achieved by occluding the feeding artery close to the aneurysm, although aneurysms in the carotid circulation are also sometimes decompressed by occlusion or compression of the carotid artery in the neck. During occlusion, the patient's blood pressure should be kept in the normal range for that patient although some practitioners prefer deliberately to increase blood pressure by 10–20% in an attempt to improve collateral blood flow.

The type of blood pressure management as well as the need for cerebral monitoring and putative cerebral protective agents should be discussed with the surgeon before the start of surgery.

Cerebral protection—This is discussed in detail in chapter 11. Specifically, in relation to aneurysm surgery, there are no adequate randomised prospective outcome studies demonstrating the efficacy of any particular technique or drug. In spite of this, the use of high dose barbiturates, propofol, etomidate, or isoflurane is common as is the use of deliberate mild hypothermia.[47] The rationale for use is that these methods may work based on deductive reasoning or laboratory data, and they do not appear to represent a great risk to the patient. Complications associated with anaesthetic overdose include the need for vasopressors and delayed awakening. Risks associated with mild hypothermia have not been defined but may include an increased incidence of myocardial ischaemia.[48]

Monitoring—During controlled hypotension and the application of temporary clips and the placement of the retractors, it would be ideal to monitor brain integrity to verify that ischaemia is not present. Modalities used include the EEG, and somatosensory and brain stem auditory evoked potentials. EEG monitoring has not proved very useful because the preoperative EEG is often abnormal, anaesthetic agents can have marked effects on the EEG, data analysis is complex, and the electrodes cannot usually be placed near the operative site, thus introducing the possibility of missing areas of focal ischaemia.

Evoked potentials may be more useful because they are not greatly influenced by intravenous anaesthetics, although they are reduced by inhalational agents. They can be used to monitor procedures involving aneurysms of both the carotid and vertebral circulations. Somatosensory evoked potential monitoring has been shown to be a better predictor of neurological deficits in patients with carotid aneurysms but has a high (43%) false positive rate with a false negative rate of 14%.[49] Brain stem auditory evoked potentials are comparable with somatosensory evoked potential monitoring in predicting neurological deficits during posterior fossa aneurysm surgery, although use of both further decreases the false negative rate.[50] Although not universally used during aneurysm surgery, the authors continue to find evoked potential monitoring useful.

Intraoperative rupture—The Cooperative Aneurysm Study quotes an intraoperative leak rate of about 6% with a frank rupture rate of 13%, for a combined incidence of 19%.[51] Most ruptures occur during dissection of the aneurysm and clip placement.[52] Not surprisingly, morbidity and mortality are increased by rupture.

Rupture at the time of induction is uncommon (0·5–5%) and can be caused or heralded by a sudden increase in blood pressure. The mortality rate is very high (50%). If rupture is suspected, the surgery should be deferred, and a CT scan done to confirm the diagnosis and determine the safety of proceeding or the need to evacuate the clot.

During aneurysmal dissection, most leaks are small and controlled by the surgeon by suctioning and the application of temporary or permanent clips. If the blood loss is more substantial, induced hypotension may reduce blood loss and improve visualisation. If the aneurysm is in the carotid circulation, manual compression of the ipsilateral carotid artery for short periods (<3 min) can provide an almost bloodless field. Concomitantly, intravascular volume must be replaced. Cerebral protective measures may also be considered (see above). Thiopentone or propofol will reduce blood pressure and vasoconstrict the cerebral vessels while perhaps protecting the neurons. Conversely, etomidate is less likely to lower blood pressure.

Recovery

In the absence of significant intraoperative complications, patients with a good neurological grade preoperatively (grades 0–2) can be extubated at the termination of the procedure. Grade 3 patients should be evaluated individually. Patients with worse neurological grades should remain intubated and be taken, while being ventilated, to an intensive care unit.

A goal of anaesthetic management for aneurysm surgery is to have the patient sufficiently awake for neurological examination as soon after the end of the procedure as possible. This allows early determination of the need for computed tomography, angiography, or reoperation.

A smooth emergence may be helped by the administration of intravenous lignocaine (lidocaine) 1·5 mg/kg 2–3 min before extubation or small doses of opioids, for example, intravenous fentanyl 25–50 μg, although both of these may deepen the level of anaesthesia.

Mild pressor responses at the time of emergence can be tolerated by the patient as long as there are no unclipped aneurysms. Some teams will allow systolic blood pressures of up to 180 mm Hg, reasoning that where the aneurysm is secured, mild hypertension may improve CBF. Anti-hypertensive agents which may be used include direct acting vasodilators such as nitroprusside, glyceryl trinitrate, and hydralazine, as well as β blockers such as esmolol, or combined α–β blockers such as labetalol.

The patient should be well oxygenated before extubation and effects of neuromuscular blocking agents reversed. After extubation, the patient should be taken to a recovery area staffed by personnel skilled in the care of neurosurgical patients. Oxygen should be administered by facemask. The patient should be nursed in a 30° head up position and adequate analgesia administered. A thorough neurological examination is usually performed by the surgical staff at this point. Vital signs and neurological status should be monitored every 15 minutes initially. Instructions should be left with the nursing staff about acceptable blood pressure parameters.

Arteriovenous malformations

Arteriovenous malformations of the brain are congenital lesions composed of a tortuous mass of arteries and veins lacking an intervening capillary bed. The resulting vascular structure shunts oxygenated blood directly into the venous system. The arteriovenous malformation is thus a high flow, low resistance circuit, resulting in a low transmural pressure: the intravascular pressure is only 45–60% that of the systemic mean arterial pressure. Occurring at a tenth the frequency of cerebral aneurysms, most arteriovenous malformations are supratentorial, with only 10% being located in the posterior fossa. There is a 4–10% prevalence rate for associated aneurysms.[53]

Arteriovenous malformations may present with spontaneous haemorrhage, seizures, headache, and/or progressive neurological deficit. Presentation usually occurs at a younger age than with cerebral aneurysm, that is, between 20 and 40 years of age. Haemorrhage is the initial presentation in 80% of patients, with an annual risk of haemorrhage from an unruptured lesion being 1–3% per year. The risk of death from the initial bleed is 10%, with the mortality rate from recurrent haemorrhage being 20% per episode.[54]

The second most common presentation, in 20–40% of patients, is seizures.[55] Arteriovenous malformations may also present during pregnancy, although the literature is divided as to whether gravid women with arteriovenous malformations are at increased risk of bleeding compared with non-gravid women.[56 57]

Treatment options

Surgery is an option for many arteriovenous malformations. Surgical risk is related to a number of factors: size, with smaller arteriovenous malformations being more amenable to total excision; location, with superficial location being favourable; the number and origin of feeding arteries and the pattern of venous drainage; the degree of eloquence (areas of cortical motor or sensory function) of the brain in which the arteriovenous malformation is located; the degree of steal from adjacent brain; and the rate of flow through the lesion.[58 59] Still the treatment of choice for arteriovenous malformations, surgical resection, almost eliminates the risk of haemorrhage and improves neurological outcome. Other treatment options include no treatment at all, radiation therapy (best results in small inoperable lesions), stereotactic radiosurgery, and endovascular embolisation. Conservative treatment is advocated for those arteriovenous malformations for which the risk of surgery outweighs the risk of no intervention. Very large arteriovenous malformations, those in areas of cortical motor or sensory function (eloquent areas) of the brain, or which involve vital structures in the brain, such as in the brain stem or hypothalamus, are often considered inoperable.

The development of microcatheters has allowed more widespread use of preoperative embolisation for decreasing the size of and blood flow to arteriovenous malformations. By rendering the arteriovenous malformation more amenable to surgery, morbidity and mortality have been reduced. Use of embolisation on its own unfortunately results in a low cure rate and its use has evolved mainly in conjunction with surgery.[60] The timing of this procedure remains controversial: post-embolisation, blood is directed to previously hypoperfused surrounding brain tissue causing a relative hyperaemia which needs time to resolve before surgery, but waiting too long increases the risk of development of deep collateral channels.

Anaesthesia

Anaesthesia may be needed either in the operating suite for surgical excision of an arteriovenous malformation or in the radiology department for embolisation. Anaesthetic techniques for embolisation have recently been extensively reviewed.[61]

For embolisation procedures in which sedation is considered, patients should be evaluated preoperatively for suitability, for example, whether or not they can lie still for many hours, the presence of a significant cough, or evidence of raised ICP, as a rise in $Paco_2$ mediated by sedative agents could worsen the neurological state. Agents useful for sedation include droperidol, midazolam, fentanyl, or propofol.

Should a general anaesthetic be required for the embolisation, the same goals apply as is the case in many intracranial procedures, that is, the need to have the patient awake as soon as possible after the end of the procedure so that it is possible to make a neurological assessment. Only light levels of anaesthesia are usually needed but immobility is required.

Preoperative evaluation

Preoperative evaluation follows the same principles as for other neurosurgical procedures. Four units of blood should be crossmatched and made available for immediate use.

Intraoperative management

Anaesthetic management follows the same principles as would be used in a patient with any highly vascular intracranial mass. Excellent vascular access, central venous, and intra-arterial monitoring are mandatory because intraoperative blood loss can be torrential. The anaesthetic technique should not increase ICP or brain bulk and should maintain haemodynamic stability. As there is a substantial pressure drop between the arterial tree and the arteriovenous malformation, increases in blood pressure are less frequently associated with rupture than with aneurysms. Conversely, sudden haemorrhage can cause precipitous and unexpected drops in blood pressure. The use of deliberate hypotension is controversial, the potential benefits being a decreased blood loss during resection and a decrease in hyperaemic complications. Against this must be balanced the risk of ischaemia from hypoperfusion.

The patient needs to regain consciousness promptly following surgery so as to permit early neurological evaluation. Hypertension during emergence needs to be avoided to prevent bleeding from the arteriovenous malformation bed. Blood pressure should be maintained in the patient's normal range with antihypertensive agents (see previous section on aneurysms).

Postoperative complications

Most postoperative complications are related either to bleeding from the arteriovenous malformation bed or to the increase in perfusion to previously hypoperfused areas of normal brain surrounding the resected arteriovenous malformation. This effect is one of the major causes of postoperative morbidity from surgery for arteriovenous malformation. After obliteration of the high flow, low pressure, vascular bed of the arteriovenous malformation, blood is rerouted through the relatively normal vessels of the surrounding brain. The resulting hyperaemia can then put the brain at risk of complications such as cerebral oedema, haemorrhage, and intracranial hypertension. This syndrome, called normal perfusion pressure breakthrough, has an estimated frequency of 2–37%, the higher occurrence being with larger arteriovenous malformations. Initially thought to result from the loss of autoregulation in surrounding vessels, recent studies do not support this contention.[62] Controversy continues to exist regarding the mechanism of this phenomenon, with many authorities even doubting its existence. Measures to prevent normal perfusion pressure breakthrough include staged procedures, induced hypotension, clamping of the carotid artery, and barbiturate coma. Staging the treatment of arteriovenous malformations has the advantage of minimising complications from normal perfusion pressure breakthrough, and is the current trend; however, this must be balanced against the risk of increased chance of haemorrhage from the arteriovenous malformation bed. Once the syndrome develops, many advocate the careful use of deliberate hypotension. Symptoms of intracranial hypertension are treated with the usual measures, that is, hyperventilation, head up position, and osmotic diuretics, with the use of barbiturates for intractable hypertension.[63]

Summary

In this chapter the salient points have been highlighted for the anaesthetic management of patients with cerebral aneurysms and arteriovenous malformations. Anaesthetic management of patients with these lesions must be smooth, and undertaken with good knowledge and understanding of the pathophysiology. For aneurysms, control of transmural pressure, avoidance of cerebral hypoperfusion, and diagnosis and management of vasospasm are essential elements. For arteriovenous malformations, the potential for massive intraoperative blood loss and postoperative hyperperfusion sequelae are the major concerns. As improvements in treatment techniques occur and understanding of the mechanisms of vasospasm continues, it is hoped that the morbidity and mortality associated with cerebral aneurysms and arteriovenous malformations will improve.

1 Chason JL, Hindman WM. Berry aneurysms of the circle of Willis: results of a planned autopsy study. *Neurology* 1958; **8**: 41–4.
2 Philips LH, Whisnant JP, O'Fallon W, Sundt TM. The unchanging pattern of subarachnoid hemorrhage in a community. *Neurology* 1980; **30**: 1034–40.
3 Kristensen MO. Increased incidence of bleeding intracranial aneurysms in Greenlandic Eskimos. *Acta Neurochir (Wein)* 1983; **67**: 37–43.
4 Locksley HB. Report on the cooperative study of intracranial aneurysms and subarachnoid hemorrhage. Section V, Part 1. Natural history of subarachnoid hemorrhage, intracranial aneurysms, and arteriovenous malformations. *J Neurosurg* 1966; **25**: 219–39.
5 Locksley HB. Report of the cooperative study of intracranial aneurysms and subarachnoid hemorrhage. Section V, Part II. Natural history of subarachnoid hemorrhage, intracranial aneurysms and arteriovenous malformations. *J Neurosurg* 1966; **25**: 321–38.

6 Voldby B, Enevoldsen EM. Intracranial pressure changes following aneurysm rupture. 1. Clinical and angiographic correlations. *J Neurosurg* 1982; **56**: 186–96.

7 Voldby B, Enevoldsen EM, Jensen FT. Cerebrovascular reactivity in patients with ruptured intracranial aneurysms. *J Neurosurg* 1985; **62**: 59–67.

8 Botterell EH, Longhead WM, Scott JW, Vanderwater SL. Hypothermia and interruption of carotid or carotid and vertebral circulation in the surgical management of intracranial aneurysms. *J Neurosurg* 1956; **13**: 1–42.

9 Hunt WE, Hess RM. Surgical risk as related to time of intervention in the repair of intracranial aneurysms. *J Neurosurg* 1968; **28**: 14–20.

10 Drake CG. Report of World Federation of Neurologic Surgeons Committee on a Universal Subarachnoid Hemorrhage Grading Scale. *J Neurosurg* 1988; **68**: 985–6.

11 Ferguson GG. Direct measurement of mean and pulsatile blood pressure at operation in human intracranial saccular aneurysms. *J Neurosurg* 1972; **36**: 560–3.

12 Cruikshank JM, Neil-Dwyer G, Stott AW. Possible role of catecholamines, corticosteroids and potassium in production of electrocardiographic abnormalities associated with subarachnoid haemorrhage. *Br Heart J* 1974; **36**: 697.

13 Manninen PJ, Gelb AW, Lam AM, Moote CA, Contreras J. Perioperative monitoring of the electrocardiogram during cerebral aneurysm surgery. *J Neurosurg Anesth* 1990; **2**: 16–22.

14 Marion DW, Segal R, Thompson ME. Subarachnoid hemorrhage and the heart. *Neurosurgery* 1986; **18**: 101–6.

15 Davies KR, Gelb AW, Manninen DH, *et al.* Cardiac function in aneurysmal subarachnoid haemorrhage: a study of electrocardiographic and echocardiographic abnormalities. *Br J Anaesth* 1991; **67**: 58–63.

16 Brazenor GA, Chamberlain MJ, Gelb AW, Manninen PH, Boughner DR, Bisnaire D. Systemic hypovolemia after subarachnoid hemorrhage. *Journal of Neurosurgical Anesthesia* 1990; **2**: 42–9.

17 Rosenfeld JV, Barnett GH, Sila CA, Little JR, Bravo EL, Beck GJ. The effect of subarachnoid hemorrhage on blood and CSF atrial natriuretic factor. *J Neurosurg* 1989; **71**: 32–7.

18 Hasan D, Wijdicks EF, Vermeulen M. Hyponatremia is associated with cerebral ischemia in patients with aneurysmal subarachnoid hemorrhage. *Ann Neurol* 1990; **27**: 106–8.

19 Rudenhill A, Gordon E, Sundqvist K, Sylven C, Wahlgren NG. A study of ECG abnormalities and myocardial specific enzymes in patients with subarachnoid haemorrhage. *Acta Anaesth Scand* 1982; **26**: 344–50.

20 Seiler RW, Grolimund P, Aaslid R, Huber P, Nornes H. Cerebral vasospasm evaluated by transcranial ultrasound correlated with clinical grade and CT-visualized subarachnoid hemorrhage. *J Neurosurg* 1986; **64**: 594–600.

21 Adams HP, Kassell NF, Torner JC, Haley EC Jr. Predicting cerebral ischemia after aneurysmal subarachnoid hemorrhage: influences of clinical condition, CT results and antifibrinolytic therapy. A report of the Cooperative Aneurysm Study. *Neurology* 1987; **37**: 1586–91.

22 Mizukami M, Takemae T, Tazawa T, Kawase T, Matsuzaki T. Value of computed tomography in the prediction of cerebral vasospasm after aneurysm rupture. *Neurosurgery* 1980; **7**: 583–6.

23 MacDonald RL, Weir BK, Runzer TD, *et al.* Etiology of cerebral vasospasm in primates. *J Neurosurg* 1991; **75**: 415–24.

24 Heros RC, Zervas NT, Varsos V. Cerebral vasospasm after subarachnoid hemorrhage: An update. *Ann Neurol* 1983; **14**: 599–608.

25 Taneda M. Effect of early operation for ruptured aneurysms on prevention of delayed ischemic symptoms. *J Neurosurg* 1982; **57**: 622–8.

26 Mizukami M, Kawase T, Usami T, Tazawi T. Prevention of vasospasm by early operation with removal of subarachnoid blood. *Neurosurgery* 1982; **10**: 301–7.

27 Ohman J, Servo A, Heiskanen O. Effect of intrathecal fibrinolytic therapy on clot lysis and vasospasm in patients with aneurysmal subarachnoid hemorrhage. *J Neurosurg* 1991; **75**: 197–201.

28 Levy ML, Giannotta SL. Cardiac performance indices during hypervolemic therapy for cerebral vasospasm. *J Neurosurg* 1991; **75**: 27–31.

29 Awad IA, Carter LP, Spetzler RF, Medina M, Williams FC Jr. Clinical vasospasm after

subarachnoid hemorrhage: response to hypervolemic hemodilution and arterial hypertension. *Stroke* 1987; **18**: 365–72.

30 Kassell NF, Peerless SJ, Durward OJ, Beck DW, Drake CG, Adams HP. Treatment of ischemic deficits from vasospasm with intravascular volume expansion and induced arterial hypertension. *Neurosurgery* 1982; **11**: 337–43.

31 Newell DW, Eskridge JM, Mayberg MR. Angioplasty for the treatment of symptomatic vasospasm following subarachnoid hemorrhage. *J Neurosur* 1989; **71**: 654–60.

32 Picard JD, Murray GD, Illingworth R, *et al.* Effect of oral nimodipine on cerebral infarction and outcome after subarachnoid haemorrhage: British aneurysm nimodipine trial. *BMJ* 1989; **298**: 636–42.

33 Petruk KC, West M, Mohr G, *et al.* Nimodipine Treatment in Poor Grade Aneurysm patients. Results of a multicentre double-blind placebo controlled trial. *J Neurosurg* 1988; **68**: 505–17.

34 Brown MF, Benzel EC. Morbidity and mortality associated with rapid control of systemic hypertension in patients with intracranial hemorrhages. *J Neurosurg Anesth* 1990; **2**: 53–5.

35 Vermeulen M, Lindsay KW, Murray GD, *et al.* Antifibrinolytic treatment in subarachnoid hemorrhage. *N Engl J Med* 1984; **311**: 432–7.

36 Kassell NF, Torner JC, Jane JA, Halrey EJ, Adams HP. The international cooperative study on the Timing of Aneurysm surgery. Part II – surgical results. *J Neurosurg* 1990; **73**: 37–47.

37 Graff-Radford NR, Torner J, Adams HJ, Kassell NF. Factors associated with hydrocephalus after subarachnoid hemorrhage. A report of the Cooperative Aneurysm Study. *Arch Neurol* 1989; **46**: 744–52.

38 Higashida RT, Halbach VV, Cahan LD, Hieshima GB, Konishi Y. Detachable balloon embolization therapy of posterior circulation intracranial aneurysms. *J Neurosurg* 1989; **71**: 512–19.

39 Casasco AE, Aymard A, Gobin YP, *et al.* Selective endovascular treatment of 71 intracranial aneurysms with platinum coils. *J Neurosurg* 1993; **79**: 3–10.

40 Hsu R, Turndorff H, Mangiardi J, *et al.* In Varkey GP (Ed.), *Anesthetic considerations in the surgical repair of intracranial aneurysms.* Vol 20, *International Anesthesiology Clinics.* Boston: Little, Brown & Co, 1982: 89–93.

41 Manninen PH, Mahendran B, Gelb AW, Merchant RM. Succinylcholine does not increase serum potassium levels in patients with acutely ruptured cerebral aneurysm. *Anesth Analg* 1990; **70**: 172–5.

42 Stirt JA, Grosslight KR, Bedford RF, Vollmer D. "Defasciculation" with metocurine prevents succinylcholine induced increases in intracranial pressure. *Anesthesiology* 1987; **67**: 50–3.

43 Manninen PH, Lam AM, Gelb AW, Brown SC. The effect of high-dose mannitol on serum and urine electrolytes and osmolality in neurological patients. *Can J Anaesth* 1987; **34**: 422–6.

44 Craen R, Gelb AW. Applications in neurosurgery. In: Ornstein E (Ed.), *Problems in anesthesia: deliberate hypotension in anesthesia and surgery*, Vol 7. Philadelphia: Lippincott, 1993: 23–30.

45 Lam AM, Gelb AW. Cardiovascular effects of isoflurane-induced hypotension for cerebral aneurysm surgery. *Anesth Analg* 1983; **62**: 742–8.

46 Puchstein C, Van Aken H, Anger C, Hidding J. Influence of urapidil on intracranial pressure and intracranial compliance in dogs. *Br J Anaesth* 1983; **55**: 443–8.

47 Craen RA, Gelb AW, Eliasziw M, Lok P. Current anesthetic practices and use of brain protective therapies for cerebral aneurysm surgery at 41 North American centers. *Anesthesiology* 1994; **81**: A209.

48 Frank SM, Beattie C, Christopherson R, *et al.* Unintentional hypothermia is associated with postoperative myocardial ischemia. The perioperative Ischemia Randomized Anesthesia Trial Study Group. *Anesthesiology* 1993; **78**: 468–76.

49 Manninen PH, Lam AM, Nantau WE. Monitoring of somatosensory evoked potentials during temporary arterial occlusion in cerebral aneurysm surgery. *J Neurosurg Anesthesiol* 1990; **2**: 97–104.

50 Manninen PH, Patterson S, Lam AH, Gelb AW, Nantau WE. Evoked potential monitoring during posterior fossa aneurysm surgery: a comparison of two modalities. *Can J Anaesth* 1994; **41**: 92–7.

51 Kassell NF, Torner JC, Jane JA, Haley EJ, Adams HP. The international cooperative study on the timing of aneurysm surgery. Part I. Overall management results. *J Neurosurg* 1990; **73**: 18–36.

52 Batjer H, Samson D. Intraoperative aneurysmal rupture: incidence, outcome, and suggestions for surgical management. *Neurosurgery* 1986; **18**: 701–7.

53 Perret G, Grip A. Report on the cooperative study of intracranial aneurysms and subarachnoid hemorrhage. Section VI. Arteriovenous malformations. An analysis of 545 cases of cranio-cerebral arteriovenous malformations and fistulae reported to the Cooperative Study. *J Neurosurg* 1966; **25**: 467–90.

54 Luessenhop AJ. Natural history of cerebral arteriovenous malformations. In: Wilson CB, Stein BM (Eds), *Intracranial arteriovenous malformations*. Baltimore: William & Wilkins, 1984: 12–23.

55 Crawford PM, West CR, Chadwich DW, Shaw MDM. Arteriovenous malformations of the brain: natural history in unoperative patients. *J Neurol Neurosurg Psychiatry* 1986; **49**: 1–10.

56 Horton JC, Chambers WA, Lyons SL, Adams RD, Kjellberg RN. Pregnancy and the risk of hemorrhage from cerebral arteriovenous malformations. *Neurosurgery* 1990; **27**: 867–71.

57 Robinson JL, Hall CS, Sedizimir CB. Arteriovenous malformations, aneurysms and pregnancy. *J Neurosurg* 1974; **41**: 63–70.

58 Spetzler RF, Martin NA. A proposed grading system for arteriovenous malformations. *J Neurosurg* 1986; **65**: 476–83.

59 Spetzler RF, Zabramski JM. Grading and staged resection of cerebral arteriovenous malformations. *Clin Neurosurg* 1990; **36**: 318–37.

60 Fox AJ, Pelz DM, Lee DH. Arteriovenous malformations of the brain: Recent results of endovascular therapy. *Radiology* 1990; **177**: 51–7.

61 Young WL, Pile-Spellman J. Anesthetic considerations for interventional neuroradiology. *Anesthesiology* 1994; **80**: 427–56.

62 Young WL, Kader A, Prohovnik I, *et al*. Pressure autoregulation is intact after arteriovenous malformation resection. *Neurosurgery* 1993; **32**: 491–7.

63 Awad IA, Magdinec M, Schubert A. Intracranial hypertension after resection of cerebral arteriovenous malformations. Predisposing factors and management strategy. *Stroke* 1994; **25**: 611–20.

213

9: Anaesthetic considerations for specific neurosurgical procedures

JAN VAN HEMELRIJCK

Paediatric neurosurgery

Paediatric neuroanaesthetic care requires knowledge of the basics of neuro-anaesthesia and of the physiological and pharmacological differences between paediatric and adult patients, and familiarity with paediatric anaesthetic equipment. Important differences exist between different age groups within the paediatric patient population. Fluid and electrolyte management, blood replacement strategies, and the maintenance of body temperature may be particularly cumbersome. Pharmacodynamic and pharmacokinetic characteristics of drugs differ widely with the patient's age.

The first section deals with some aspects of intracranial physiology that are specific for paediatric patients. Subsequently, some important aspects of the anaesthetic management are discussed. Finally, specific problems related to some common surgical procedures are presented. The anaesthetic management for neuroradiology is discussed in chapter 3.

Children are born with a relatively immature central nervous system (CNS). At birth the number of neurons is almost complete but the glial growth, dendritic arborisation, synapse formation, and myelinisation continue during the first two years of life. The development of the cerebellum is completed within the first year, before the cortex and the brain stem. Data on cerebral blood flow (CBF) in children are sparse in the literature (table 9.1). CBF in normal neonates and pre-term infants averages about 40 ml/min per 100 g, which is lower than in adults.[1][2] In children between six months and 12

Table 9.1   Cerebral blood flow (CBF) and cerebral metabolism for oxygen ($CMRO_2$) in paediatric and adult patients

	CBF (ml/min per 100 g)	$CMRO_2$ (ml O_2/min per 100 g)
Neonates and infants	40	2·5
1–12 years	100	5
Adults	50–80	3–3·5

214

years of age, CBF is considerably higher than in adults, namely about 100 ml/min per 100 g.[3] The average cerebral metabolic rate for oxygen (CMR_{O_2}) is presumably relatively low in newborns, although cerebral metabolism has been extensively studied only in newborn animals. Between two weeks and 12 months of age, the CMR_{O_2} was measured as 2·3 ml O_2/100 g per min.[4] Between three and 11 years of age it increases to 5 ml O_2/100 g per min, and it progressively decreases again to 3–3·5 ml O_2/100 g per min in adults.[3] The cerebrovascular constriction in response to hyperoxia may be greater in neonates than in the more mature brain. Hypoxia results in vasodilatation at similar values to the adult brain.[5] Cerebral blood flow is reactive to changes in carbon dioxide concentration but the responsiveness may be attenuated in newborns.

Autoregulation of the CBF to changes in cerebral perfusion pressure (CPP) is normal in healthy infants and children. The perfusion pressure limits for normal autoregulation are, however, probably different from the limits in adults. A mean arterial pressure (MAP) of 60 mm Hg is not commonly seen in younger children, which would imply that, according to the criteria for adults, blood pressure in children is always below the autoregulation limits. Cerebral autoregulation has been found to fail in newborns with respiratory distress syndrome or perinatal asphyxia.[6] This may explain the high incidence of intracranial bleeding observed in these infants.

Normal intracranial pressure (ICP) in children is between 0 and 15 mm Hg. Increases in ICP may decrease CPP, and cause brain ischaemia and herniation of brain tissue by the same mechanism as in adults.[7] In infants, however, the fontanelles and non-fused bone sutures can separate, providing relative protection against changes in ICP with gradual changes in intracranial volume. Acute volume changes are not, however, well absorbed by this mechanism. An increased ICP, resulting from an obstructive hydrocephalus or from the presence of large cysts, does not usually respond very well to therapeutic manoeuvres other than the removal of cerebrospinal fluid (CSF) or the content of the cyst.

Preoperative evaluation

The preoperative evaluation of a child should include a full neurological history and examination. Signs of increased ICP should especially be looked for. In small children the tonus of the fontanelles gives a good indication of the ICP; increased ICP can cause somnolence although children may look remarkably alert. An important sign is the presence of persistent vomiting. Electrolyte abnormalities may be present, and preoperative blood cell count may reveal anaemia as a result of a chronic infection or poor intake. The preoperative visit also gives the opportunity to evaluate the psychological condition of the child, which is an important factor in deciding on the anaesthetic induction technique. Alleviation of parental anxiety will be

215

automatically transmitted to the child, and may result in a valuable sedative effect. Sedative premedication should be used cautiously in patients suspected of having increased ICP. Hypercapnia, eventually associated with the administration of sedative agents, may cause a dangerous increase in ICP and even brain coning. Sedative agents may therefore only be administered if the child remains under the close supervision of the anaesthetist.

Anaesthetic technique

Induction of anaesthesia should be smooth, avoiding struggling, crying, respiratory obstruction, and breath holding, especially in children with compromised intracranial compliance. Ideally these goals can be achieved by intravenous induction agents. Intravenous cannulation before induction should not, however, be attempted in the anxious child because this will predictably produce crying, excitation, blood pressure and central venous pressure increases, and a dangerous increase in ICP. Inhalational induction may be preferable in such cases. Although isoflurane is generally considered a more suitable agent for neuroanaesthesia than halothane, the use of isoflurane for inhalational induction is associated with increased airway reactivity leading to an unacceptable incidence of coughing and laryngospasm.[8] Halothane is therefore preferred if inhalational induction is necessary.

As soon as possible ventilation can be manually assisted, although hyperventilation does not predictably prevent the cerebrovasodilatory effects of volatile anaesthetics in the presence of brain pathology.[9][10] Inhalational induction with desflurane has a similar profile to isoflurane.[11][12] Sevoflurane may become the inhalational agent of choice in neuroanaesthesia in view of its favourable induction characteristics, although its effects on cerebral physiology are similar to those of isoflurane.[13-18] As soon as the child is unresponsive, venous access can be acquired, anaesthesia deepened with intravenous agents, and intubation facilitated with neuromuscular blocking agents.

Anaesthesia can be maintained with a balanced or total intravenous technique. The possible presence of an increased ICP is the primary consideration that dictates choice of anaesthetic technique. A combination of intravenous opioids, a moderate concentration of isoflurane (0·5–1 vol %), with intermittently higher concentrations if required, and muscle relaxation is a valuable choice.[19] Nitrous oxide can be used in the absence of air pockets, although the possibility that CBF could be increased must be taken into consideration.[20]

Total intravenous anaesthesia with propofol, opioids, and a neuromuscular blocking agent is a good alternative, although the use of propofol infusions in children is questionable, especially in infants. Although the movement disorders occasionally observed during induction of anaesthesia with propofol are probably not epileptogenic in origin,[21] longer lasting neurological dysfunction has been described following the termination of propofol

216

infusions used for sedation in intensive care, as well as after use of a brief period of anaesthesia in an 18 year old patient.[22][23] Five cases of metabolic acidosis and fatal myocardial failure have been reported in children with respiratory infections who received prolonged, high dose infusions of propofol for sedation during mechanical ventilation.[24] Prolonged propofol infusions should probably not be used in paediatric patients until more data on safety are available, and careful attention to aseptic technique is required if a propofol infusion is used. Induction with propofol produces a smaller blood pressure decrease in children than in adults, and likewise blood pressure is better maintained during induction with propofol compared with halothane, although the incidence of respiratory obstruction is lower.[25] Nevertheless, concomitant use of propofol, alfentanil, and suxamethonium (succinylcholine) warrants careful monitoring for hypotension and bradycardia.[26] Vagal mediated reflexes to surgical stimulation may be prominent.[27]

The fast recovery and the low incidence of postoperative vomiting are beneficial characteristics of propofol anaesthesia in neurosurgery. The use of total intravenous anaesthesia may also be advantageous when space for anaesthesia machines is limited and during patient transportation.[28] The pharmacokinetic and pharmacodynamic properties of propofol are somewhat different from the properties in adults. When compared with adults, this translates not only into higher induction and maintenance blood concentrations, but also into relatively higher dose and infusion rate requirements to obtain these concentrations.[29] When using computer controlled infusion devices, these need to be programmed using pharmacokinetic data from a similar age population to avoid systematic overprediction of propofol blood concentrations.[30]

Although fentanyl is still widely used, the pharmacokinetic properties of alfentanil and sufentanil make these drugs more suitable for continuous intravenous administration as a component of a total intravenous anaesthetic technique. Alfentanil has been demonstrated not to increase ICP in children with hydrocephalus during isoflurane–nitrous oxide anaesthesia.[31] Vecuronium provides excellent cardiovascular stability and produces little histamine release, but the dose–response relationship might be a little unpredictable in smaller children, necessitating the use of neuromuscular monitoring for guidance of dosing. Atracurium has a very predictable elimination and duration of action, and is an excellent choice in infants.

Ideally, normothermia (36·0–36·5°C) should be maintained by preventing heat loss, warming of respirator gases, use of hot air mattresses, and inline perfusion warming devices. When surgical difficulties are expected, however, lowering brain temperature to 33–34°C may have a cerebral protective effect in the event of compromised cerebral perfusion.[32][33] This degree of hypothermia can be easily achieved by avoiding measures to prevent heat loss. Hyperthermia must be avoided, because it has been demonstrated that it increases neurological deficit in the presence of brain ischaemia in animal studies.[32] [34] [35]

Neurosurgical procedures in children often involve large amounts of blood loss, as a result of the relatively large size of the head. On the other hand, blood loss is often difficult to measure during neurosurgery. Large transfusions are not uncommon and sufficient care must be taken to replace clotting factors and to avoid hyperkalaemia and hypocalcaemia. Rapid transfusion of large amounts of blood may produce severe hypothermia, making the use of blood warming devices mandatory.

Hyperglycaemia has been associated with adverse outcome in the presence of brain ischaemia. In adult patients sugar containing solutions are often avoided during neurosurgery. In children, who often have depleted glycogen stores as a result of preoperative vomiting and fasting, this practice may provoke hypoglycaemia. Careful monitoring of the glycaemia and the administration of appropriate glucose containing solutions is necessary.[36]

Neurosurgical procedures in infants and children

The most commonly performed neurosurgical procedures in neonates (less than 44 weeks' gestation) are closure of spina bifida or encephaloceles, drainage of hydrocephalus, and elevation of fractures caused by delivery (table 9.2). Although emergency surgery for neural tube defects is unnecessary, unless for uncovered lesions, early surgery is recommended to diminish the risk of rupture of the coverings and infection. Care should be taken to

Table 9.2 Common paediatric neurosurgical problems and associated anaesthetic considerations

Age group	Neurosurgical lesion	Anaesthetic problem
Neonatal	Intaventricular haemorrhage Skull fracture	Prematurity Associated oedema
Infant	Meningocele, meningomyelocele, encephalocele	Positioning, blood loss, hypothermia, postoperative ICP increase
	Arnold–Chiari malformation	Brain stem compression, high ICP
	Craniosynostoses, craniofacial dysostoses	Long procedures, high blood loss, hypothermia, venous air embolism, brain tissue damage
	Vascular malformations	High blood loss, hypothermia, deliberate hypotension
	Trauma, haematoma, brain oedema	Antioedema therapy, deliberate moderate hypothermia (?)
Older children	Posterior fossa tumours	High ICP, brain stem compression, haemodynamic instability, respiratory control, cranial nerve dysfunction, sitting versus prone position, venous air embolism

avoid pressure on the lesion during intubation and installation of the patient. Tube defects may cause considerable fluid losses, which should be taken into account when calculating intraoperative fluid requirements. The administration of glucose containing fluids is necessary to avoid hypoglycaemia. The use of opioids should be avoided, because the risk of postoperative apnoea, which is already elevated in infants, may be increased by the neurological condition of the patient. Hydrocephalus often develops following closure of spinal defects, necessitating secondary interventions.

Surgical treatment of hydrocephalus is the most common neurosurgical intervention in children. Hydrocephalus is often secondary to intracranial infection or haemorrhage. Ventriculoperitoneal shunt insertion is the treatment of choice. In the presence of intraperitoneal pathology, temporary external drainage may be indicated. Ventriculoatrial shunts are seldom used because of the risk of bacterial endocarditis in the event of shunt infection.

Malignant tumours of the CNS are the second most frequent malignancy in children. Most brain tumours occur in the posterior fossa. Although in many centres these procedures are performed in the prone position, many surgeons prefer the sitting position, because of the decrease in blood loss as a result of the improved venous drainage. The sitting position carries an increased risk for venous air embolism and mandates the use of monitoring techniques that are sensitive enough to detect its development at an early stage. The incidence of emboli causing cardiovascular instability can be considered sufficiently low to justify the continued use of the sitting position.[37]

Craniosynostosis is the result of the premature fusion of bone sutures, and can be treated by surgical correction of the cranial vault, usually during the first six months of life. These procedures often involve major blood loss. When the base of the skull or the facial bones are involved in the process, perioperative airway management can be extremely cumbersome. Postoperative treatment in a paediatric intensive care unit is mandatory for complex cases.

Trans-sphenoidal hypophysectomy

Endocrine dysfunction

Pituitary pathology causes overproduction and/or decreased secretion of hormones. Symptoms are usually caused by disturbances in the production of hormones by those organs that are dependent on the regulatory influence of the pituitary gland. Suprasellar involvement may cause visual disturbances. Excessive production of growth hormone can result in hypertension, cardiomyopathy, and diabetes mellitus. Airway management may be difficult in acromegalic patients. Cushing's disease is the result of excessive secretion of cortisol secondary to the excessive production of adrenocorticotrophic hormone (ACTH), and may cause diabetes mellitus, hypertension, secondary hyperaldosteronism with electrolyte disturbances, and mild congestive heart failure. Any hypertension, diabetes, or electrolyte disturbances secondary to hormonal abnormalities should be corrected before surgery. Patients with pituitary hormone deficiencies will usually be on replacement therapy when presenting for surgery. In the event of hyposecretion of ACTH, glucocorticoid replacement should be started preoperatively and continued during the whole perioperative period.

Hypocortisolaemia predisposes to hypoglycaemia, hypotension, and hypothermia. Regular blood sugar monitoring is mandatory. Intraoperative thyroid hormone replacement is rarely needed, and treatment may be interrupted during the period in which oral intake is not permitted. If necessary, triiodothyronine 5–20 μg may be administered intravenously and repeated every 12 hours. Although hormonal substitution therapy for the pituitary dependent organs will be required following hypophyseal resection, administration of cortisol is usually sufficient in the early postoperative phase.[38] Additional hormone substitution is usually necessary after the first 48 hours.

Deficient secretion of antidiuretic hormone can cause the development of diabetes insipidus, particularly when the resection involves the suprasellar region. The diagnosis should be suspected if urine production is abnormally large (table 9.3). Clinical confirmation can be obtained when the high urine output persists whereas the infusion of fluids is temporarily restricted. A ratio of urine and serum osmolality lower than 1, and urine osmolality lower than 50–100 mosmol/kg, are typical findings. Postoperative diabetes insipidus occurs in 10–20% of the patients and is usually a self limiting condition. Adequate fluid replacement is often the only therapy required. The volume of fluids to be administered per hour is the sum of the normal maintenance requirement plus the previous hour's urine output. If plasma hyperosmolality is already present, the water deficit should be calculated. Replacement of half the deficit should proceed, after which the need for further therapy is re-evaluated. Hormonal treatment may be necessary if the pathological condition is prolonged. The parenteral administration of 2–4 μg desmopressin acetate, repeated 12 hourly, is usually efficacious.[39]

Table 9.3 Diagnosis of diabetes insipidus

Clinical signs	Polyuria (>200–300 ml/h)
Laboratory investigations	Hypernatraemia ($Na^+ > 150$ mmol/l)
	Serum hyperosmolality (>300 mosmol/kg)
	Decreased urine osmolality (50–100 mosmol/kg)
	Specific gravity of urine $1\cdot001$–$1\cdot005$

Surgical technique and anaesthetic management

The trans-sphenoidal approach to the sella turcica and the immediate suprasellar region has greatly facilitated the surgical treatment of hypophyseal tumours (fig 9.1). Specific problems of the trans-sphenoidal approach involve the position of the airway near the surgical field, the use of adrenaline (epinephrine) containing solutions to improve haemostasis, the proximity of the optic chiasma, and the position of the carotid arteries just lateral to the surgical site, particularly in the suprasellar area. As the airway is located close to the surgical field, the use of a reinforced or preformed endotracheal tube, secured to the lower jaw, is recommended. Aspiration of blood and debris from the pharynx into the lower airways can be prevented by "packing" the throat with gauzes and carefully clearing the mouth and pharynx before extubation. The use of anaesthetic agents that increase the sensitivity of the myocardium to catecholamines should be avoided. In the absence of signs of increased ICP, manoeuvres to decrease brain volume are usually unnecessary with the trans-sphenoidal approach, and may even be contraindicated because they could cause the pituitary gland to retreat upwards out of the sella. Surgical damage to the optical tract is less likely during trans-sphenoidal surgery, because extrasellar invasion of the tumoral process is less

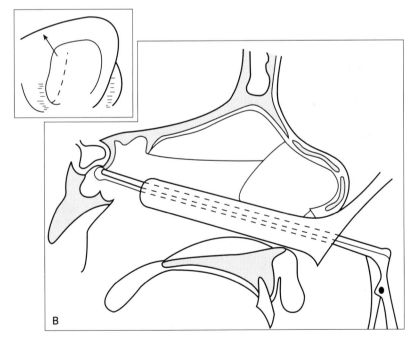

Fig 9.1 Trans-sphenoidal approach to the sella turcica. (Reproduced with permission from Aranciba CU, Frost EAM, Transsphenoidal access. In: Frost EAM, ed, *Clinical anesthesia in neurosurgery*. Borough Green: Butterworths, 1984)

likely. Although very sensitive to the effects of anaesthetic agents, visual evoked potential monitoring may be helpful for the early detection of visual tract damage during pituitary surgery.[40] Intracranial carotid artery bleeding is a rare, though often fatal, complication of trans-sphenoidal surgery.

Infratentorial surgery

The infratentorial part of the brain includes the midbrain, the pons, the medulla, the brain stem, the fourth ventricle with the respiratory and cardiovascular centres in its floor, the lower cranial nerves, and the cerebellum (fig 9.2). Posterior fossa pathology may interfere with the circulation of the CSF and thereby cause supratentorial hydrocephalus. Ultimately, extension of the volume of the infratentorial content will cause coning, most often into the foramen magnum. Less commonly, reverse coning occurs where the posterior fossa content is displaced upward through the tentorial hiatus.

Anaesthetic management

The anaesthetic management of posterior fossa surgery follows the general principles of neuroanaesthesia. Special considerations for infratentorial surgery, however, pertain to the region of the CNS involved and to the positioning of the patient during surgery. Surgery involves brain areas that

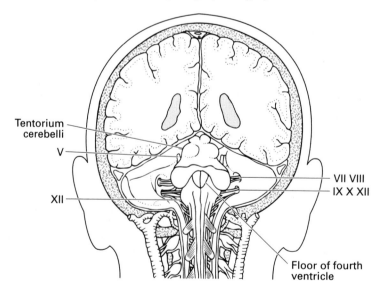

Fig 9.2 Contents of the posterior fossa (posterior view with the cerebellum removed). (Reproduced with permission from Ingram GS, Walters FJM. Anaesthesia for posterior fossa surgery. In: *Anaesthesia and intensive care for the neurosurgical patient*, 2nd edn. Oxford: Blackwell Scientific, 1994: 213)

control the airway, respiration, and the autonomic nervous system (fig. 9.3). Sudden haemodynamic instability and disturbance of the cardiac rhythm may occur as a result of surgical manipulations of the vagal nerve, and of the autonomic nervous centres in the floor of the fourth ventricle and the medullary reticular formation. Hypertension may also result from stimulation of the trigeminal nerve. The need for prompt detection necessitates the use of invasive blood pressure monitoring. Interrupting surgical manipulation is usually efficacious although drug treatment could be required. Respiratory regulation centres are situated in the vicinity of the cardiovascular centre and damage may result in apnoea or inadequate breathing. To avoid intraoperative damage some surgeons prefer to perform the critical parts of the operation while the patient is breathing spontaneously, breathing pattern abnormalities serving as a warning sign. The inevitable increase in carbon dioxide tension may, however, result in poor operative conditions. Brain stem auditory evoked potentials may also be used as an intraoperative monitor of brain stem function.[41]

After the operation, consciousness and respiratory function should be carefully evaluated before extubation. The function of the cranial nerves involved in airway patency and airway reflexes should be tested. The possibility of a necessary reintubation must be envisaged.

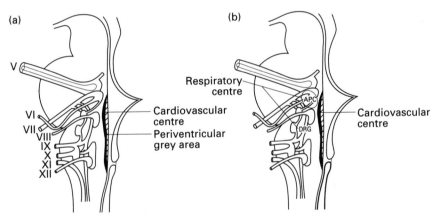

Fig 9.3 The pons and medulla containing the fifth to twelfth cranial nerves and nuclei, the cardiovascular centre and the respiratory centre represented by the apneustic centre (APC) and the dorsal group of neurons (DRG). (Reproduced from Ingram GS, Walters FJM. Pons and medulla. In: *Anaesthesia and intensive care for the neurosurgical patient*, 2nd edn. Oxford: Blackwell Scientific, 1994: 230)

Position of the patient

Infratentorial surgery can be performed in the prone, lateral, or sitting position. When the prone position is used, care must be taken to ensure free

223

movement of the abdomen to decrease the risk of venous thrombosis, to decrease intrathoracic pressure, and to promote venous return. Surgical access to the midline structures is good, but visibility may be obscured by blood running down in the surgical field. The lateral position is usually referred to as the "park-bench position." It is indicated particularly for surgery of the cerebellopontine angle. Traction is often exerted on the upper arm to improve access, although excessive traction may cause injury to the brachial plexus. The neck is flexed and rotated, excessive rotation of the head possibly causing obstruction of venous drainage.

Although the sitting position offers the advantage of excellent surgical exposure and improved venous drainage, it imposes specific risks.[42–44] Moving the patient into the sitting position may cause haemodynamic instability, especially in older patients with cardiovascular disease. Postoperative quadriplegia is a rare complication, but may result from extreme flexion of the neck or insufficient intraoperative CPP.[45] Pneumocephalus is defined as the presence of air in the cranium and is often present in the cerebral convexity when the sitting position is used. This condition may develop into a tension pneumocephalus, when the intracranial content expands, or when the air pocket expands as a result of diffusion of nitrous oxide.[46–48] Tension pneumocephalus can cause intraoperative intracranial hypertension, delayed awakening, or postoperative deterioration of the neurological condition.

Venous air embolism

The most feared complication of the sitting position is, however, venous air embolism, which can be detected in as many as 40% of the patients.[42–44] Although venous air embolism may develop into a life threatening condition, mortality or the postoperative morbidity associated with it is relatively infrequent if all measures for a timely detection and adequate treatment are used.[49]

Venous air embolism results from entrainment of air into open vessels, especially non-collapsed veins, and may occur whenever the venous pressure is lower than the atmospheric pressure. Typically, venous air embolism is the result of the continuous entrapment of repeated small quantities of air. As the entrapment of air bubbles continues, pulmonary artery pressure increases. Eventually an airlock of right ventricular outflow develops. Failure of the right ventricle ultimately impairs left ventricular function. In patients with a patent foramen ovale, air may pass into the left ventricle and the cerebral or coronary circulation, if the right atrial pressure increases above the left atrial pressure.[50] This condition is known as paradoxical air embolism and can be detected by transoesophageal echocardiography in 15% of cases of venous air embolism.[51] Although paradoxical air embolism may result in brain infarction or myocardial ischaemia, the consequences are benign in most cases.

The relative sensitivity of the available monitors to detect venous air embolism is described in fig 9.4. The most sensitive methods are the use of precordial Doppler ultrasonography and transoesophageal echocardiography.[52–54] Although changes in haemodynamic and respiratory parameters are insensitive indicators of early venous air embolism, invasive arterial monitoring and right atrial catheterisation are necessary tools to evaluate the haemodynamic consequences of extensive venous air embolism. Arterial desaturation and a sudden, important decrease in end expiratory carbon dioxide tension, which are readily detectable by pulse oximetry and capnography, are relatively early predictors of an impending haemodynamic catastrophe. Treatment of venous air embolism consists of flooding the operation wound with saline, discontinuing the administration of nitrous oxide, and aspirating the right atrial catheter. By this last manoeuvre it is sometimes possible to remove a quantity of air out of the right heart. The usefulness and safety of applying positive end expiratory pressure (PEEP) and bilateral jugular compression to increase the intracranial venous pressure is debated.[55 56] If the entrapment of air continues or leads to major haemodynamic instability the patient should be moved into the horizontal position.

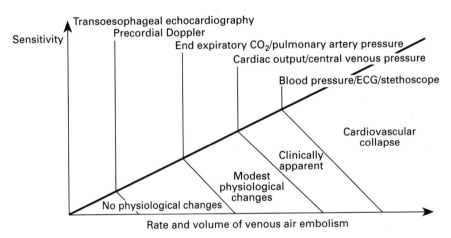

Fig 9.4 Relative potency of the available monitors for the detection of venous air embolism

Stereotactic procedures

Stereotactic surgical techniques are increasingly employed to obtain biopsies from tissues in deep or functionally important areas of the brain, and

225

to make discrete neural lesions for pain relief, for control of movement disorders, or, rarely, for treatment of psychiatric disorders. Other indications include implantation of dopamine secreting neurons for Parkinson's disease and of electrostimulation electrodes for intractable pain. During stereotactic surgery, instruments are directed to specific areas of the brain using the relationship of the position of the target zone to intracerebral landmarks or an extracranial reference device. Often intraoperative radiological procedures, for example, computed tomography or magnetic resonance imaging, are needed, necessitating patient transport to the radiology facilities.

Anaesthetic management

Most stereotactic procedures are performed under local anaesthesia in the conscious patient, the role of the anaesthetist being confined to providing mild sedation and monitoring for adverse reactions.[57-59] General anaesthesia is an alternative, and a total intravenous anaesthetic technique can greatly facilitate patient transportation. Moreover, increases in ICP can be avoided in patients with brain tumours and decreased intracranial compliance.

Total intravenous anaesthesia obviates the need for nitrous oxide, which is a definite advantage for operations in the sitting position, which carry an increased risk of venous air embolism, or when air encephalography is used to identify the lateral ventricles. The most frequently observed adverse reactions are vagal overstimulation and orthostatic hypotension. Convulsions, venous air embolism, and intracranial haemorrhage with neurological deterioration are rare events needing prompt treatment. Pulse oximetry, non-invasive blood pressure measurement, electrocardiography, and venous access are mandatory. Capnography is required for procedures under general anaesthesia. The precordial Doppler monitor is a useful tool to detect venous air embolism for procedures in the sitting position. Equipment for emergency airway control must always be available.

During some stereotactic procedures under general anaesthesia, it may be required to wake the patient up for neurological evaluation. Intravenous anaesthesia with propofol and alfentanil, eventually in combination with nitrous oxide, is a valuable technique for this purpose. The infusions of propofol and alfentanil are titrated to the minimum requirements. When it is time to wake the patient up, the administration of propofol and nitrous oxide is discontinued. If necessary, depending on the intensity of pain, the infusion of alfentanil may be continued, eventually at a lower infusion rate. This technique allows communication with a fully cooperative and calm patient 10 minutes after stopping the propofol infusion.

Thermocoagulation of Gasser's ganglion

Thermocoagulation of Gasser's ganglion is often an efficient therapy for neuralgia of the trigeminal nerve. Usually short repeated periods of unconsciousness are required, the patient being cooperative intermittently for the purpose of testing the electrode position. In addition, access to the airway is limited and endotracheal intubation unnecessary. Introduction of the electrode into the ganglion may provoke pronounced sympathetic and vagal pain reactions, which can be blunted by administering catecholamine receptor blocking drugs, for example, labetalol, and atropine. Intermittent unconsciousness is produced by a short acting hypnotic, for example, propofol or methohexitone (methohexital).

Neuroradiological procedures

The role of the anaesthetist in the neuroradiology department involves providing life support for injured or intensive care patients and sedation or anaesthesia during diagnostic or interventional procedures. Anaesthesia and sedation techniques for neuroradiology must be based on the same principles as anaesthesia for neurosurgery, because most of these patients are subject to the same pathophysiological changes. Although neuroradiology of the brain used to be confined to air encephalography, contrast ventriculography, and angiography, computed tomography has become the most important diagnostic tool since its introduction in 1973. Improvements in catheter technology have opened the rapidly developing field of interventional, therapeutic procedures during the last decade. Since the late 1980s magnetic resonance imaging (MRI) has become more widely available, providing an invaluable diagnostic tool for many pathological conditions. Interventional neuroradiology and the special environment of the MRI setting generate the greatest challenges for the anaesthetist. This discussion will focus on the special problems related to these two subjects.

Interventional neuroradiology

Although the principles of endovascular treatment of neurovascular lesions have been described more than 20 years ago, during the past decade the development of novel materials and techniques has opened the way for enormous progress in the field of interventional neuroradiology. Interventional neuroradiology includes therapeutic embolisation of cerebral aneurysms and cerebral or spinal arteriovenous malformations, sclerotherapy of venous angiomas, ballon angioplasty of occlusive cerebrovascular disease or vasospasm secondary to aneurysmal subarachnoid haemorrhage, embolisation for epistaxis, and intra-arterial chemotherapy of head and neck tumours.[60–68]

Anaesthetic management
Anaesthetic considerations for interventional neuroradiology have recently

227

been reviewed.[69] Many procedures can be performed under local anaesthesia and sedation, although for some procedures general anaesthesia is preferred. The role of the anaesthetist is not, however, confined to providing sedation or anaesthesia. The neuroanaesthetist has a key role in manipulating systemic and cerebral haemodynamics. An important role for the anaesthetist therefore lies in the prevention and management of morbidity and mortality associated with interventional neuroradiology. The risks are very similar to the risks encountered during neurosurgical procedures, for example, aneurysmal rupture, intracerebral bleeding, vasospasm, and cerebral ischaemia. Although the neurological complication rate differs with the kind of procedure, the risk of single cerebral angiography has been estimated at between 1% and 10%.[70 71]

Important aspects of the preanaesthetic evaluation include history of allergic reactions, especially to contrast material, and anticoagulant therapy. A full neurological history and examination are mandatory. As manipulation of the blood pressure may be required, the patient's normal blood pressure should be assessed.

Premedication with anxiolytic drugs can be considered in patients with normal consciousness. The addition of antiemetic drugs is useful because nausea and vomiting can interfere dramatically with the procedure, especially in sedated patients.

Although this practice has not yet been documented as effective, prophylaxis of cerebral ischaemia and prevention of cerebral vasospasm with nimodipine are possible options, because of the possible benefit in the event of ischaemic stroke and subarachnoid haemorrhage.[72–75]

As many of these procedures take several hours, it is essential to get the patient in a comfortable position. Monitoring includes five lead ECG, automated blood pressure monitoring, and pulse oximetry. A pulse oximeter probe placed on the toe of the leg with the femoral artery catheter can give an early indication of femoral artery obstruction or embolisation. Capnography serves as a warning sign of airway obstruction in sedated patients and is considered mandatory in anaesthetised patients. As manipulation of systemic haemodynamics with vasoactive drugs is often necessary, invasive blood pressure monitoring is advisable for many procedures. This can be obtained from the introducer sheath placed in the femoral artery by the radiologist or from a separate radial artery cannulation. Additionally, the pressure tracing from the coaxial catheter in the carotid or vertebral artery can be monitored to detect thrombus formation and vascular spasm. Monitoring the pressure from the tip of the superselective or balloon catheter can be useful during embolisation of intracranial arteriovenous malformations and during carotid occlusions ("stump pressure").

Repeated assessment of the neurological condition is the simplest method of detecting problems caused by vessel manipulation or temporary or permanent embolisation. The basic anaesthetic approach is therefore conscious sedation. When the procedure is performed under general anaesthesia, it is often required to wake the patient up during the procedure. Intravenous anaesthesia with propofol, eventually in combination with alfentanil, is a valuable technique for this purpose, allowing fast and smooth awakening of the patient. Alternatively or additionally, some method of CNS monitoring may be used. Technical modalities depend on the indication for the procedure and may include EEG, sensory and motor evoked potentials, transcranial Doppler ultrasonography, and CBF measurement.

Sedative techniques are aimed at alleviating anxiety and discomfort, improving patient immobility, and decreasing pain. The level of sedation should be readily reversible, and all patients should receive supplemental oxygen. A sedative infusion of propofol 10–50 μg/kg per min, for example, may provide suitable conditions. Alternatively, midazolam 3–5 mg and droperidol 2·5–5 mg may be used. A small dose of an opioid, for example, fentanyl 2–4 μg/kg, may be added before infiltration with local anaesthetic or injection of contrast, which usually causes some discomfort. Dysphoria or disorientation is a potential problem with sedative techniques and may greatly interfere with the requirement of immobility. Airway obstruction must be avoided.

The choice of general anaesthesia is dictated by the patient's age and general condition; in addition, some procedures are preferably performed under general anaesthesia. In view of its rapid reversibility and its suitable neurophysiological qualities, intravenous anaesthesia with propofol is a reasonable choice.[76 77] The possible presence of air bubbles in the arterial circulation can be considered a relative contraindication for the use of nitrous oxide, although hard data to support this argument are lacking.

For some procedures movement caused by positive pressure ventilation may interfere with high quality imaging. This problem can be circumvented by intermittent apnoea or by low tidal volume, high rate ventilation. If available, high frequency jet ventilation may offer an ideal solution.

Anticoagulation

To prevent thromboembolic complications, partial heparinisation is usually required during the procedure. The dose of heparin can be adjusted with the help of repeated measurements of the activated clotting time. The target is a two or threefold prolongation of the baseline activated clotting time. It may be necessary to continue the antithrombotic treatment during the first night after the procedure. The femoral introducer sheath is best left in place until normalisation of coagulation.

Haemodynamic interventions

Controlled hypotension is sometimes requested, for example, to test the safety of carotid occlusion or to keep the glue in place during the obliteration of arteriovenous malformations. Hypotensive agents used should have minimal effects on the cerebral vessels. Both sodium nitroprusside and glyceryl trinitrate (nitroglycerin) have the theoretical potential to introduce cerebral steal. Both drugs interfere with normal autoregulation, and may increase ICP in patients with a pre-existing reduction of intracranial compliance, thereby decreasing CPP, especially as the skull remains closed.[78-82]

Esmolol, which for the purpose of inducing deliberate hypotension may be administered, for example, as a bolus of 1 mg/kg followed by a continuous infusion at 0·5 mg/kg per min, is free of cerebral vasodilating properties.[83-85] Labetalol can be used as an adjunct or an alternative.[86] A useful and safe adjunctive treatment is urapidil;[87-89] it is a relatively short acting α receptor blocking agent with central nervous system serotonin (5-hydroxytryptamine) $5HT_{1A}$ receptor activity, which attenuates reflex tachycardia.

In the event of cerebral ischaemia it may be useful to augment the blood pressure by 30–40% compared with baseline (deliberate hypertension) in an attempt to increase the collateral flow through the circle of Willis and through the pial to pial anastomoses.[90] Augmentation of the collateral flow through the circle of Willis may increase the flow to an ischaemic zone when a carotid or vertebral artery is obstructed. An increase of flow through the pial to pial anastomoses may increase the perfusion of watershed areas, which are the boundary zones between vascular territories. Phenylephrine (1 μg/kg followed by a titrated infusion), eventually in combination with dopamine or dobutamine 2–10 μg/kg per min is usually effective. Deliberate hypertension may produce imbalance of the myocardial oxygen supply/demand ratio, and the patients should be carefully monitored for myocardial ischaemia.

Hypercapnia is sometimes useful to increase intracranial venous outflow when agents are injected into the venous circulation. It must be avoided in patients with decreased intracranial compliance.

Complications

Success of the management of neurological catastrophes depends largely on the communication of the anaesthetist, radiologist, and neurologist or neurosurgeon, and on the availability of a preplanned strategy.[91-93] When neurological problems are suspected, the anaesthetist should immediately alert the radiologist. The first priority is to secure the airway and preserve gas exchange. Eventually, thiopentone (thiopental) and a neuromuscular blocking agent are administered if the patient has not been intubated. The first branch in the decision making tree is to decide whether the problem is haemorrhagic or occlusive—this is usually obvious from the radiological image. If the problem is bleeding, blood pressure should be lowered immediately and anticoagulation reversed.

Thiopentone is a good choice as a first line, pressure lowering agent because it prevents seizures. The potential neuroprotective effect of thiopentone is debatable. When the bleeding is stopped, for example, by obliteration of the bleeding vessel, blood pressure normalisation, or even augmentation, should be considered, because the condition may revert to ischaemia. In the situation of vascular occlusion, blood pressure augmentation should be attempted to increase distal flow. Eventually, the radiologist may succeed in reopening the vessel by thrombolysis. The possibility of urgent neurosurgical treatment of the lesion must be considered. Further therapy includes placing the patient in a neutral 15° head up position and administering intravenous antiepileptic agents. Hyperventilation to $Paco_2$ of 2·66–2·46 kPa (26–20 mm Hg), intravenous mannitol, and a thiopentone infusion to produce EEG burst suppression may be used to decrease ICP. Lowering the body temperature to 33–34°C may offer some degree of neuroprotection.[32-33]

Complications may not only arise during the procedure but are not infrequent during the first 24 hours. Therefore, those patients who have undergone intracranial procedures should be observed in the intensive care unit during the first night. The neurological status should be followed rigorously and the haemodynamic and antithrombotic therapy continued if necessary.

Magnetic resonance imaging

Atoms with a net electrical charge, for example, hydrogen, are aligned in the presence of an extrinsic magnetic field (0·15–2 tesla or T). When the atoms are then subjected to a radiofrequency pulse, the orientation of the atoms is deflected. When the radiofrequency pulse is removed, the nuclei rotate back into alignment with the static magnetic field and the energy is released. This released energy is translated into the magnetic resonance image (MRI). As MRI requires immobility of the patient, deep sedation or anaesthesia is necessary for uncooperative patients.

Technical considerations

The presence of high strength magnetic fields imposes specific challenges with regard to electrical monitors and anaesthesia equipment.[94-96] Additional problems are the noise and poor access to the patient. The presence of non-compatible anaesthesia equipment can greatly disturb the quality of the images. Electrical connections to the patient and wire leads act as antennas and introduce radiofrequency signals that can distort the image. Another source of image distortion are the magnetic fields created by the electronics within the monitors.

All ferromagnetic material components will be propelled and may endanger the patient and personnel. All necessary equipment that contains ferromagnetic elements must be firmly secured to the walls or the floor and be kept as distant as possible from the magnet. Safe metals include nickel, stainless steel, alloys, tantalum, and titanium.

A potential problem is radiofrequency heating from induced currents.

231

Although no clinical signs of core body heating have been reported, voltage induced in wire leads and skin electrodes has been reported to cause severe burns.

Monitors are affected by the magnetic field that distorts and displaces the image of the display. Most ECG artefacts cannot be eliminated. Several compatible monitoring systems with good artefact suppression as well as non-ferromagnetic respirators are now commercially available. New technology is mostly based on fibreoptic signal transmission, the use of non-ferromagnetic materials (for example, graphite), "signal gating," and the use of signal filters. Infusion pumps may be subject to malfunction; they should be placed as far as possible from the magnet and secured firmly. The unavailability of special magnetic resonance compatible equipment must never be a reason for unsafe anaesthetic practice. If a particular monitor is judged to be mandatory for safe anaesthetic practice in the operation room, it should also be used in the radiology department, especially as access to the patient and visibility are limited.

Anaesthetic technique

Every anaesthetic technique that is suitable for the neuropathological condition of the patient can be applied. Sedation techniques are often adequate. Care must, however, be taken to prevent respiratory depression, especially in neurosurgical patients. Airway management is often easier and safer under general anaesthesia than under deep sedation. Nevertheless, even in children, light propofol anaesthesia without intubation can be used safely, if performed by an anaesthetist and if the patient is monitored extensively.[97 98] Only a non-ferromagnetic (plastic) laryngoscope should be used for intubation. A laryngeal mask may offer a suitable alternative to orotracheal intubation in anaesthetised patients.[99] A long Mapleson D circuit provides the best conditions for artificial ventilation because of its light weight and flexibility.

Spinal surgery

Spinal surgery involves surgical procedures on the spinal nervous system and the vertebral column, which are of common interest to orthopaedic surgeons and neurosurgeons. Special anaesthetic problems relate to patient positioning, intubation of patients with cervical spine pathology, and anaesthesia for patients with muscle paralysis.

When the anterior approach is used for surgery on the cervical spine, possible complications include vagal nerve stimulation, damage to the laryngeal recurrent nerve, swallowing disturbances, and tracheal compression caused by haematoma formation. Interventions in the thoracic or lumbosacral area are mostly performed with the patient in the prone position.

232

Rarely, the "park bench position" is preferred. Thoracic disc pathology might necessitate an anterior approach through a thoracotomy or a costo-transversectomy. The risks of installing an unconscious patient in the prone position should not be underestimated.[100] Some have therefore advocated getting the patients to position themselves before inducing anaesthesia, especially in the presence of an unstable cervical spine.[101] This practice does not, however, prevent damage resulting from prolonged malpositioning.

The prone position carries an increased risk of eye damage. The eyes should be taped with waterproof tape to prevent direct contact with the cornea and conjunctiva. Any pressure on the eyeball must be scrupulously avoided because it may result in blindness. Hyperextension of the neck must be avoided because it could cause cervical spine compression. Excessive torsion of the neck may result in jugular compression or carotid artery obstruction. The abdominal contents should hang freely to avoid increases in the venous pressure in the lumbar venous plexus. Venous air embolism appears to be extremely rare during spinal surgery. Prolonged pressure on peripheral nerves can result in postoperative paresis or paralysis.

The unstable cervical spine

Injury to the spinal cord during intubation and positioning is a major concern in patients with pathology of the cervical spine.[102–105] Some advocate conscious fibreoptic intubation. This approach may not, however, be necessary in every patient. If normal active mobilisation of the cervical spine is possible and there are no airway abnormalities or radiological signs of spine displacement, normal induction and intubation can be performed, eventually with simple axial traction. If difficulties with airway management are expected, however, conscious fibreoptic intubation is preferable. In the presence of a truly unstable spine, intubation under general anaesthesia with traction in the direction of the normal spinal axis, carefully avoiding extension of the neck, may be employed, although the safety of this technique is debatable.[106] Alternatively, blind nasotracheal or fibreoptic intubation can be performed either under local anaesthesia with sedation or under general anaesthesia. It may be necessary to reawaken the patient and re-evaluate the neurological condition before proceeding with surgery.

Quadriplegia

The intraoperative management of quadriplegic patients with symptoms of spinal shock necessitates the use of invasive haemodynamic monitoring, and involves correction of the intravascular volume, judicious use of cardiosupportive medication, and vasopressors. Stimulation under the level of spinal cord transection may elicit massive autonomic responses, causing severe hypertension, often accompanied by reflex bradycardia. Sometimes the autonomic response is associated with vasoconstriction below and vasodilatation above the lesion. Pulmonary oedema, arrhythmias, myocardial ischaemia, and acute heart failure may occur. A sufficient level of anaesthesia is usually adequate in preventing autonomic hyperreflexia. Locoregional anaesthesia has also been advocated.[107-109] The use of depolarising neuromuscular blocking agents in patients with muscle denervation may result in a rise in serum potassium concentration sufficient to cause cardiac arrest.[110]

Monitoring of neuronal integrity

Somatosensory and motor evoked potentials can be useful tools to evaluate the integrity of the neuronal pathways during manipulation of an unstable spine or during surgery of the spinal cord or its blood supply. Volatile anaesthetics profoundly interfere with reliable evoked potential monitoring. Intravenous anaesthetic techniques using propofol and opioids yield more satisfactory recordings.[111 112]

Summary

Paediatric patients are scheduled for a wide variety of neurosurgical interventions. The anaesthetist should be familiar with paediatric anaesthesia as well as with the age related differences in neurophysiology.

Diaseases of the pituitary gland cause endocrine abnormalities which should be carefully assessed preoperatively, and detected and treated postoperatively. Although it is a relatively non-invasive surgical technique, the trans-sphenoidal approach imposes some specific anaesthetic requirements.

Important aspects of infratentorial surgery are the involvement of essential brain areas and the choice of position of the patient. Venous air embolism is a possible life threatening complication of the sitting position.

Stereotactic procedures are greatly facilitated by an easily reversible sedative or anaesthetic technique. The development of short acting drugs, in particular propofol, has greatly enhanced the ability of anaesthetists to fulfil these requirements.

One of the most important recent developments in the field of neurosurgery is the introduction of new diagnostic and interventional radiological techniques. The special environment of MRI and the radiological treatment of cerebrovascular disease impose new challenges on anaesthetic management.

Careful patient positioning, intubation technique for patients with an unstable cervical spine, and the management of patients with extensive dysfunction of the spinal cord deserve special attention.

1 Cross KW, Dear PRF, Hathorn MKS, *et al.* An estimation of intracranial blood flow in the new-born infant. *J Physiol* 1979; **289**: 329–45.
2 Younkin DP, Reivich M, Jaggi J, Obrist W, Delivoria-Papadopoulos M. Noninvasive method of estimating human newborn regional cerebral blood flow. *J Cereb Blood Flow Metab* 1982; **2**: 415–20.
3 Kennedy C, Sokoloff L. An adaptation of the nitrous oxide method to the study of the cerebral circulation in children: normal values of cerebral blood flow and cerebral metabolic rate in childhood. *J Clin Invest* 1957; **36**: 1130–7.
4 Settergren G, Lindblad BS, Persson B. Cerebral blood flow and exchange of oxygen, glucose ketone bodies, lactate, pyruvate and amino acids in infants. *Acta Paediatr Scand* 1976; **65**: 343–53.
5 Rahilly PM. Effects of 2% carbon dioxide 0.5% carbon dioxide, and 100% oxygen on cranial blood flow of the human neonate. *Pediatrics* 1980; **66**: 685–9.
6 Lou HC, Lassen NA, Friis-Hansen B. Impaired autoregulation of cerebral blood flow in the distressed newborn infant. *J Pediatr* 1979; **94**: 118–21.
7 Bruce DA, Berman WA, Schut L. Cerebrospinal fluid pressure monitoring in children: physiology, pathology, and clinical usefulness. *Adv Pediatr* 1977; **24**: 233–90.
8 Friesen RH, Lichtor JL. Cardiovascular effects of inhalation induction with isoflurane in infants. *Anesth Analg* 1983; **62**: 411–14.
9 Shah N, Long C, Marx W, *et al.* Cerebrovascular response to CO_2 in edematous brain during either fentanyl or isoflurane anesthesia. *J Neurosurg Anesthesiol* 1990; **2**: 11–15.
10 Scheller MS, Todd MM, Drummond JC, Zornow MH. The intracranial pressure effects of isoflurane and halothane administered following cryogenic brain injury in rabbits. *Anesthesiology* 1987; **67**: 507–12.
11 Taylor RH, Lerman J. Induction, maintenance, and recovery characteristics of desflurane in infants and children. *Can J Anaesth* 1992; **39**: 6–13.
12 Zwass MS, Fisher DM, Welborn LG, *et al.* Induction and maintenance characteristics of anesthesia with desflurane and nitrous oxide in infants and children. *Anesthesiology* 1992; **76**: 373–8.
13 Doi M, Ikeda K. Sevoflurane irritates airway least among four anesthetic agents: halothane, enflurane, isoflurane, sevoflurane (abstract). *Anesthesiology* 1992; **77**: A335.
14 Scheller MS, Tateishi A, Drummond JC, Zornow MH. The effects of sevoflurane on cerebral blood flow, cerebral metabolic rate for oxygen, intracranial pressure, and the electroencephalogram are similar to isoflurane in the rabbit. *Anesthesiology* 1988; **68**: 548–51.
15 Scheller MS, Nakakimura K, Fleisher JE, Zornow MH. Cerebral effects of sevoflurane in the dog: comparison with isoflurane and enflurane. *Br J Anaesth* 1990; **65**: 388–92.
16 Kleinman S, Lerman J, Yentis S, Sikich N. Induction and emergence characteristics of and hemodynamic responses to sevoflurane in children (abstract). *Can J Anaesth* 1992; **39**: A100.
17 Levine M, Sarner J, Lerman J, *et al.* Emergence characteristics after sevoflurane anesthesia in children: a comparison with halothane (abstract). *Anesth Analg* 1993; **76**: S221.
18 Lerman J, Sikich N, Kleinman S, Yentis S. The pharmacology of sevoflurane in infants and children. *Anesthesiology* 1994; **80**: 814–24.
19 Bisonnette B, Leon JE. Cerebrovascular stability during isoflurane anaesthesia in children. *Can J Anaesth* 1992; **39**: 128–34.
20 Leon JE, Bisonnette B. Transcranial doppler sonography: nitrous oxide and cerebral blood flow velocity in children. *Can J Anaesth* 1991; **38**: 974–9.
21 Borgeat A, Dessibourg C, Popovic V, Meier D, Blanchard M. Propofol and spontaneous movements: an EEG study. *Anesthesiology* 1991; **74**: 24–7.
22 Trooter C, Serpell MG. Neurological sequelae in children after prolonged propofol infusion. *Anaesthesia* 1992; **47**: 340–2.
23 Reynolds LM, Koh JL. Prolonged spontaneous movement following emergence from propofol/nitrous oxide anesthesia. *Anesth Analg* 1993; **76**: 192–3.

24 Parke TJ, Stevens JE, Rice ASC, *et al*. Metabolic acidosis and fatal myocardial failure after propofol infusion in children; five case reports. *BMJ* 1992; **305**: 613–16.
25 Martin TM, Nicolson SC, Bargas MS. Propofol anesthesia reduces emesis and airway obstruction in pediatric outpatients. *Anesth Analg* 1992; **76**: 144–8.
26 Hiller A, Saarnivaara L. Injection pain, cardiovascular changes and recovery following induction of anaesthesia with propofol in combination with alfentanil or lignocaine in children. *Acta Anaesth Scand* 1992; **36**: 564–8.
27 Larsson S, Asgerisson B, Magnusson J. Propofol–fentanyl anaesthesia compared to thiopentone–halothane with specific reference to recovery and vomiting after pediatric strabismus surgery. *Acta Anaesth Scand* 1992; **36**: 182–6.
28 Martin LD, Pasternak LR, Pudiment MA. Total intravenous anaesthesia with propofol in pediatric patients outside the operating room. *Anesth Analg* 1992; **74**: 609–12.
29 Browne BL, Prys-Roberts C, Wolf AR. Propofol and alfentanil in children; infusion and dose requirements for total i.v anaesthesia. *Anaesthesia* 1992; **69**: 570–6.
30 Marsh B, White M, Morton N, Kenny GN. Pharmacokinetic model driven infusion of propofol in children. *Br J Anaesth* 1991; **67**: 41–8.
31 Markowitz BP, Duhaime AC, Sutton L, Schreiner MS, Cohen DE. Effects of alfentanil on intracranial pressure in children undergoing ventriculo-peritoneal shunt revision. *Anesthesiology* 1992; **75**; 71–6.
32 Busto R, Dietrich WD, Globus MY-T, Valdes I, Scheinberg P, Gingsberg MD. Small differences in intraischemic brain temperature critically determine the extent of ischemic neuronal injury. *J Cereb Blood Flow Metab* 1987; **7**: 729–38.
33 Ridenour TR, Warner DS, Todd MM, McAllister AC. Mild hypothermia reduces infarct size resulting from temporary but not permanent focal ischemia in the rat. *Stroke* 1992; **23**: 733–8.
34 Dietrich WD, Busto R, Valdes I, Loor Y. Effects of normothermia versus mild hyperthermic forebrain ischemia in rats. *Stroke* 1990; **21**: 1318–25.
35 Chen H, Chopp M, Welch KMA. Effect of mild hyperthermia on the ischemic infarct volume after middle cerebral artery occlusion in the rat. *Neurology* 1991; **41**: 1133–5.
36 Sieber FE, Smith DS, Traytsman RJ, Wollman H. Glucose: a reevaluation of its intraoperative use. *Anesthesiology* 1987; **67**: 72–81.
37 Cucchiara RF, Bowen B. Air embolism in children undergoing suboccipital craniectomy. *Anesthesiology* 1982; **57**: 338–9.
38 Cobb WE. Endocrine management after pituitary surgery. In: Post KD, Jackson IMD, Reichlin S (Eds), *The pituitary adenoma*. Plenum Press: New York, 1980: 417–35.
39 Cusick JF, Hagen TC, Findling JW. Inappropriate secretion of antidiuretic hormone after transsphenoidal surgery for pituitary tumours. *N Engl J Med* 1984; **311**: 36–8.
40 Nuwer MR. Evoked potential monitoring in the operating room. New York: Raven Press, 1986.
41 Grundy BL. Monitoring of sensory evoked potentials during neurosurgical operations: Methods and applications. *Neurosurgery* 1982; **11**: 556–75.
42 Standifer M, Bay JW, Trusso R. The sitting position in neurosurgery: a retrospective analysis of 488 cases. *Neurosurgery* 1984; **14**: 649–58.
43 Matjasko J, Petrozza P, Cohen M, Steinberg P. Anesthesia and surgery in the seated position: analysis of 554 cases. *Neurosurgery* 1985; **17**: 695–702.
44 Black S, Ockert DB, Oliver WC Jr, Cucchiara RF. Outcome following posterior fossa craniectomy in patients in the sitting or horizontal positions. *Anesthesiology* 1988; **69**: 49–56.
45 Wilder BL. Hypothesis: the etiology of midcervical quadriplegia after operation with the patient in the sitting position. *Neurosurgery* 1982; **11**: 530–1.
46 Kitahata LM, Katz JD. Tension pneumocephalus after posterior fossa craniotomy, a complication of the sitting position. *Anesthesiology* 1976; **44**: 448–50.
47 Artru AA. Nitrous oxide plays a direct role in the development of tension pneumocephalus intraoperatively. *Anesthesiology* 1982; **57**: 59–61.
48 Goodbie D, Traill R. Intraoperative subdural tension pneumocephalus arising after opening of the dura. *Anesthesiology* 1991; **74**: 193–5.
49 Young ML, Smith DS, Murtagh F, Vasquez A, Levitt J. Comparison of surgical and

anesthetic complications in neurosurgical patients experiencing venous air embolism in the sitting position. *Neurosurgery* 1986; **18**: 157–61.

50 Black S, Cucchiara RF, Nishimura RA, Michenfelder JD. Parameters affecting occurrence of paradoxical air embolism. *Anesthesiology* 1989; **71**: 235–41.

51 Black S, Muzzi DA, Nishimura RA, Cucchiara RA. Preoperative and intraoperative echocardiography to detect right-to-left shunt in patients undergoing neurosurgical procedures in the sitting position. *Anesthesiology* 1990; **72**: 436–8.

52 Michenfelder JD, Miller RH, Gronert GA. Evaluation of an ultrasonic device (precordial Doppler) for the diagnosis of venous air embolism. *Anesthesiology* 1972; **36**: 164–7.

53 Gildenberg PL, O'Brien RP, Britt WJ, Frost EAM. The efficacy of precordial Doppler monitoring for the detection of venous air embolism. *J Neurosurg* 1981; **54**: 75–8.

54 Cucchiara RF, Nugent M, Seward JB, Messick JM. Air embolism in upright neurosurgical patients: detection and localization by two-dimensional transesophageal echocardiography. *Anesthesiology* 1984; **60**: 353–5.

55 Perkins-Pearson NAK, Bedford RF. Hemodynamic consequences of PEEP in seated neurological patients—implications for paradoxical air embolism. *Anesth Analg* 1984; **63**: 429–32.

56 Pfitzner J, McLean AG. Controlled neck compression in neurosurgery: studies in venous air embolism in upright sleep. *Anaesthesia* 1985; **40**: 624–9.

57 Girvin JP. Neurosurgical considerations and general methods for craniotomy under local anaesthesia. *Int Anesth Clin* 1986; **24**: 89–114.

58 Lanier WL, Hool GJ, Faust RJ. Sedation for stereotactic headframe application; a randomized comparison of two techniques. *Appl Neurophysiol* 1987; **50**: 227–32.

59 Perkins WJ, Kelly PJ, Faust RJ. Stereotactic surgery. In: Cucchiara RF, Michenfelder JD (Eds), *Clinical neuroanaesthesia*, New York: Churchill Livingstone, 1990: 379–419.

60 Brown MM. Surgery, angioplasty, and interventional neuroradiology. *Curr Opin Neurol Neurosurg* 1993; **6**: 630–2.

61 Eskridge JM. Interventional neuroradiology. *Radiology* 1989; **172**: 991–1006.

62 Halbach VV, Higashida RT, Hieshima GB. Interventional neuroradiology. *AJR Am J Roentgenol* 1989; **153**: 467–76.

63 Setton A, Berenstein A. Interventional neuroradiology. *Curr Opin Neurol Neurosurg* 1992; **5**: 870–80.

64 Higashida RT, Halbach VV, Cahan LD, *et al*. Transluminal angioplasty for treatment of intracranial vasospasm. *J Neurosurg* 1989; **71**: 648–53.

65 Yamamoto Y, Smith RR, Bernanke DH. Mechanism of action of balloon angioplasty in cerebral vasospasm. *Neurosurgery* 1992; **30**: 1–6.

66 Kerber C. Use of balloon catheters in the treatment of cranial arterial abnormalities. *Stroke* 1980; **11**: 210–16.

67 Debrun G, Vinuela F, Fox A, Drake CG. Embolization of cerebral arteriovenous malformations with bucrylate. *J Neurosurg* 1982; **56**: 615–27.

68 Higashida RT, Halbach VV, Dowd CF, Barnwell SL, Hieshima GB. Intracranial aneurysms: interventional neurovascular treatment with detachable balloons – Results in 215 cases. *Radiology* 1991; **178**: 663–70.

69 Young WL, Pile-Spellman J. Anesthetic considerations for interventional neuroradiology. *Anesthesiology* 1994; **80**: 427–56.

70 Earnest F 4th, Forbes G, Sandok BA, *et al*. Complications of cerebral angiography: prospective assessment of risk. *AJR Am J Roentgenol* 1984; **142**: 247–53.

71 Dion JE, Gates PC, Fox AJ, Barnett HJM, Rita JB. Clinical events following neuroangiography: a prospective study. *Stroke* 1986; **18**: 997–1004.

72 Gelmers HJ, Gorter K, De Weerdt CJ, Wiezer MJ. A controlled trial of nimodipine in acute ischemic stroke. *N Engl J Med* 1988; **318**: 203–7.

73 Mee E, Dorrance D, Lowe D, Neil-Dwyer G. Controlled study of nimodipine in aneurysm patients treated early after subarachnoid hemorrhage. *Neurosurgery* 1988; **22**: 484–91.

74 Ohman J, Heiskanen O. Effect of nimodipine on the outcome of patients after aneurysmal subarachnoid hemorrhage and surgery. *J Neurosurg* 1988; **69**: 683–6.

75 Pickard JD, Murray GD, Illingworth R, *et al*. Effect of oral nimodipine on cerebral infarction and outcome after subarachnoid hemorrhage: British aneurysm nimodipine trial. *BMJ* 1989; **298**: 636–42.

237

76 Van Hemelrijck J, Fitch W, Mattheussen M, Van Aken H, Plets C, Lauwers T. Effect of propofol on the cerebral circulation and autoregulation in the baboon. *Anesth Analg* 1990; **71**: 49–54.

77 Van Hemelrijck J, Van Aken H, Merckx L, Mulier J. Anesthesia for craniotomy: total intravenous anesthesia with propofol and alfentanil compared to anesthesia with thiopental, isoflurane, fentanyl and nitrous oxide. *J Clin Anesth* 1991; **3**: 131–6.

78 Turner JM, Powell D, Gibson RM, McDowall DG. Intracranial pressure changes in neurosurgical patients during hypotension induced with sodium nitroprusside or trimethaphan. *Br J Anaesth* 1977; **49**: 419–25.

79 Cottrell JE, Patel KP, Turndorf H, Ransohoff J. Intracranial pressure changes induced by sodium nitroprusside in patients with intracranial mass lesions. *J Neurosurg* 1978; **48**: 329–31.

80 Fitch W, Arendt I, Pichard JD, Graham DI. Autoregulation of cerebral blood flow. Effects of nitroprusside and nitroglycerine. In: Vickers MD, Lunn JM (Eds), *Mortality in anaesthesia. Proceedings of the European Academy of Anaesthesiology.* New York: Springer-Verlag, 1982: 120.

81 Rogers MC, Hamburger C, Owen K, Epstein MH. Intracranial pressure in the cat during nitroglycerine-induced hypotension. *Anesthesiology* 1979; **51**: 227–9.

82 Cottrell JE, Gupta B, Rappaport H, Turndorf H, Ransohoff J, Flamm ES. Intracranial pressure during nitroglycerine-induced hypotension. *J Neurosurg* 1980; **53**: 309–11.

83 Turlapaty P, Laddu A, Muthy VS, Singh B, Lee R. Esmolol: a titratable short-acting intravenous beta-blocker for acute critical care settings. *Am Heart J* 1987; **114**: 866–85.

84 Ornstein E, Matteo RS, Weinstein JA, Schwartz A. A controlled trial of esmolol for the induction of deliberate hypotension. *J Clin Anaesth* 1988; **1**: 31–5.

85 Ornstein E, Young WL, Ostapovich N, Matteo RS, Diaz J. Deliberate hypotension in patients with arteriovenous malformations: esmolol compared with isoflurane and sodium nitroprusside. *Anesth Analg* 1991; **72**: 639–44.

86 Van Aken H, Puchstein C, Heinecke A. Effect of labetalol on intracranial pressure in dogs with and without intracranial hypertension. *Acta Anaesthesiol Scand* 1982; **26**: 615–19.

87 Puchstein C, Van Aken H, Anger C, Hidding J. Influence of urapidil on intracranial pressure and intracranial compliance in dogs. *Br J Anaesth* 1983; **55**: 443–8.

88 Anger C, Van Aken H, Feldhaus P. Permeation of the blood-brain barrier by urapidil and its influence on intracranial pressure in man in the presence of compromised intracranial dynamics. *J Hypertens* 1988; **6**: S63–4.

89 Sicking K, Puchstein C, Van Aken H. Blutdrucksenkung mit Urapidil: Einfluss auf die Hirndurchblutung. *Anesth Intensivmed* 1986; **27**: 147–51.

90 Young WL, Cole DJ. Deliberate hypertension: rationale and applications for augmenting cerebral blood flow. *Prob Anaesth* 1993; **7**: 140–53.

91 Purdy PD, Batjer HH, Samson D. Management of hemorrhagic complication from preoperative embolization of arteriovenous malformations. *J Neurosurg* 1991; **74**: 205–11.

92 Drummond JC. Cerebral ischemia: state of the art management. *Anesth Analg* 1992; **74** (suppl): 120–8.

93 Brian JE Jr, Eleff S, McPherson RW. Immediate hemodynamic management following subarachnoid hemorrhage during embolization of cerebral vascular abnormalities. *J Neurosurg Anesth* 1989; **1**: 63–7.

94 Patteson SK, Chesney JT. Anesthetic management for magnetic resonance imaging: problems and solutions. *Anesth Analg* 1992; **74**: 121–8.

95 Menon D, Peden C, Hall A, Sargentoni J, Whitwam JG. Magnetic resonance for the anaesthetist. Part I: physical principles, applications, safety aspects. *Anaesthesia* 1992; **47**: 240–55.

96 Menon D, Peden C, Hall A, Sargentoni J, Whitwam JG. Magnetic resonance for the anaesthetist. Part II: Anaesthesia and monitoring in MR units. *Anaesthesia* 1992; **47**: 508–17.

97 Vangerven M, Van Hemelrijck J, Wouters P, Vandermeersch E, Van Aken H. Light anaesthesia with propofol for paediatric MRI. *Anaesthesia* 1992; **47**: 706–7.

98 Frankville DD, Spear RM, Dyck JB. The dose of propofol to prevent children from moving during magnetic resonance imaging. *Anesthesiology* 1993; **79**: 953–8.

99 Rafferty C, Burke AM, Cossar DF, Farling PA. Laryngeal mask and magnetic resonance imaging. *Anaesthesia* 1990; **45**: 590–1.

100 Anderton JM. The prone position for the surgical patient: a historical review of the principles and hazards. *Br J Anaesth* 1991; **67**: 452–63.

101 Lee C, Barnes A, Nagel EL. Neuroleptanalgesia for awake pronation of surgical patients. *Anesth Analg* 1977; **56**: 276–8.

102 Fraser A, Edmonds-Seal J. Spinal cord injuries: a review of the problems facing the anaesthetist. *Anaesthesia* 1982; **37**: 1084–98.

103 Crosby ET, Lui A. The adult cervical spine: implications for airway management. *Can J Anaesth* 1990; **37**: 77–93.

104 Hastings RH, Marks JD. Airway management for trauma patients with potential cervical spine injuries. *Anesth Analg* 1991; **73**: 471–82.

105 Wood PR, Lawler PGP. Managing the airway in cervical spine injury. A review of the Advanced Trauma Life Support Protocol. *Anaesthesia* 1992; **47**: 798–801.

106 Turner LM. Cervical spine immobilization with axial traction: a practice to be discouraged. *J Emerg Med* 1989; **7**: 385–6.

107 Frazer A, Edmonds-Seal J. Spinal cord injuries. A review of the problems facing the anaesthetist. *Anaesthesia* 1982; **37**: 1084–98.

108 Alderson JD. Spinal cord injuries. *Anaesthesia* 1983; **38**: 605–8.

109 Barker L, Alderson J, Lydon M, Franks CI. Cardiovascular effects of spinal subarachnoid anaesthesia. A study in patients with chronic spinal cord injuries. *Anaesthesia* 1985; **40**: 533–6.

110 Brooke MM, Donovan WH, Stolov WC. Paraplegia: succinylcholine-induced hyperkalemia and cardiac arrest. *Arch Phys Med Rehab* 1978; **59**: 306–9.

111 Macon JB, Poletti CE, Sweet WH, Ojemann RG, Zervas NT. Conducted somatosensory potentials during spinal surgery. Part 1: Clinical applications. *J Neurosurg* 1982; **57**: 354–9.

112 Jellinek D, Platt M, Jewkes D, Symon L. Effects of nitrous oxide on motor evoked potentials recorded from skeletal muscle in patients under total anaesthesia with intravenously administered propofol. *Neurosurgery* 1992: **29**; 558–62.

10: Management of acute head injury

GLENDA J OLDROYD, N MARK DEARDEN

Over the past two decades there has been considerable improvement in the outcome from severe head injury as a result of the recognition and prevention of disorders leading to secondary brain injury.

The true incidence of head injury is unknown. The most reliable guide is from the accident and emergency department attendance rates and hospital admissions, although these will vary according to local facilities and policies.[1]

Head injury accounts for nine deaths per 10^5 population each year in Britain, which is less than 1% of all deaths. In the age group 15–24 years, however, head injuries represent 15% of all deaths. Adult head injury is two to four times more common in males than in females, whereas in children the sex difference is less marked.[1]

The aetiology of acute head injury will vary with the population: road traffic accidents and assaults are more common in young male patients; falls and pedestrian accidents are more likely in elderly people.[2]

The anaesthetist with expertise in airway skills, resuscitation, and intensive therapy has a crucial role to play in the management of patients with severe head injury. To optimise this role it is essential to have a good understanding of the pathophysiology of head injury.

Pathophysiology

Primary traumatic injury occurs immediately on impact; its severity depends on the cause and force of the inciting injury. Little can be done to alter the detrimental effects of such primary mechanical injury other than preventive measures. The use of car seat belts and the wearing of bicycle helmets have significantly reduced the morbidity and mortality from severe head injury.[3 4]

Acute cerebral trauma also initiates a cascade of ionic and metabolic changes which render the brain particularly susceptible to secondary insults. These secondary insults result in reduction of blood supply and/or oxygen to the already injured brain and are adversely associated with neurological outcome.

240

Head injuries may be associated with skull fractures, focal brain injury, diffuse brain injury, and secondary brain injury.

Skull fractures

Skull fractures are common but do not, in isolation, cause disability. The presence of a skull fracture should, however, alert the physician to the possibility of the presence, or development, of an intracranial haematoma. All patients with a skull fracture should be admitted to hospital for neurological observation.

Linear non-depressed fracture

No specific treatment is indicated, except neurological observation and management of any underlying brain injury. If the fracture occurs across a suture line or vascular groove, there is an increased risk of developing an extradural haematoma.

Depressed skull fracture

Management is directed at the underlying brain injury. Operative elevation is usually indicated if the fragment is depressed more than the thickness of the skull. Over 75% of depressed skull fractures are compound and require early surgery to facilitate surgical toilet, elevation of the depressed bone fragment, and evaluation of the underlying dura and brain. Delay in surgical toilet and dural closure (>24 h) is associated with significant risk of infection.

Basal skull fractures

These fractures are often difficult to see on plain skull radiographs, although intracranial air, a fluid level in the sphenoid sinus, or an opaque sphenoid sinus may be useful clues. Basal skull fractures are usually diagnosed by clinical findings, which are often delayed, and confirmed by computed tomography. The following are the clinical findings associated with basal skull fractures:

1 Cerebrospinal fluid (CSF) leakage from the ear (otorrhoea) or nose (rhinorrhoea). If the CSF is mixed with blood, it can be detected by allowing a drop of the fluid to separate on a piece of tissue paper. A "ring sign" develops because the CSF produces one or more concentric rings around the blood which stays centrally.
2 Battle's sign (bruising in the mastoid region).
3 Haemotympanum (blood behind the tympanic membrane visible on auroscopy).
4 Racoon eyes (periorbital bruising without extending to the eyebrows, caused by cribriform plate fracture).

241

Focal brain injury

This is a localised brain injury and may be a contusion, haemorrhage, or haematoma. Focal brain injuries may require urgent surgical intervention because of their mass effect and must be recognised early during resuscitation of the patient.

Contusions (fig 10.1)

These may be single or multiple, large or small, and may or may not be associated with skull fractures. Contusions occur beneath any areas of impact (coup contusions) or in areas remote from injury (*contre coup* contusion) in association with the bony ridges of the base of the skull. The neurological effects on the patient vary with the severity of injury, from mild concussion to focal neurological deficits, to prolonged coma. These patients should be

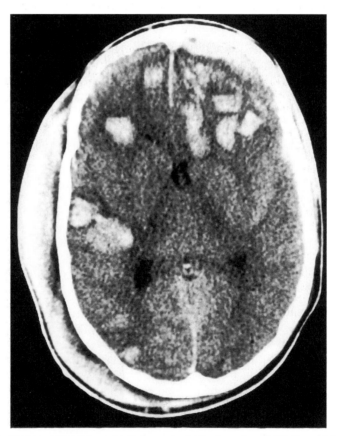

Fig 10.1 CT scan showing multiple intracerebral contusions following a high speed rapid deceleration brain injury

242

admitted to hospital for observation because of the risk of delayed neurological deterioration.

Extradural haematoma (fig 10.2)

Extradural haematomas may be rapidly fatal. These usually result from a tear in a dural artery, usually the middle meningeal artery, or rarely from a dural sinus tear. In both adults and children, there is a high association with a linear skull fracture, particularly in the parietal or temporal regions. The classic presentation of an acute extradural haematoma consists of an initial period of loss of consciousness (concussion) followed by an intervening lucid interval (although this may not be a return to full consciousness), with a secondary depression of consciousness, ipsilateral pupillary dilatation, and the development of a contralateral hemiparesis. With computed tomography (CT) and the association with a fracture, however, this presentation should rarely be seen and patients should be treated whenever possible before neurological deterioration occurs. Prognosis from this lesion is usually

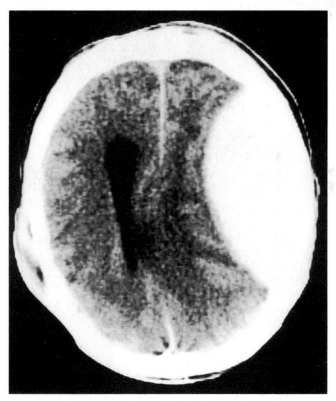

Fig 10.2 CT scan of an acute large left sided extradural haematoma exerting significant mass effect with contralateral ventricular dilatation

excellent, provided early surgical evacuation of the haematoma is performed, because the underlying brain injury is relatively minor.

Acute subdural haematoma (fig 10.3)

Acute subdural haematomas are more common, usually associated with underlying brain contusions, and carry a poorer prognosis than extradural haematomas. These haematomas are caused by lacerations of the cerebral cortex, or by rupture of bridging veins between the dura and cerebral cortex.

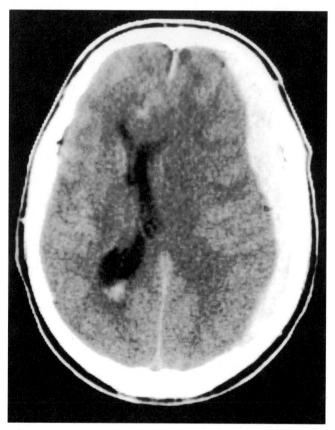

Fig 10.3 CT scan of an acute left sided subdural haematoma. There is marked shift to the right

Intracerebral haematoma

These may occur in any location and in association with brain contusions. Intraventricular and intracerebellar haemorrhages both carry a very high mortality rate.

Diffuse brain injury (fig 10.4)

Diffuse brain injury results from rapid movement of the head (acceleration or deceleration) and causes widespread interruption of brain function. The neurological disturbance may be temporary, causing concussion (a brief period of confusion or unconsciousness), or more severe, causing prolonged coma—an injury referred to as diffuse axonal injury. Diffuse axonal injury is strictly a pathological condition which can only be diagnosed microscopically. When diffuse head injury is associated with the CT scan findings of compression or obliteration of the mesencephalic cisterns and/or slit like third ventricle, raised intracranial pressure (ICP) is likely to ensue.[5] Diffuse brain injury is twice as common in children as in adults, occurring in up to 20% of cases with severe head injury.[6] Neurological deterioration is usually seen in the first 48 hours following injury. As with the adult population, systemic insults (hypoxaemia or hypotension) are important in the pathogenesis of diffuse brain injury. The mesencephalic cisterns are usually well imaged in children, therefore compression or obliteration of these cisterns on CT scan indicates the presence of brain swelling.[7]

Secondary brain injury

Secondary brain injury may be caused by extracranial or intracranial conditions (table 10.1) and may occur minutes, hours, or days after the primary injury. Under normal circumstances cerebral blood flow (CBF) and cerebral metabolism are coupled through autoregulation of cerebral vasculature. Cerebral resistance vessels are sensitive to both metabolic stimuli and changes in cerebral perfusion pressure (CPP), which is the difference between mean arterial pressure (MAP) and mean ICP. After severe head injury autoregulatory mechanisms may become deranged and CBF becomes dependent on CPP. In the management of severe head injury, avoiding factors that compromise cerebral oxygen delivery is therefore paramount. The occurrence of both hypotension and hypoxia is associated with a doubling of mortality after head injury.

Initial management

The primary goal of management is the prevention, recognition, and treatment of conditions known to cause secondary brain injury, including identification and evacuation of surgically remediable compressive lesions.

Initial management of a trauma patient involves taking a history, assessment, and simultaneous resuscitation. The history may be obtained from the patient or more commonly from the attending ambulance crew. An accurate account of the timing and mechanism of injury enables the physician to have a high index of suspicion for specific injuries. For example, if a patient falls

245

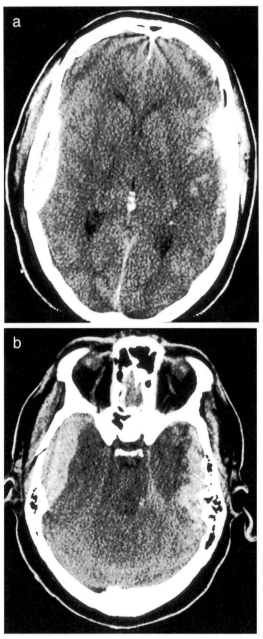

Fig 10.4 (a) CT scan of the head at the level of the third ventricle in a patient with a right sided extradural haematoma and a left sided subdural haematoma associated with underlying brain contusion. The slit like compressed third ventricle indicates that ICP either is or will soon become raised. (b) CT scan at the level of the basal cisternae in the same patient showing effacement of the perimesencephalic cisternae

Table 10.1   Causes of secondary brain injury: systemic secondary insults and their potential causes

Secondary insult	Cause
Hypoxaemia	Respiratory arrest
	Airway obstruction
	Aspiration
	Pneumothorax
	Haemothorax
	Anaemia
	Carbon monoxide poisoning
Hypotension	Hypovolaemic shock
	Tension pneumothorax
	Cardiac contusion
	Cardiac tamponade
	Spinal cord injury
	Myocardial infarction
Hypercapnia	Airway obstruction
	Respiratory depression
	Respiratory arrest
Other	Severe hypocapnia (spontaneous hyperventilation)
	Hypo/hyperglycaemia
	Hyponatraemia
	Hyperthermia
	Intracranial haematoma (extradural, subdural, intracerebral)
	Cerebrovascular engorgement
	Increased brain water content (cerebral oedema)
	Acute hydrocephalus
Others	Seizures
	Vasospasm
	Intracranial infection

from a height there is a fourfold risk of having an intracranial haematoma. The initial roadside assessment, including the cardiorespiratory and neurological status, is important because it provides a baseline for subsequent reassessment.

The assessment and management of a trauma patient on arrival in the accident and emergency department start with a primary survey to identify life threatening conditions which should be treated immediately. All trauma patients should receive supplemental oxygen, particularly those with head injury, because hypoxaemia is a common cause of secondary brain injury.

Primary survey

The primary survey should include the following factors:

A Airway maintenance with cervical spine control
B Breathing and ventilation
C Circulation with haemorrhage control
D Disability: neurological status
E Exposure: completely undress the patient.

During assessment and maintenance of the airway, consideration must be given to the possibility of a cervical spine injury. Patients with a clinically significant head injury have a 4·5% overall risk of an accompanying cervical spine injury; this risk is increased to 7·3% in patients with severe head injury associated with a Glasgow coma score (GCS) of 8 or less.[8] If such an injury cannot be excluded, the cervical spine should be assumed to be fractured, and treated as such, until proved otherwise. This involves secure immobilisation of the cervical spine in a neutral position with a hard cervical collar (which should not impede cerebral venous drainage), sand bags placed either side of the head, and strapping applied across the forehead to the trolley, as described in the Advanced Trauma Life Support (ATLS) course manual.[9] If airway manoeuvres are required, in particular intubation, the cervical spine must be immobilised by a trained member of staff performing manual inline immobilisation, preventing flexion, extension, or rotation of the neck.

Adequacy of ventilation should be quickly assessed, including arterial blood gas analysis, and assisted if necessary. The indications for intubation and ventilation of a head injured patient are shown in table 10.2. Chest trauma is particularly detrimental in head injured patients because of the risk of hypoxia, hypotension, and raised intrathoracic pressure. Tension pneumothorax should be treated by immediate decompression.

If intubation should be required, a rapid sequence induction, with preoxygenation and cricoid pressure, must be performed to reduce the risk of regurgitation and aspiration. The patient should be intubated via the oral route as a basal skull fracture cannot be excluded. The endotracheal tube should be secured with adhesive strapping to the face rather than to the neck, to avoid causing potential cerebral venous engorgement. Repeated visualisation of chest movement and auscultation should be performed to confirm correct positioning of the endotracheal tube and to allow early detection of a pneumothorax, which is likely to be exacerbated by positive pressure

Table 10.2   Indications for intubation and ventilation of head injured patients in the accident and emergency department

---

Immediately
   Inability to maintain or protect airway
   Associated injuries requiring ventilation, for example, chest injury
   Coma (not obeying commands, speaking, or eye opening)
   GCSS $\leqslant 8$
   Hypoxaemia ($Pao_2 < 9$ kPa on air; < 13 kPa on oxygen)
   Hypoventilation ($Paco_2 > 6$ kPa)
   Spontaneous hyperventilation ($Paco_2 < 3\cdot5$ kPa)
   Respiratory arrhythmia

Before transfer
   Significant deterioration in conscious level
   Potential airway compromise (bleeding, fractured mandible)
   Convulsions (in addition to starting anticonvulsant therapy)

GCSS, Glasgow coma sum score.

248

ventilation. An orogastric tube should be inserted because gastric distension is common following severe trauma, which increases the risk of regurgitation and aspiration, and may raise ICP secondary to autonomic stimulation.

The anaesthetic drugs used, for sedation, analgesia, and neuromuscular blockade, will be influenced by the cardiovascular status of the patient. It is desirable to obtund the hypertensive response to laryngoscopy and intubation. Suxamethonium (succinylcholine) should be used to facilitate intubation and to ensure adequate and rapid muscle relaxation, in spite of the shortlived rise in ICP that this may cause.

During assessment of the circulation, intravenous access should be gained with two large bore cannulas, necessary blood samples taken for laboratory investigations, and intravenous fluids started, guided by the clinical signs. In children and healthy young adults, the pulse rate, respiratory rate, and capillary refill times are more accurate signs of the degree of hypovolaemia than the blood pressure. The presence of hypovolaemia should alert the clinician to consider early provision of direct arterial pressure monitoring to assist resuscitation. Fluid resuscitation is initially started with crystalloid solutions, such as physiological saline (0·9%); colloid solutions and blood products are administered when indicated. Dextrose containing intravenous fluids should be avoided as these can be detrimental to the injured brain. The use of hypertonic saline in head injury is being investigated.

All sources of blood loss must be identified and controlled. Significant blood loss is usually caused by thoracoabdominal injury and pelvic or long bone fractures. If intra-abdominal haemorrhage cannot be excluded, particularly in the unconscious patient, a diagnostic peritoneal lavage should be performed, because the clinical signs may be obtunded or delayed. If hypovolaemic shock persists, in spite of continuing fluid resuscitation, immediate laparotomy or thoracotomy should be considered. Application of external fixation for an unstable pelvic fracture may be required in the resuscitation room.

A diagnosis of spinal cord transection should be considered in the patient with persistent hypotension following apparently adequate fluid resuscitation. If the lesion occurs in the high thoracic or cervical region, a bradycardia is likely to be present.

A rapid neurological assessment is made at the end of the primary survey, establishing the patient's level of consciousness, using the AVPU method, and examining the pupillary size and reaction to light.

A	**A**lert
V	responds to **V**ocal stimuli
P	responds to **P**ainful stimuli
U	**U**nconscious

249

Alteration of consciousness is the hallmark of brain injury and may indicate intracranial pathology or inadequate cerebral perfusion or oxygenation, necessitating immediate reassessment of the patient's oxygenation, ventilation, and circulatory status. The mini-neurological examination should reveal any gross neurological deficit.

Secondary survey

After the initial primary survey is complete and appropriate resuscitation initiated, the secondary survey is performed. The secondary survey is a thorough examination of the patient from head to toe which includes "log-rolling" the patient to inspect the dorsal surface of the body as well as the spine.

Specific assessment of head injuries

Documentation of neurological examination should always be accompanied by the cardiorespiratory status because these may profoundly influence each other. Severe systemic hypoxaemia or hypotension may render a patient (without head injury) unconscious.

Never presume that brain injury is the cause of hypotension; this is a terminal event resulting from brain stem failure. Intracerebral bleeding alone, except very rarely in infants, cannot produce hypovolaemic shock. It is possible for young children and elderly people, however, to become shocked by excessive bleeding from scalp lacerations. Hypertension associated with tachycardia and reduced respiratory rate (Cushing's response) is a potentially terminal event caused by a severe rise in ICP and may be associated with an expanding intracranial haematoma. Evacuation of the haematoma, and consequent reduction in ICP, may unmask hypovolaemia and lead to a sudden drop in blood pressure.

Neurological examination is directed to assess the following:

1 Level of consciousness
2 Pupillary signs
3 Lateralised extremity weakness.

Level of consciousness

The Glasgow coma scale (GCS) provides a quantitative measure of the patient's level of consciousness.[10] The Glasgow coma sum score (GCSS) is the sum of scores for three areas of assessment of the GCS: eye opening, motor response, and verbal response (table 10.3). The maximum score is 15, the minimum 3. If the patient is intubated and paralysed, this should be documented. Painful stimuli should be applied to the face (supraorbital or

Table 10.3   Glasgow coma scale for assessment of level of consciousness

---

Eye opening (E score)
If the eyes are unable to open as a result of swelling, this must be documented and the E score is invalid

Spontaneous	E = 4
To speech (not necessarily a request for eye opening)	E = 3
To pain (stimulus should not be applied to face)	E = 2
None	E = 1

Best motor response (M score)
The best response from the upper limb is recorded. For patients not responding to verbal command, a graded painful stimulus is applied to the nail bed, followed by pressure applied more centrally, over the supraorbital nerve or angle of the jaw, to assess localisation of the stimulus

Obeys commands	M = 6
Localises (purposeful movement towards the stimulus)	M = 5
Normal flexion (withdraws from painful stimulus)	M = 4
Abnormal flexion (decorticate posture)	M = 3
Extension (decerebrate posture)	M = 2
No movement	M = 1

Verbal response (V score)
If speech is impossible, for example, the patient is intubated, this must be documented

Oriented (knows name, age)	V = 5
Confused (still answers questions)	V = 4
Inappropriate words (recognisable words produced)	V = 3
Incomprehensible sounds (grunts/groans, no actual words)	V = 2
None	V = 1

Paediatric GCS
The motor and verbal scores of the GCS have to be modified for young children:

	Best motor response	*Best verbal response*
<6 months	Flexion	Smiles and cries
6–12 months	Localisation	Smiles and cries
1–2 years	Localisation	Sounds and words
2–5 years	Obeys commands	Words and phrases

---

mastoid process pressure) as well as to the limbs (heavy pressure to the nail beds) to facilitate detection of a spinal lesion.

The GCSS should be recorded as early as possible and repeated frequently, especially during the first hour after injury.

Coma is defined as the following:

E = 1: a patient with no eye opening
M = 1–5: inability to follow commands
V = 1–2: no word verbalisation.

Coma is therefore defined as a patient with a GCSS of 8 or less, with E = 1.

The GCSS can be used to categorise the severity of head injury:

Severe head injury	GCSS ≤ 8
Moderate head injury	GCSS = 9–12

Minor head injury   GCSS = 13–15

Pupillary function

Pupil size and light reflex, in the absence of eye pathology, are important diagnostic signs and may be valuable in localising the injury. A difference in pupil diameter of more than 1 mm is abnormal. Pupil signs may be associated with other neurological signs, for example, an expanding supratentorial mass (haematoma or cerebral oedema) will usually cause an ipsilateral fixed dilated pupil and contralateral limb weakness.

Occasionally, hemiplegia and third nerve palsy may present on the same side. The ipsilateral weakness results from rapid shift of the brain stem by the hippocampus, causing compression of the contralateral corticospinal tract against the opposite tentorial edge. Unilateral third nerve palsy almost always occurs on the same side as the lesion, as a result of compression of the oculomotor nerve against the incisura by uncal (temporal lobe) herniation, and as such is a more reliable indicator than hemiplegia in determining the side of the lesion. Damage to the optic nerve, by orbital trauma, also results in loss of the ipsilateral direct light reflex; however, the consensual light reflex will also be absent, unlike damage to the oculomotor nerve, when the consensual reflex is preserved. Bilateral loss of pupillary response is indicative of brain stem injury. Pinpoint pupils are seen with pontine injury and are believed to result from autonomic dysfunction.

Lateralised extremity weakness

The GCS only records the best motor response, but the worst response is also important. All movements are observed for equality; a delay in onset of movement, reduced movement, or need to apply a greater stimulus to one side is significant. A lateralised weakness is strongly suggestive of an intracranial mass lesion, but may also be seen in a postictal period.

If the patient has been sedated and paralysed, the only clinical neurological assessment possible is the pupillary size and response to light. This must not be forgotten during the transfer of patients or during operative treatment for extracranial injuries.

If the patient has seizures, anticonvulsant drugs should be administered such as diazepam or thiopentone (thiopental), and care should be taken to avoid respiratory, cardiovascular, and neurological depression. If repeated convulsions occur, consideration should be given to starting treatment with phenytoin 5–10 mg/kg by slow intravenous injection. Continuous electrocardiography (ECG) monitoring and regular blood pressure recording are required because of the risk of dysrhythmias and hypotension. Repeated convulsive activity is considered by many to be an indication for long term (at least six months) administration of anticonvulsant therapy.

It is important to reassess and document the neurological status of the patient regularly in addition to the cardiorespiratory status, to ensure early detection of neurological deterioration and initiation of appropriate treatment without delay. The cause of deterioration may be hypoxaemia, hypotension, or the development of an expanding intracranial haematoma or raised ICP.

Significant neurological deterioration is defined as the following:

- Deterioration in the GCSS of two or more points
- Development of pupillary abnormality
- Development of focal neurological signs.

Monitoring

The following are the aims of monitoring patients with severe head injury:

1 To establish completion of resuscitation measures
2 To ensure and maintain adequate cerebral perfusion and oxygenation
3 Early detection, prevention, and treatment of remediable causes of secondary brain injury
4 Early detection of deterioration in neurological status
5 To monitor effects of treatment administered.

Monitoring should be instituted as soon as practicable after injury and continued until intensive therapy is no longer required.

The recommendations, published by the Association of Anaesthetists for the minimal standards of monitoring that are required for anaesthesia, apply equally to the resuscitation and transfer of severely head injured patients.[11]

All patients with severe head injury should be monitored by clinical observation and with continuous ECG, pulse oximetry, blood pressure, and ventilation monitoring (capnography, if available, is highly recommended). The use of invasive arterial pressure monitoring should be encouraged early in the management of the patient, so as to detect hypotension or hypertension accurately; either of these may be deleterious if left untreated. This also enables repeat blood gas analysis to be carried out which is essential to confirm satisfactory oxygenation and arterial carbon dioxide tension ($Paco_2$). The use of non-invasive blood pressure monitoring has been shown to be unreliable during transfer of patients.[12] Central venous access can be used for administration of intravenous fluids, particularly in the multiply injured patient in whom intravenous access may be difficult, and to monitor central venous pressure for assessing adequacy of fluid resuscitation. All patients should be catheterised and hourly urine output measured. An accurate record of fluid balance should be kept. Neurological assessment (GCS, pupil response) should be recorded with the other observations on an appropriately designed observation chart. In the operating room, capnography and core temperature should also be monitored. Additional monitoring required on the intensive care unit is discussed later.

253

Investigations

All multiply injured or unconscious patients must have chest, lateral cervical spine, and pelvic radiographs. The indications[13] for a skull radiograph are:

- Loss of consciousness at any time
- Neurological symptoms or signs
- CSF or blood from nose or ear
- Suspected penetrating injury
- Scalp bruising and swelling.

If a CT scan is indicated clinically, a skull radiograph is not usually required. The indications for a CT scan are:

- Patients in coma (GCSS ≤ 8)
- Patients with skull fracture and altered conscious level or seizures or focal neurological deficit
- Depressed skull fracture
- Suspected basal skull fracture
- Suspected penetrating injury (spike or gunshot)
- Neurological deterioration
- Localising neurological deficit
- Convulsions
- To rule out intracranial pathology in patients with altered conscious level and multiple injuries requiring urgent surgery under general anaesthesia (only if cardiovascularly stable)
- GCSS < 15 for longer than 24 hours.

Computed tomography has revolutionised the management of head injury by providing a non-invasive, high accuracy technique for identifying and demonstrating the location, nature, and effect of intracranial pathology. Computerised tomography is capable of differentiating cerebral oedema, contusion, and haematoma. It provides more accurate information regarding bony injury, particularly basal skull fractures, than plain radiographs. Obtaining a CT scan must not take priority over resuscitation or delay referral to a neurosurgeon. A normal CT scan obtained early after injury does not exclude the occurrence of delayed brain swelling or haematoma formation which may result in a fatal outcome.

Magnetic resonance imaging (MRI) seems to be more accurate than computed tomography in detecting early cerebral oedema and focal contusion. It is also a better predictor of delayed traumatic intracerebral haematoma. It does not, however, detect more lesions amenable to emergency surgery, it is a slower technique, and it does not allow more extensive investigation of bony injuries. In addition, it is not as readily available at present and problems exist regarding anaesthetic equipment and monitoring.

Table 10.4   Referral to the neurosurgeon

Immediately after initial assessment and resuscitation
Fractured skull with:
    any alteration of concious level
    focal neurological signs
    convulsions
    any other neurological symptoms or signs
Coma persisting after adequate resuscitation ⎱
Deterioration of conscious level   Even without a skull fracture
Focal pupil signs
Focal neurological signs ⎰
Urgently
Confusion or other neurological disturbance persisting after six hours, even without a skull fracture
Compound depressed skull fracture
Penetrating head injury
Suspected basal skull fracture
Persistent or worsening headache or vomiting (especially in children)

Referral to the neurosurgeon

The criteria for referral to a neurosurgeon are listed in table 10.4. Consultation with a neurosurgeon should not be considered until the initial assessment and resuscitation are complete. All of these patients will require a CT scan which may be available at the referring hospital or may require transfer to the neurosurgical centre. Very early CT scans may mislead the clinician as to the severity of an intracranial haematoma which could still be evolving.[15]

The patient should *never* leave the accident and emergency department for any investigation, treatment, or transfer to a neurosurgical centre, until the airway is secure, ventilation adequate, and cardiovascular stability has been assured. The only exception to this rule is when a patient requires immediate transfer to the operating room, for laparotomy or thoracotomy, to identify and control continuing major blood loss.

Not all patients with neurological symptoms and signs will need to be transferred to a neurosurgical centre, and can be managed on a general intensive care unit or surgical ward in a district general hospital, particularly if computed tomography is available locally. Some centres have image transfer systems enabling the neurosurgeon to view the CT scan from the referring hospital and thus may avoid unnecessary transfers. Should neurological deterioration occur, immediate transfer to the neurosurgical centre can be organised. The final decision and timing of transfer is a neurosurgical one.

When the decision to operate for an intracranial haematoma is made by the neurosurgeon, or raised ICP is diagnosed on the CT scan, 1 g/kg 20% mannitol should be given intravenously to minimise the rise in ICP during transfer of the patient. The patient must be catheterised. Colloids should be administered during the diuresis to maintain the circulating blood volume.

Transfer

Most patients in the United Kingdom with an acute head injury who require a neurosurgical opinion during their initital management will need to be transferred from the primary hospital to a neurosurgical unit. This system inevitably leads to delay in neurosurgical intervention and avoidable deaths,[16] which occur either from failure to appreciate the need for transfer from the primary hospital or from failure to institute appropriate treatment, often for non-cranial injuries, before or during transfer. Transfer time itself contributes little to avoidable deaths.[17] Even if the patient is admitted to a neurosurgical unit initially, transfer of the patient to the CT scanner will be required. The standard of transfer of acutely head injured patients, both between and within hospitals, is suboptimal in up to 50% of cases.[16 18 19] Several factors contribute to this suboptimal care: inexperienced staff, infrequent exposure to multiply injured patients, anxiety, urgency for transfer, low input by senior medical staff, inadequate airway management, and inadequate equipment and monitoring.[19] All of these factors are potentially avoidable.

The occurrence of secondary insults, in particular systemic hypoxaemia or hypotension, is associated with poor outcome.[16] Pre-transfer insults and a high injury severity score are predictive of further secondary adverse events during and after transfer, highlighting the necessity for adequate resuscitation before transfer.[18] Detection and treatment of raised ICP before transfer appear to prevent further ICP insults during transfer.[18]

Detailed guidelines should be agreed locally to minimise the hazards of transfer of unconscious patients between hospitals.[14 16 20] These guidelines should make clear to junior staff what has been agreed, and should include a protocol for the practical steps necessary to ensure the safe transfer of patients by appropriately trained medical and nursing personnel. New staff must be informed of the guidelines and know when to seek advice. Routine audit of all transfers should be performed to facilitate revision of local guidelines as required.

All patients with severe brain injury should be anaesthetised, intubated, and ventilated before transfer to a neurosurgical unit or CT scanner. It is crucial that the neurological status of the patient is properly assessed before anaesthetising the patient and documented clearly in the notes, along with all drugs and intravenous fluids administered.

Most transfers between hospitals in Britain are by road in an ambulance. Care must be taken to avoid excessive heat loss by using space blankets. All lines should be clearly labelled and secured, before moving the patient.

The importance of adequate and continuous assessment, resuscitation, and monitoring, especially in patients with multiple injuries, cannot be over-emphasised.

Surgical intervention

Indications

Evacuation of haematoma—A traumatic intracranial haematoma should be suspected in the following patients:

1 If the neurological state deteriorates
2 If the neurological state fails to improve with resuscitation
3 The presence of a skull fracture
4 The presence of a skull fracture with altered level of consciousness.

The combination of a skull fracture and altered level of consciousness is associated with a 1:4 chance of an intracranial haematoma.[21] These patients require an urgent CT scan after necessary initial resuscitation. The presence or absence of a skull fracture is a crucial piece of information in the management of head injured patients. Any delay in the diagnosis and treatment of a traumatic intracranial haematoma reduces the chance of survival and a good neurological recovery.

The degree of urgency of surgical evacuation depends on the following:[22 23]

Type of haematoma	Extradural/subdural/intracerebral
Size	>25 ml
Degree of midline shift	>15 mm
Age of patient	Younger
Extracranial injuries	Severity and urgency of treatment

If an extracerebral haematoma is considered too small to warrant surgical evacuation on initial computed tomography, a repeat CT scan should be carried out a few hours later because a significant proportion of these haematomas will have expanded and thus require surgical intervention.[15] Early evacuation of extracerebral haematomas is associated with a significant improvement in outcome,[22 23] although it remains controversial, the usual management being to monitor ICP and repeat computed tomography to detect those who may benefit from surgery. Some centres favour evacuation of haematoma if the ICP is more than 25 mm Hg, whereas others only do so when a sustained ICP of more than 30 mm Hg is unresponsive to medical treatment.

Depressed skull fractures—Surgical toilet, assessment of the dura, and elevation of depressed skull fractures should be performed within six hours of injury to reduce the risk of infection.

Insertion of intracranial pressure monitoring—The fibreoptic catheters can now be inserted on the intensive care unit into the subdural space or brain tissue. The tip of the catheter acts as a transducer. Intraventricular catheters are usually inserted in the operating room.

Talk and deteriorate

Of patients with a severe head injury 12–32% talk at some point before deteriorating into coma. These patients represent a potentially salvageable group. Four of every five of these patients who become comatose after a seemingly minor or moderate head injury have a mass lesion potentially requiring neurosurgical intervention.[22] The shorter the lucid interval, the higher the probability that an extradural haematoma is present. Mortality rates are higher in patients with focal pathology. Subdural haematoma carries the highest mortality rate (54·3%), followed by brain contusion/haematoma (38·2%), and extradural haematoma (19·6%). More severe lesions occur with greater frequency in patients over 40 years of age. The mortality rate for this group of patients is 30–40%. The findings differ in children: diffuse brain swelling is the most frequent cause of secondary deterioration following a lucid period. The following are independent outcome predictors (in order of significance): GCS score following deterioration into coma; the highest ICP recording during the patient's course; the degree of midline shift on CT scan; the type of intracranial lesion; and the age of the patient.[22 23] Outcome in patients with an acute subdural haematoma is worse if surgery is delayed beyond four hours.

The following are factors that contribute to mortality in the group of patients who talk and deteriorate:

- Advanced age
- Shift of midline on CT scan > 15 mm on initial scan
- Presence of a subdural haematoma.

As the overwhelming majority of patients with marked shift on CT scan have surgical lesions, early operative intervention is strongly recommended in these patients before their inevitable deterioration.

The higher mortality rate of head injury patients who become comatose after showing a lucid period indicates that intracranial complications are often not recognised or treated quickly enough.

Patients with minimal or no changes on the initial CT scan, but who show persistent neurological impairment, may benefit from sequential computed tomography or MRI.

Care must be taken when anaesthetising head injured patients for treatment of extracranial lesions—vigilance must be maintained about the possibility of perioperative development of an intracranial haematoma. The use of a neuroanaesthetic technique must be employed and the patient observed postoperatively for neurological function and any deterioration.

Diffuse brain swelling is the most frequent cause of secondary deterioration in children showing a lucid period after head injury. All children with abnormal neurological examination (including GCS score and mental status) should be observed initially for 48 hours. If the admission CT scan shows loss of the third ventricle and/or basal cistern effacement, ICP monitoring and assisted ventilation should be considered.[22]

Intensive therapy unit

Indications
The following are the indications for intensive care management:

1 Postcraniotomy in a patient who was comatose preoperatively
2 Patients requiring intubation and ventilation as indicated in table 10.2
3 Patients with raised ICP
4 Patients with multiple injuries requiring ventilation
5 Patients with continued coma following adequate resuscitation.

Monitoring—All patients with severe head injury should be monitored continuously as previously stated, by ECG, pulse oximetry and of invasive intra-arterial pressure, and central venous and pulmonary artery pressure (if indicated). Ventilation monitoring should include regular arterial blood gas analysis. Core and peripheral temperatures should be recorded along with hourly urine output, and fluid and electrolyte balance. Neurological assessment includes hourly GCS motor score, including assessment of inequality of movement, and pupillary response to light. Appropriate haematological, biochemical, and bacteriological investigations should be conducted.

Additional monitoring used in some centres include cerebral electrical activity (cerebral function monitor, EEG), direct ICP and hence CPP, jugular venous oxygen saturation (Sjo_2), and transcranial Doppler ultrasonography.

Continuous monitoring of cerebral electrical activity is particularly useful in patients who are paralysed with neuromuscular blocking agents, in whom the only clinical neurological assessment possible is pupillary response to light. Cerebral function monitoring or EEG monitoring may allow detection of seizure activity or may indicate a reduction in cerebral activity. These measurements can be influenced by administration of drugs.

Measurement of ICP enables calculation of the CPP. The most accurate assessment of ICP is to measure it directly using a subdural, intracerebral, or intraventricular device with either a fluid filled or a fibreoptic system. CPP should be calculated as mean arterial pressure minus ICP, measured with a 15–30° head up tilt, with the zero reference for both transducers at the external auditory meatus. Complications associated with these procedures are blockage of the catheter, haemorrhage, haematoma formation, infection, and epilepsy.

Continuous Sjo_2 monitoring is performed using a fibreoptic catheter placed in the jugular bulb as described by Andrews *et al.*[24] Monitoring of Sjo_2 allows

259

calculation of the cerebral arteriovenous difference in oxygen content and assessment of global cerebral perfusion (hyperaemia or ischaemia) and oxygenation. Additional information regarding cerebral ischaemia can be gained by estimating the lactate oxygen index. This figure is calculated from the arteriojugular difference in lactate concentration and the arteriojugular difference in oxygen content. Sjo_2 monitoring may also prove useful in determining prognosis from severe head injury.

Transcranial Doppler ultrasonography is used to measure blood flow velocity, intermittently or continuously, usually in the middle cerebral artery. This technique measures the pulsatility index which is a dimensionless figure derived from the difference between systolic and diastolic flow velocity divided by mean flow velocity. As CPP decreases, the mean velocity decreases and the pulsatility index increases, alerting the clinician about the possibility of inadequate cerebral perfusion. This technique is also useful in identifying cerebral vasospasm; a unilateral increase in insonated cerebral artery flow velocity is seen when the CPP is adequate.

Basic management—The aims of management of patients with head injury are to provide the optimal conditions for recovery of the injured brain. It is essential to identify risk factors and to monitor the patient closely to prevent, to detect, and to treat causes of secondary brain injury.

All patients with severe head injury will be sedated, intubated, and ventilated. Patients should be nursed with the head in a neutral position and 15–30° head up. The endotracheal tube should be secured with adhesive strapping to the face to avoid potential cerebrovascular engorgement if neck tapes are used. Continuous intravenous infusion of sedatives, analgesics, and neuromuscular blocking agents (if required) should be administered to maintain cardiovascular stability. Additional boluses of intravenous sedatives or analgesics may be required before therapeutic interventions which could increase ICP, such as physiotherapy.

Patients are ventilated to ensure optimal oxygenation and Pao_2 above 13 kPa, and to maintain $Paco_2$ in the range 3·5–4·5 kPa. Adequate oxygenation is paramount; the use of positive and expiratory pressure to achieve this, if required, should not be deleterious provided that the patient is nursed 30° head up, and the mean arterial pressure and CPP are maintained. Regular chest physiotherapy is essential, particularly in paralysed patients.

Arterial pressure should be maintained with appropriate intravenous fluids and inotropes if indicated. The most common causes of hypotension are inadequate fluid resuscitation and the administration of sedative drugs, in particular propofol.

Intracranial pressure—Raised ICP is associated with significant morbidity and mortality after severe head injury. Fifty to seventy per cent of patients with severe head injury develop raised ICP at some time.[25] The causes of raised ICP are the following:

- Intracranial haematoma (extradural, subdural, intracerebral)
- Cerebrovascular engorgement
- Increased brain water content (cerebral oedema)
- Acute hydrocephalus.

Intracranial haematoma may be extradural, subdural, or intracerebral, and can also be associated with cerebral oedema. Cerebrovascular engorgement may occur as a result of convulsions, active cerebral arterial vasodilatation (secondary to a reduction in CPP, elevation of $Paco_2$, or reduction of Pao_2), passive distension of vessels associated with an increased arterial pressure in the presence of impaired autoregulation, or obstruction of cerebral venous outflow (PEEPs, excessive flexion/rotation of the neck, pneumothorax, elevated central venous pressure, or coughing/straining). Cerebral oedema may be caused by vasogenic, cytotoxic, hydrostatic, osmotic, or interstitial mechanisms.[26] Acute hydrocephalus results from impaired CSF drainage secondary to haematoma, cerebral oedema, or blood in the ventricles.

If the cerebral compliance is reduced, any increase in volume within the vault (blood, brain, CSF) may result in a significant increase in ICP, leading to a critical reduction in CPP, cerebral ischaemia, and potential cell death.

The presence of raised ICP is often very difficult to detect clinically. Papilloedema seldom occurs after head injury, even in patients with elevated ICP. The CT scan findings of cerebral oedema are areas of radiolucency with a shift in the surrounding structures. Signs indicating raised ICP include the pattern of diffuse brain swelling with loss of the appearance of the third ventricle and the perimesencephalic CSF cisternae, or of mass effect with compression of one lateral ventricle and enlargement of the opposite ventricle (see figs 10.2 and 10.4).

The most accurate assessment of ICP is to measure it directly as discussed previously. The indications for monitoring ICP are the following:

1 Coma with intracranial haematoma or contusion
2 Coma with loss of third ventricle and perimesencephalic cistern on computed tomography
3 Coma with abnormal motor responses (GCSS < 6)
4 Tight brain at operation for evacuation of intracranial haematoma
5 Multiple injuries requiring the patient to be ventilated.

Continuous monitoring of ICP and CPP allows early detection and correction of adverse events, and monitoring of the effects of therapeutic intervention. Treatment is usually started if the mean ICP exceeds 25 mm Hg during the first 48 hours after injury and is above 30 mm Hg thereafter.

It is important to be aware of the possible causes of intracranial hypertension and for therapy to be guided by the underlying pathophysiological process.[25] [26]

Treatment of raised ICP

1 Specific therapy for raised ICP should only be implemented after measures have been taken to correct remediable causes.
2 Hyperventilation to Pa_{CO_2} of about 3·0–3·5 kPa; the effect is only short lived and may produce sufficient cerebral vasoconstriction to cause ischaemia.
3 Diuretic therapy, for example, intravenous mannitol 0·5 g/kg over 15 minutes; the rapid action of mannitol is thought to result from the reduction in blood viscosity which leads to cerebral vasoconstriction to maintain constant CBF. The prolonged effect of mannitol is explained by the reduction in brain water content. Colloids should be given subsequently to maintain circulating blood volume. Frusemide (furosemide) given after the mannitol potentiates the effect on ICP.
4 Hypnotic drugs control ICP by reducing cerebral metabolism and affecting CBF. Their effect is dependent on persistence of cerebral vascular reactivity to carbon dioxide. During treatment with hypnotic drugs it is important not to reduce the CPP secondary to a reduction in mean arterial pressure; this problem is accentuated by hypovolaemia. Suitable drugs could be intravenous thiopentone (thiopental) 5 mg/kg over 5 minutes or propofol 1·5 mg/kg.
5 Drain CSF via ventricular drain.
6 Surgical decompression.
7 Increase systemic arterial pressure with intravenous fluids and/or inotropes to raise CPP (pulmonary artery pressure monitoring is essential in this group of patients).

Remediable causes of raised ICP include:

- Airway obstruction
- Hypoxia
- Hypercapnia
- Hypertension/hypotension
- Neck flexion/rotation
- Inadequate sedation/analgesia
- Inadequate neuromuscular blockade
- Coughing/spontaneous respiratory effort against the ventilator
- PEEP
- Pyrexia
- Pain
- Hyponatraemia
- Hypoproteinaemia.

Steroid therapy failed to reduce the incidence or severity of intracranial hypertension after head injury and was associated with a higher morbidity and mortality in patients with raised ICP.[27]

Most patients with head injury are nursed with a 10–15° head up tilt to aid venous and CSF drainage. Further head elevation can be useful in patients with raised ICP, although maintenance of an adequate CPP is necessary. Feldman et al[28] demonstrated that head elevation to 30° significantly reduced ICP without reducing CPP or CBF.[28]

Alteration in CBF and Sjo_2 during ICP treatment correlates better with changes in the CPP than with the ICP, suggesting that CPP is the crucial parameter to monitor. Chan et al[29][30] demonstrated that below a critical CPP of 70 mm Hg, resulting either from an increase in ICP or from a decrease in mean arterial pressure, there was a linear relationship of CPP, Sjo_2, and the transcranial Doppler pulsatility index. Above this critical CPP, Sjo_2 and pulsatility index were unaltered by a further rise in CPP. Ideally, to ensure adequate cerebral oxygen supply a CPP of at least 70 mm Hg must be maintained. Close monitoring of the CPP and Sjo_2 allows the optimal CPP to be individually determined, and indicates when treatment has been effective, thus avoiding potentially harmful therapeutic interventions.[24][29][30] The choice of treatment for raised ICP should be based on whether the main cause is vascular or cerebral oedema.

Hypnotics appear to be more effective in patients with diffuse brain injury, associated with vascular swelling, mannitol being more effective in cases of focal brain injury (contusions or after haematoma removal).[26]

Outcome

Outcome is assessed using the Glasgow outcome scale (table 10.5).[31] The following factors have a significant adverse effect on outcome:

- **Age**:[2][32][33] older patients have a higher overall mortality as a result of age related effects on the pathophysiological response of the CNS to severe trauma. The age effect seems to be independent of factors such as pre-

Table 10.5   Glasgow outcome scale (GOS)[30]

1	Death
2	Persistent vegetative state (unresponsive and speechless)
3	Severe disability (conscious but disabled)
4	Moderate disability (disabled but independent)
5	Good recovery (resumption of normal life)

The time of the assessment should be stated, as during the first year following head injury some patients will improve their Glasgow outcome score and others, in the persistent vegetative state or severe disability, will die.

existing medical status, occurrence of multiple injuries, and injury severity, although the mechanism of injury, and greater incidence of hypoxaemia and hypotension, in this group may play an additional role in outcome

- **Admission motor score**[33]
- **Abnormal pupils**:[32 33] patients who have abnormal pupil reactivity following resuscitation, in particular bilaterally, have a much greater chance of death or persistent vegetative state
- **Intracranial pressure**: proportion of hourly ICP readings greater than 20 mm Hg[33]
- **Hypotension**: proportion of hourly systolic blood pressure readings less than 80 mm Hg[32]
- **Intracranial pathology**
- **Mass lesion**: determinants of outcome in patients with traumatic intracranial haematoma are: GCSS on admission to the neurosurgical unit, pupillary abnormalities, number (reflecting diffuse nature of injury), site (central haematomas < 20% good outcome) and size (associated with late deterioration) of haematoma, necessity for airway/ventilation intervention (emphasising the importance of early intubation and ventilation to avoid secondary insults) and surgical removal[34]
- **Secondary insults**: hypotension and hypoxia have a major influence on outcome
- **Mechanism of injury**: this relates to intracranial pathology, associated injuries, and patient age.[2 32]

It is generally recognised that patients with diffuse brain injury have a lower mortality rate than patients with mass lesions. Marshall *et al*[35] devised a new classification of head injuries based on the initial CT findings and found that specific subsets of patients with diffuse brain injury have a similar outcome when compared with patients with mass lesions. Therefore, patients considered to be low risk on clinical examination can be identified as being high risk on the CT scan. Patients with diffuse injuries associated with a midline shift of more than 5 mm have a higher incidence of developing intracranial hypertension and a mortality rate of more than 50%. Although the incidence of diffuse head injury with midline shift is relatively low, it has a very high mortality rate, suggesting that this group of patients represents a target group in which innovative therapies might first be tested.[35]

Diffuse brain injury in children is associated with a high mortality rate, 53% as compared with 15% in all other paediatric head injury.[6]

Recent evidence suggests that the outcome of a substantial proportion of patients with severe head injury can be expected to improve significantly up to six months after injury, suggesting that decisions regarding the withdrawal of treatment in vegetative patients should be delayed until the six month time period.[36]

Future

Improved outcome after brain trauma will depend on two main strategies. The first relates to improved early management aimed at preventing avoidable causes of secondary insults and to the development of new methods of monitoring patients to detect these insults. The second relates to provision of new therapeutic regimens aimed at countering the damaging biochemical cascades that follow brain injury.

There is little doubt that improved resuscitation and avoiding management errors would influence outcome favourably. Institution of more universally agreed methods of assessment and diagnostic categories would permit more meaningful comparisons between published series and might allow definition of appropriate subsets of patients who can be investigated for the potential benefit of targeted treatment regimens.[32] New technologies such as the near infrared spectroscope may soon permit continuous non-invasive monitoring of cerebral oxygen usage. Novel therapies directed at reducing neuronal injury secondary to ischaemic insults are currently the subject of frantic activity in the pharmaceutical world. Although studies with the calcium channel blocker nimodipine have shown no benefit after brain injury,[37] other phase three studies are currently investigating whether the free radical scavenger polyethylene glycol superoxide dismutase, several N-methyl-D-aspartate (NMDA) receptor antagonists, 21 aminosteroids, and N channel calcium entry blockers are beneficial after brain trauma. It is hoped that these strategies will allow further inroads into reducing mortality and morbidity after this crippling disorder of predominantly young adults.

1 Jennett B, MacMillan R. Epidemiology of head injury. *BMJ* 1981; **282**: 101–4.
2 Vollmer DG, Torner JC, Jane JA, *et al*. Age and outcome following traumatic coma: why do older patients fare worse? *J Neurosurg* 1991; **75**: S37–49.
3 Lestina DC, Williams AF, Lund AK, Zador P, Kuhlmann TP. Motor vehicle crash injury patterns and the Virginia seat belt law. *JAMA* 1991; **265**: 1409–13.
4 Thomas S, Acton C, Nixon J, Battistutta D, Pitt WR, Clark R. Effectiveness of bicycle helmets in preventing head injury in children: case-control study. *BMJ* 1994; **308**: 173–6.
5 Teasdale E, Cardoso E, Galbraith S, Teasdale G. A new CT scan appearance with raised intracranial pressure in severe diffuse head injury. *J Neurol Neurosurg Psychiatry* 1984; **47**: 600–3.
6 Aldrich EF, Eisenberg HM, Saydjari C, *et al*. Diffuse brain swelling in severely head-injured children. *J Neurosurg* 1992; **76**: 450–4.
7 Zimmerman RA, Bilaniuk LT, Bruce D, Dolinskas C, Obrist W, Kuhl D. Computed tomography of pediatric head trauma: acute general cerebral swelling. *Radiology* 1978; **126**: 403–8.
8 Hills MW, Deane SA. Head injury and facial injury: is there an increased risk of cervical spine injury? *J Trauma* 1993; **34**: 549–53.
9 American College of Surgeons Committee on Trauma. *ATLS course manual*. Chicago: American College of Surgeons, 1993.
10 Teasdale G, Jennett B. Assessment of coma and impaired conciousness. *Lancet* 1974; **ii**: 81–4.
11 Association of Anaesthetists of Great Britain and Ireland. *Recommendations for standards of monitoring during anaesthesia and recovery*. London: Association of Anaesthetists, 1988.
12 Runcie CJ, Reeve WG, Reidy J, Dougall JR. Blood pressure measurement during transport. A comparison of direct and oscillotonometric readings in critically ill patients. *Anaesthesia* 1990; **45**: 659–65.

13 Briggs M, Clarke P, Crockard A, et al. Guidelines for initial management after head injury in adults. BMJ 1984; 288: 983–5.

14 Gentleman D, Dearden NM, Midgeley S, Maclean D. Guidelines for resuscitation and transfer of patients with serious head injury. BMJ 1993; 307: 547–52.

15 Knuckey NW, Gelbard S, Epstein MH. The management of 'asymptomatic' epidural haematomas. A prospective study. J Neurosurg 1989; 70: 392–6.

16 Gentleman D, Jennett B. Audit of transfer of unconscious head-injured patients to a neurosurgical unit. Lancet 1990; 335: 330–4.

17 Marsh H, Maurice-Williams RS, Hatfield R. Closed Head Injuries: where does delay occur in the process of transfer to neurosurgical care? Br J Neurosurg 1989; 3: 13–20.

18 Andrews PJD, Piper IR, Dearden NM, Miller JD. Secondary insults during intrahospital transport of head-injured patients. Lancet 1990; 335: 327–30.

19 Lambert SM, Willett K. Transfer of multiply-injured patients for neurosurgical opinion: a study of the adequacy of assessment and resuscitation. Injury 1993; 24: 333–6.

20 Guidelines for the transfer of critically ill patients. Crit Care Med 1993; 21: 931–7.

21 Mendelow AD, Teasdale G, Jennett B, Bryden J, Hessett H, Murray G. Risk of intracranial haematoma in head injured adults. BMJ 1983; 287: 1173–6.

22 Lobato RD, Rivas JJ, Gomez PA, et al. Head-injured patients who talk and deteriorate into coma. J Neurosurg 1991; 75: 256–61.

23 Marshall LF, Toole BM, Bowers SA. The National Traumatic Coma Data Bank. Part 2: Patients who talk and deteriorate: Implications for treatment. J Neurosurg 1983; 59: 285–8.

24 Andrews PJD, Dearden NM, Miller JD. Jugular bulb cannulation: Description of a cannulation technique and validation of a new continuous monitor. Br J Anaesth 1991; 67: 553–8.

25 Miller JD, Dearden NM, Piper IR, Chan KH. Control of intacranial pressure in patients with severe head injury. J Neurotrauma 1992; 9: S317–26.

26 Miller JD, Dearden NM. Management of brain edema in head injury. In: Takeshita H, Siesjo BK, Miller JD (Eds), Advances in brain resuscitation, vol 17. Springer Verlag: Tokyo, 1991: 221–32.

27 Dearden NM, Gibson JS, McDowall DG, Gibson RM, Cameron MM. Effect of high dose dexamethasone on outcome from severe head injury. J Neurosurg 1986; 64: 81–8.

28 Feldman Z, Kanter MJ, Robertson CS, et al. Effect of head elevation on intracranial pressure, cerebral perfusion pressure, and cerebral blood flow in head-injured patients. J Neurosurg 1992; 76: 207–11.

29 Chan KH, Dearden NM, Miller JD, Andrews PJD, Midgley S. Multimodality monitoring as a guide to treatment of intracranial hypertension after severe brain injury. Neurosurgery 1993; 32: 547–53.

30 Chan KH, Miller JD, Dearden NM, Andrews PJD, Midgley S. The effect of changes in cerebral perfusion pressure upon middle cerebral artery blood flow velocity and jugular bulb venous oxygen saturation after severe brain injury. J Neurosurg 1992; 77: 55–61.

31 Jennett B, Bond M. Assessment of outcome after severe brain damage. A practical scale. Lancet 1975; i: 480–4.

32 Marshall LF, Gautille T, Klauber MR, et al. The outcome after severe closed head injury. J Neurosurg 1991; 75: S26–36.

33 Marmarou A, Anderson RL, Ward JD, et al. Impact of ICP instability and hypotension on outcome in patients with severe head trauma. J Neurosurg 1991; 75: S59–66.

34 Choksey M, Crockard HA, Sandilands M. Acute traumatic intracranial haematomas: determinants of outcome in a retrospective series of 202 cases. Br J Neurosurg 1993; 7: 611–22.

35 Marshall LF, Marshall SB, Klauber MR, et al. A new classification of head injury based on computerized tomography. J Neurosurg 1991; 75: S14–20.

36 Choi SC, Barnes TY, Bullock R, Germanson TA, Marmarou A, Young HF. Temporary profile of outcomes in severe head injury. J Neurosurg 1994; 81: 169–73.

37 Teasdale G, Bailey I, Bell A, et al. The effect of nimodipine on outcome after head injury: a prospective randomised control trial. The British/Finnish Co-operative Head Injury Trial Group. Acta Neurochirurg suppl, 1990; 51: 315–16.

11: Brain protection and brain death

MARLEEN VERHAEGEN, DAVID S WARNER

Brain ischaemia research has produced a recent explosion of information regarding the pathophysiology of this disorder. Indeed, we are in the midst of a theoretical revolution which yields real hope that physicians will soon be able to offer safe and effective therapy to patients with an ischaemic insult. In spite of this, current approaches to reducing permanent injury from perioperative cerebral ischaemia have remained largely unchanged over the past few decades. The few clinical advances that have occurred largely involve recognition of the importance of physiological variables (which the anaesthetist can easily control) on the pathogenesis of and outcome from cerebral ischaemia. The goal of this chapter is to review the scientific basis of our current clinical practices and also to set the stage for therapies that are likely to become clinically available in the next few years.

Although many topics are candidates for discussion, four seem of greatest relevance to the neurosurgical patient. The first is the role of balancing metabolic supply and demand during ischaemia by the use of drugs that reduce cerebral metabolic rate. This approach has been largely discredited but continues to dominate clinical practice. Second, hypothermia has re-emerged as a protective strategy for the neurosurgical patient. Emphasis has now been placed on the effects of mild reductions in body temperature which have been found to be highly protective without apparent substantive risk. Third, the effects of glucose on the ischaemic brain have generally been found to be adverse. This imposes on the anaesthetist a responsibility for monitoring and regulating plasma glucose concentrations. Finally, the concept of glutamatergic excitotoxicity, although still experimental, promises in the near future to allow new approaches to care of patients who might endure an ischaemic insult.

After the above points have been discussed, this chapter will turn its attention to a related topic. Coexistent with advances made in the field of brain protection and resuscitation, equally important advances have occurred with respect to maintaining viability of other organ systems. Consequently the clinical presentation of brain death in the context of an otherwise living human body has become a common reality which presents both medical and ethical dilemmas. A discussion of the procedures for and the limitations of clinical evaluation of brain death presents an argument for a thorough history and physical examination supplemented by laboratory and technical tests to confirm this diagnosis.

Brain protection

Definitions

Cerebral ischaemia is a haemodynamic insult resulting in reduction of cerebral blood flow (CBF) to values which, if sustained, will cause irreversible neuronal injury. Outcome from this insult can be quantified on either a histological or neurological basis. Two forms of ischaemia are often discussed:

1 Global ischaemia is classically associated with events such as cardiac arrest resulting in hypoperfusion of the entire organ. This term is sometimes also applied to states of regional hypoperfusion where there is no potential for recruitment of collateral flow.
2 Focal ischaemia, in contrast, represents occlusion of an artery distal to the circle of Willis such as the middle cerebral artery. As collateral flow can occur, brain tissue sustains graded degrees of hypoperfusion resulting in a densely ischaemic core (pathophysiologically resembling global ischaemia) surrounded by a penumbral zone. In the penumbra, the fate of neurons is precarious but presumably more salvageable than is the case for the ischaemic core.

Cerebral protection involves interventions instituted before the ischaemic insult which result in an improved tolerance of the brain to that insult. In contrast, cerebral resuscitation refers to intervention instituted after onset of the ischaemic insult. On a mechanistic basis, the goal of cerebral protection is to prevent ischaemic initiation of pathophysiological processes. The goal of cerebral resuscitation is to interrupt those processes.

Balancing substrate demand with delivery

The concept is simple. Ischaemia reduces supply of metabolic substrates including glucose and O_2. Abrupt cessation of flow leads to an isoelectric EEG within 20–30 s and high energy phosphate stores are fully depleted within 2 min. Drugs that decrease metabolic demand should influence energy balance favourably and allow prolonged tolerance to and improved outcome from a discrete and temporary ischaemic insult (fig 11.1). This subject will be covered in detail because the story is now nearly complete with respect to the potential for this mechanism of action to provide a strategy for brain protection.

Modern theory and practice were heavily influenced by a clinical report

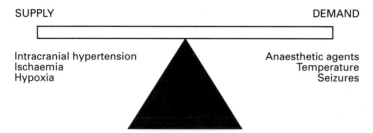

SUPPLY   DEMAND

Intracranial hypertension   Anaesthetic agents
Ischaemia   Temperature
Hypoxia   Seizures

Fig 11.1 Classic concept of cerebral energetics: the balance between metabolic supply and demand can be influenced favourably or unfavourably by a variety of factors

made in 1963 by vascular surgeons who observed decreased incidence of neurological complications from carotid endarterectomy in patients who received general as opposed to local anaesthesia for the procedure.[1] That study would not have met current methodological standards and the true role of anaesthesia regarding outcome from carotid endarterectomy is not yet defined. Nevertheless, given the information then available, it was reasonable to attempt to define which aspect of the anaesthetic was purportedly responsible for the protection. This was addressed with a canine study from the same group (again methodologically flawed) which discerned that neurological outcome from hypoxia was substantially improved by barbiturates but not by procaine, 100% O_2, or morphine.[2]

Barbiturate therapy thus became the focus of both laboratory and clinical studies. The most pertinent are the following. First, it was recognised that barbiturates reduce cerebral metabolic rate by about 50%. This reduction is accompanied by a progressive electroencephalographic (EEG) quiescence. When the EEG trace becomes isoelectric, no further reduction of cerebral metabolic rate (CMR) can be achieved by additional doses of the drug.[3] It was concluded that barbiturate reduction in CMR was linked to inhibition of synaptic neurotransmission and hence preservation of energy. Thus the mechanism by which barbiturates were thought to offer protection limited the possible scenarios where protection could be expected.

An experimental depiction of the above theory is as follows. Dogs were randomised to receive high dose thiopentone (thiopental) or no treatment before either haemorrhagic hypotension or anoxia.[4] Cortical high energy phosphate concentrations were determined during these insults. The hypotensive insult was mild enough to allow persistent but attenuated EEG activity in the absence of the barbiturate. In this case, there was opportunity for thiopentone to suppress neurotransmission and reduce energy requirements. A substantial slowing in the deterioration of adenosine triphosphate (ATP) stores was observed. In contrast, when the anoxic insult was applied in the absence of barbiturates, an isoelectric EEG rapidly developed. There was no EEG activity for thiopentone to suppress and predictably the decay of ATP concentration was uninfluenced by thiopentone.

269

These observations led to a conclusion which has pervaded research and practice concerning effects of anaesthetics on ischaemic brain damage for over two decades. Drugs that reduce CMR by virtue of reduction in EEG activity can only be effective in conditions in which the ischaemic insult is mild enough to allow some EEG activity to persist. An example would be in the penumbra of a focal ischaemic insult. In contrast, if the insult is so severe that it produces an isoelectric EEG trace, as might occur during global ischaemia, there would be no mechanism for such drugs to offer benefit and no protection could be expected. This theory predicted the results of many experiments in both laboratory animals and humans, which observed a consistent benefit from barbiturates during focal ischaemia[5-7] and failure of these drugs to improve outcome from global insults.[8-10] Clinically, barbiturates would be expected to work only during conditions such as temporary intracranial vascular occlusion for intracranial aneurysm surgery or for open cardiac procedures, such as valve surgery, which carry a major risk of arterial emboli.

Eventually, other drugs became available which reduced CMR as effectively as the barbiturates but had shorter durations of action, thereby allowing the sedative side effects to be present only during surgical procedures. Presumably these drugs would be superior intraoperative neuroprotectants because patients could be more readily awakened for neurological examination after the surgical procedure. This list includes etomidate, propofol, isoflurane, and sevoflurane. Isoflurane drew the largest interest because it is routinely used, rapidly eliminated, and EEG burst suppression can be achieved with clinically relevant doses. To the surprise of many, isoflurane did not offer unique protection as opposed to other anaesthetic agents, even during focal insults.[11-14] As isoflurane is a cerebral vasodilator, it was speculated that this drug results in a cerebrovascular steal which might counteract the favourable energetics associated with it. When CBF was compared during a focal ischaemic insult in rats receiving isoflurane or a barbiturate anaesthetic, however, perfusion was best with isoflurane.[15] Etomidate, although seeming to allow good outcome from aneurysm surgery,[16] has never met the scrutiny applied to barbiturates in controlled primate or human studies. Etomidate thus remains a distant competitor as an intraoperative protective agent. Similarly, propofol and sevoflurane have also failed to provide a greater degree of protection than provided by halothane anaesthesia in rat models of focal ischaemia.[17 18]

The results with isoflurane and other anaesthetic depressants of CMR were troublesome because the idea of balancing demand and supply could not be extended to drugs other than the barbiturates. Two recent studies in the rat can help provide a perspective on this. The first study examined the role of CMR reduction in delaying onset of terminal depolarisation. Terminal depolarisation is an electrophysiological response to profound ischaemia identified as a shift in the resting direct current potential between brain and body. This resting potential normally represents a mass of polarised tissue. When energy failure ensues, neurons depolarise (ionic gradients deteriorate) in mass and this event can be easily detected by cortical microelectrodes. The effects of isoflurane anaesthesia, in a dose resulting in a reduction of metabolic rate of about 40%, were compared with those from a dose of halothane which resulted in a reduction of metabolic rate of about 10%. Onset of terminal depolarisation occurred about 90 s earlier in rats anaesthetised with halothane.[19] Presumably the prolongation of time to depolarisation in the isoflurane group was attributable to the reduction in energy requirement. To place this 90 s in context, however, when an identical ischaemic insult is applied to halothane anaesthetised rats which are allowed to recover and survive, histological changes are not evident unless the duration of ischaemia exceeds 4 min. Even at 10 min, there is only restricted histological damage and few neurological changes.[20 21] The effect of reducing the duration of ischaemia by 90 s on histological outcome is therefore not discernible with current animal models. The limited effect of anaesthetic agents on the rate of cerebral energy failure may explain why an effect on outcome from global ischaemia has never been observed in well controlled studies.

That conclusion was punctured by the following study. Rats underwent 10 min of global ischaemia while receiving either halothane (minimal effect on CMR) or isoflurane anaesthesia (major effect on CMR). The halothane group was subdivided on the basis of the intraischaemic pericranial temperature (38°C or 35°C). Histological outcomes were compared. In both the isoflurane–38°C and halothane–38°C groups, severe damage was observed without a difference between groups. In contrast, the halothane–35°C group had only minimal injury.[22] Thus mild hypothermia (which causes a reduction in CMR of about 15%) was far more protective than a reduction in CMR of about 50% provided by isoflurane.

There are several conclusions which can be drawn from extant evidence. First, the "time bought" by CMR reduction is probably irrelevant and suggests little clinical importance for this mechanism of brain protection. Second, the mechanism by which hypothermia protects the brain is probably other than simple reduction of metabolic rate (see below). Third, the neuroprotection afforded by barbiturates is also likely to be attributable to mechanisms of action other than reduction in metabolic rate.

This last point concerning barbiturates draws special interest when the following question is asked. Is there direct evidence that barbiturates reduce focal ischaemic brain damage in a dose dependent manner? If indeed the mechanism of action is a reduction in metabolic rate, it should be the case that progressively larger doses of barbiturates (and the corresponding progressive reduction in metabolic rate) are associated with progressively smaller infarcts. Several early studies have addressed this issue,[5 23] the best controlled of which is the following.[5] Baboons were subjected to permanent middle cerebral artery occlusion. The dose of pentobarbitone (pentobarbital) was graded although EEG activity was not monitored. Indeed, when all subjects were considered, a dose dependent reduction in cerebral infarct size was observed. As data for each animal were provided in the article it is possible, however, to examine for outliers retrospectively. In fact, one outlier was found in the lowest dosage group. If that animal is not included in the analysis, a very different conclusion can be drawn. Pentobarbitone reduced cerebral infarct volume (when compared with halothane anaesthesia), but the maximal effect occurred at doses lower than those that produced maximal reduction in metabolic rate (fig 11.2). Therefore, the best evidence available that barbiturate protection is mediated by reduction of CMR is equivocal.

The above cited studies do not necessarily mean that anaesthetics other than barbiturates offer no protection against ischaemic insults in the central nervous system (CNS). There are numerous studies which suggest the contrary. Cole et al[24] demonstrated superior neurological function during recovery from transient spinal cord compression when rats were anaesthetised (regardless of anaesthetic) versus those animals sustaining the insult with no anesthetic. Other investigators, using very lightly anaesthetised control groups, have consistently observed improved neurological/histological outcome in more deeply anaesthetised rats undergoing incomplete hemispherical ischaemia—but this also appears to be independent of anaesthetic agent.[25–28] Subsequent work has associated this improved outcome with reduced concentrations of circulating catecholamines and possibly decreased central adrenergic neurotransmitter activity, suggesting a potential mechanism of action.[29] Finally, others have shown that rats anaesthetised

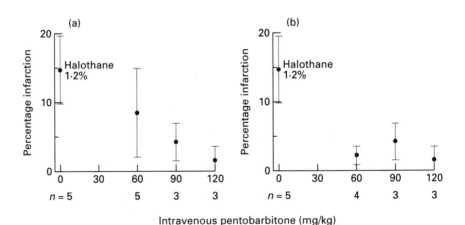

Fig 11.2 (a) Example of dose–response relationship between a barbiturate and percentage of ipsilateral hemisphere infarcted as a result of middle cerebral artery occlusion in the baboon. (b) The dose–response relationship dissipates, however, with the exclusion of one animal (outlier) from the lowest dose group. Sample sizes (n) are given. (Recreated from Hoff et al[5])

with either sevoflurane or halothane experience substantially better histological and neurological outcomes from focal insults than do rats kept conscious.[17] This effect persists even when pericranial temperature is strictly controlled at normothermia.[30] Clearly, further work is necessary for an explicit definition of the role of anaesthesia in the pathophysiology of ischaemic brain damage.

Hypothermia

Hypothermia has been invoked as an intraoperative neuroprotection strategy for over 30 years.[31] For most of that time, the mechanism of action was thought to be attributable to a reduction in CMR. Indeed CMR undergoes a log-linear reduction as brain temperature is progessively reduced (but see Michenfelder and Milde[32]).[33] Corresponding to this is the dramatic protection observed during cardiac arrest for paediatric cardiac surgical procedures. Even adults undergoing repair of giant intracranial aneurysms tolerate prolonged intervals of arrested circulation (reported durations of up to 51 min) when body temperature is reduced to 17–20°C.[34] In spite of these clear benefits, however, it became obvious that deep hypothermia with obligatory cardiopulmonary bypass and anticoagulation is a therapy that presents serious hazards. In fact, adverse effects of only moderate hypothermia induced by surface cooling (about 29°C) were found to outweigh neuroprotective benefits in primates,[35 36] leading to the near total abandonment of this therapy in all but a very few selected cases in the neurosurgical population.

More recently, renewed interest in intraoperative hypothermia has emerged but this time attention has been focused on only mild reductions in body temperature.[37] This renaissance is directly attributable to the development of rodent models of cerebral ischaemia. When attempting to account for variable outcome from standardised insults, it was recognised that the rodent head cools quickly when deprived of blood flow. Systematic reduction of brain temperature by only a few degrees centrigrade was found to result in substantial protection.[38] At the same time numerous new strategies were being investigated for cerebral protective efficacy (see below). None offered the magnitude of protection afforded by simply cooling the brain 2–3°C. Indeed, even global ischaemia was found to be amenable to protection by mild hypothermia, although this form of ischaemia had been entirely resistant to most other forms of therapy. Further, a mildly hypothermic state was found to reduce ischaemic injury even if administered after reperfusion of the brain had occurred in the rat.[39 40] More recently, benefits of mild hypothermia have been extended to the condition of head injury.[41–44] The above outlined observations were of special interest to anaesthetists who frequently encounter mild hypothermia as a simple (and otherwise undesirable) byproduct of general anaesthesia.

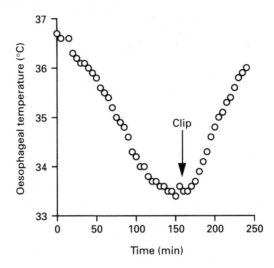

Fig 11.3 Example of intraoperative oesophageal temperature profile during induced hypothermia and rewarming in a patient undergoing cerebral aneurysm clipping

The mechanism of action by which mild hypothermia ameliorates ischaemic brain damage is not clear. Most probably, the process is multifactorial. It is highly unlikely that the minor reduction in CMR accounts for the protective effect. Other proposed mechanisms include changes in ion permeability,[45] protein synthesis,[46] free radical reactions and membrane lipid peroxidation,[47] blood–brain barrier permeability,[48] regulation of protein kinase C,[49] and time to terminal depolarisation.[50]

Unfortunately, there are no outcome studies to guide us in the conduct of intraoperative induced mild hypothermia. It certainly is feasible to provide hypothermia with the appropriate level of rewarming in the neurosurgical patient (fig 11.3).[51] Further, it seems likely that properly conducted clinical trials will identify value for mild hypothermia in selected neurosurgical procedures. Preliminary studies performed in head injured patients support this expectation.[42–44] Problems that must be resolved include temperature measurement sites,[52] magnitude of hypothermia offering best risk/benefit ratio,[53] and methods of rapid rewarming to provide near normothermic temperatures at emergence from anaesthesia without burn injury or myocardial ischaemia.[53 54]

Hyperglycaemia

Research over the past two decades has presented a paradox to those dealing with cerebral ischaemia, that is, although the normal brain is almost totally dependent on a continuous delivery of exogenous glucose for maintenance of cellular energy requirements, the ischaemic or hypoxic brain finds continued glucose availability to be detrimental. Pursuit of an explanation for this has yielded a large body of information, some of which has direct clinical relevance.

The initial observation that preischaemic glucose infusion worsens ischaemic outcome was serendipitous. Myers and Yamaguchi[55] had designed an experiment using fasted primates to assess the effects of a brief cardiac arrest on learned visual tasks. They had recognised that successful cardiac resuscitation could be enhanced by prearrest intravenous volume loading. The investigators were not, however, consistent with the types of fluids administered. Although most of the animals recovered from ischaemia and went on to have visual cortical function assessed, two monkeys developed seizures and died early after reperfusion. In retrospect, the investigators recognised that those two monkeys had received dextrose in their fluid bolus, although those that survived had not. This association between glucose infusion and worsened outcome from global ischaemia was soon validated under more controlled conditions in the same laboratory, and has subsequently been repeated with remarkable consistency in numerous models, species, and research centres (fig 11.4).[56–60]

Before this discovery, other investigators had suggested an unfavourable relationship between cerebral acidosis and ischaemic injury.[61] It was not long until that acidosis was linked to glucose administration.[62] As we know, in the absence of sufficient oxygen supply, cellular energy requirements may be partially supported by anaerobic glycolysis. Under conditions of hypoxaemia or ischaemia, a relative hyperglycaemia would be expected to allow some ATP production at the cost of an enhanced accumulation of lactate, the end product of glycolysis. Lactate has a pK_a of 3·83, meaning that at physiological

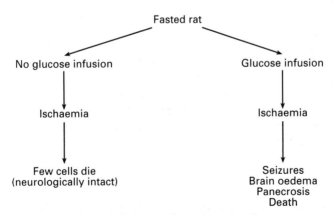

Fig 11.4 Intravenous glucose infusion can have dramatic effects on outcome from 10 min of severe forebrain ischaemia in the rat

pH virtually all of it will be ionised. The predicted effect of preischaemic glucose infusion would therefore be an intracellular acidosis. This acidosis is believed to be the cause of the worsened outcome.[63]

In the case of focal ischaemia, such as occurs during occlusion of a major intracranial vessel, the effect of glucose administration on outcome is not as clear. Mixed experimental results have been obtained.[64-68] To the authors' knowledge, a satisfactory explanation as to why there has not been the same uniformity of results as has been seen in global ischaemia has not been provided. It has been speculated, however, that these discrepancies are attributable to variations in collateral flow to the ischaemic penumbra. Injury in the ischaemic core is thought to be enhanced by hyperglycaemia whereas damage in the penumbra may be reduced.[69]

The interest in glucose effects on focal ischaemia in large part has been held by neurologists who frequently treat non-operative stroke patients. In an effort to determine if animal investigations have anything to do with the human condition, numerous studies have been reported comparing blood glucose values at the time of hospital admission with outcome from stroke[70-73] and head trauma.[74] Most of these studies did find a correlation. Patients who do the worst neurologically also have the highest glucose values on admission to the hospital. It has not been determined, however, if elevated glucose values represent a reactive hyperglycaemia, or rather are coincidental and truly cause a worsened outcome. Several recent studies have examined this question but a consensus remains evasive.[75 76]

With respect to spinal cord ischaemia, several studies have evaluated the effects of hyperglycaemia on outcome.[77-79] In a study by Drummond and Moore[79] rabbits underwent a transient infrarenal balloon occlusion of the aorta. Before ischaemia, either Ringer's lactate solution or 5% dextrose in water was infused for 90 min. A significantly higher plasma glucose concentration was observed in those rabbits receiving the dextrose which corresponded to a significantly worsened neurological outcome.

Most clinicians have accepted the above information and assume that hyperglycaemia during a potential ischaemic insult is undesirable. As anaesthetists, however, we may still be uncertain as to how this information should guide our clinical practice. It can be argued that laboratory protocols were designed to produce maximal effects, that is, in most studies preischaemic hyperglycaemia was severe (>300 mg/dl). Does this have anything to do with a modest glucose infusion such as would occur with 1 litre of dextrose containing solution at the start of a surgical procedure? Lanier et al[59] addressed this question by administering 5% dextrose in water to monkeys (in a volume equivalent to giving 1 litre of the same to a 70 kg human) before inducing a reversible global ischaemic insult. Neurological outcome in those monkeys was compared with that in a group that had received the same volume of physiological saline instead. Of note, dextrose infusion failed to produce a significant increase in blood glucose. Nevertheless a significantly worsened neurological outcome was observed in the animals receiving dextrose. Thus severe hyperglycaemia is not necessary to elicit the glucose effect and, as far as this primate model can predict, small doses of glucose may predispose patients to a worsened outcome.

It is interesting to note that coincidence may have provided the surgical patient with a safeguard. Elective procedures are most likely to be performed on fasted patients. This tends to minimise any ability to mount a hyperglycaemic response to the stress of anaesthesia and surgery. On the other hand, does withholding dextrose predispose the fasted patient to the risk of hypoglycaemia? This has been addressed in a study examining patients undergoing craniotomy for supratentorial tumours.[80] Eight fasted patients received 5% dextrose in physiological saline whereas another eight patients received physiological saline without dextrose as intraoperative fluids. Throughout the procedure and for 24 h postoperatively the patients were monitored for plasma glucose and evidence of starvation by serially measured free fatty acids, ketone bodies, arterial blood base excess/pH, and urinary nitrogen. Intraoperatively, no patients in either group became hypoglycaemic although a difference in plasma glucose was identified between the groups (physiological saline = 120–160 mg/dl; 5% dextrose in physiological saline = 200–242 mg/dl). No differences in base excess or pH were observed. Free fatty acids and ketones were modestly elevated intraoperatively in those not receiving dextrose, as was urinary nitrogen. By 24 h, however, all values had normalised without any residual differences between groups. These results support the conclusion that although our metabolic machinery recognises the absence of intraoperative dextrose, the price to be paid for withholding dextrose is small and justifiable in neurosurgical patients. The obvious exceptions to this are diabetic individuals and neonates, in whom onset of hypoglycaemia may be rapid and have severe consequences. In these patients it is the authors' practice to monitor blood glucose more frequently and to weigh the apparent probability of cerebral ischaemia against the risk of withholding dextrose.

One question often asked is if insulin should be administered to correct hyperglycaemia when ischaemia seems likely. To date there are no human studies completed to support this practice. Accumulating laboratory evidence, however, supports the concept that preischaemic correction of hyperglycaemia with insulin administration improves ischaemic outcome in a variety of animals and experimental conditions.[81–84] The concern with insulin administration is inadvertent induction of profound hypoglycaemia which may in and of itself augment ischaemic brain damage.[85] Fortunately, most anaesthetists are comfortable with acute corrections of plasma glucose concentrations. Thus before high risk neurovascular procedures, correction of substantial hyperglycaemia with insulin should be entertained.

Given the above information it appears prudent to minimise any hyperglycaemic challenge to an ischaemic or traumatic brain insult. As discussed above, the elimination of glucose (dextrose) containing solutions from routine intraoperative administration is safe. In some scenarios, close monitoring of plasma glucose concentrations is indicated particularly in diabetic subjects and neonates. Most drugs can be mixed with physiological saline instead of 5% dextrose in water (although this probably is not necessary—see Longstreth et al[86]). With respect to plasma glucose concentration, the threshold for hyperglycaemia augmented ischaemic brain damage in humans is not clearly defined. Several pieces of evidence suggest that clinical outcomes begin to worsen discernibly with values exceeding 200 mg/dl,[74] although animal work suggests that even immeasurable changes in plasma glucose are relevant.[59] It seems unlikely that a definitive answer will ever be obtained given the ethical constraints against performing the necessary study in humans. At present, therefore, it remains for the practitioner to decide when it is appropriate to intervene.

Excitotoxicity

People dealing with non-operative stroke generally find discussions regarding anaesthetic effects on ischaemic brain damage uninteresting. This is for several reasons. First, the disease is different. Non-operative stroke patients frequently present many hours after onset of symptoms, although time to hospital admission from onset of symptoms is improving.[87] The opportunity to balance supply and demand has long past. Further, risks and complications arising from administration of large doses of anaesthetics were recognised early making this approach clinically unfeasible outside the operating room. It is thus no surprise that a different approach to the problem of treating ischaemic insults evolved.

Two concepts were appreciated in the mid-1980s. The first is *selective vulnerability*. Selective vulnerability refers a heterogeneous sensitivity of different brain regions to brief episodes of ischaemia (similar to differential sensitivity of plants in a garden to the first frost). Even within regions such as the hippocampus, a graded sensitivity by cell type can be observed.[88] Particularly sensitive are pyramidal cells in the CA1 sector. A standardised insult can result in near total obliteration of this population whereas pyramidal neurons in the CA3 sector (only micrometres away) are totally spared. This could not be accounted for by differences in intraischaemic blood flow.[20] What does distinguish these neurons is the degree of glutamatergic afferentation, the CA1 sector having by far the richest supply. Similar findings are observed in the caudoputamen, layers III–V of the cortex, and Purkinje neurons of the cerebellum.

The second concept is that of *delayed neuronal necrosis* (fig 11.5). Neuropathologists have long known that if a postmortem examination is carried out immediately after cardiac arrest, little or no light microscopic changes can be detected in the brain. Modern cardipulmonary resuscitation techniques have, however, allowed postmortem examinations to be performed on individuals who have survived for several days after a cardiac arrest. By this time neurohistological changes not only become evident but also the pattern of injury is consistent with the phenomenon of selective vulnerability discussed above.[89] Thus, the final extent of histological damage cannot be observed until many hours to days after the insult has occurred.

In the mid-1980s major progress was made with the development of rodent models of ischaemia which allowed prolonged recovery from the ischaemic insult so that delayed neuronal necrosis could be accounted for.[90-92] The importance of delayed neuronal necrosis is enormous. Although resumption of ATP synthesis, correction of intracellular acidosis, and partial recovery of EEG activity occur within minutes of the onset of reperfusion, it is clear that some mechanism(s) are initiated by the ischaemic insult which requires time to result in cell death. The interval between reperfusion and cell death represents a potential therapeutic window. If the pathological cascades can be identified, pharmacological intervention seems possible even for the patient with delayed entry to medical care (or for the patient whose intraoperative ischaemic event is appreciated only after emergence from anaesthesia).

Several breakthroughs followed. It was shown with microdialysis studies

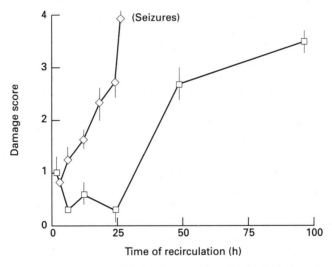

Fig 11.5 Rats undergoing 10 min of severe transient forebrain ischaemia underwent histological evaluation of extent of neuronal necrosis in selectively vulnerable regions at different intervals after reperfusion of the brain. In this case damage in the CA1 sector of the hippocampus is depicted. Open squares depict results from animals run in parallel which were infused with glucose before onset of ischaemia. A damage score of 0 indicates no histological changes whereas a score of 4 indicates infarct. Note the accelerated rate of delayed neuronal necrosis and onset of seizures at about 24 hours postischaemia in the hyperglycaemic group. □ Normoglycaemia; ◇ hyperglycaemia. (Recreated from Smith et al[88a])

that extracellular glutamate concentrations in the selectively vulnerable CA1 sector of the hippocampus become massively increased during ischaemia and the immediate recirculation period.[93][94] Ischaemia also induces a surge of spontaneous neuronal activity in the same region consistent with an abundance of excitatory neurotransmission.[95] In cell culture models, glutamate was shown to result in cell death in concentrations similar to those found in vivo during ischaemia.[96] Finally, the extent of cell death was related to the concentration of extracellular calcium in the culture medium.[97]

Calcium had earlier been proposed to play an integral role in the pathophysiology of cerebral ischaemia.[98] The extracellular : intracellular ratio of calcium is about 10 000 : 1. Maintenance of this gradient is tightly regulated and requires a constant energy supply. Calcium performs many intracellular functions including the role of secondary messenger. Calcium, when bound to the intracellular protein calmodulin, results in activation of protein kinases which, in turn, cause phosphorylative activation of a variety of enzymes. Perturbation of these functions by elevated intracellular calcium is thought to be lethal to the neuron. (For an excellent review of the role of calcium as well as excitotoxicity in cerebral ischaemia, the reader is referred to Siesjö.[99])

There are numerous mechanisms by which intracellular calcium can become increased. First, the voltage dependent calcium channels are considered. The L type voltage dependent calcium channels are postsynaptic low conductance channels opened by depolarisation of the neuron. Calcium entry through this portal can be antagonised non-competitively by a variety of compounds, the best known of which are the dihydropyridines nimodipine and nicardipine. Such compounds have been found to have modest efficacy in the treatment of both cerebral vasospasm and stoke in humans.[100–103] The same compounds have, however, generally been found to have no efficacy against global insults.[104]

Alternatively, calcium may enter the cell via agonist operated calcium channels. These channels have a greater ionic conductance than the voltage dependent calcium channels and are activated by glutamate. In fact, there are numerous postsynaptic glutamate receptor subtypes (N-methyl-D-aspartate or NMDA, α-amino-3-hydroxyl-5-methyl-4-isoxazole-propionic acid or AMPA, and trans-1-aminocyclopentane-1S,3R-dicarboxylic acid or tACPD), so named for the antagonists used to identify them. The most pertinent with respect to calcium entry is the NMDA receptor. Agonism of the NMDA glutamate receptor is allosterically facilitated by the amino acid glycine which, in and of itself, is probably not a neurotransmitter but, instead, a ubiquitous cofactor present in the synaptic cleft. When glycine and glutamate bind to the receptor during depolarisation, a magnesium ion block is alleviated in the associated NMDA ionophore and influx of Ca^{2+}, Na^+, and water ensue.[105][106] Thus antagonism of NMDA gated Ca^{2+} influx is possible by a variety of mechanisms, including competitive antagonism of the glycine or glutamate receptors or non-competitive antagonism of the NMDA ionophore.

In contrast, the AMPA receptor associated ionophore is normally impermeable to divalent cations such as calcium. The role of the AMPA receptor in ischaemia is still unclear. The AMPA receptor, however, allows fast excitation, presumably being the focus of Na^+ flux allowing depolarisation which in turn contributes to the release of the Mg^{2+} blockade in the NMDA ionophore and opening of that channel to Ca^{2+}.

Finally, we consider the tACPD receptor. This receptor is metabotrophic in the sense that it does not operate by means of a transmembrane ion flux. In contrast, the tACPD receptor stimulates synthesis of inositol triphosphate (via a G protein linked mechanism) which activates release of calcium stores from intracellular organelles and effectively increases free intracellular calcium concentration.[107]

Dramatic results have been achieved in focal ischaemia with NMDA receptor antagonists. Both competitive antagonists such as CGS 19755 and non-competitive antagonists such as MK-801 have been shown to reduce infarct volumes by about 50%, even if given at substantial intervals after onset of focal ischaemia in laboratory animals.[108] These same compounds are, however, entirely ineffective against global insults.[109 110] The reason for this is still not clear. One hypothesis is that with single drug therapy, antagonism of either the voltage dependent or agonist operated calcium channels leaves calcium flux through the remaining channel type unopposed.

A more attractive theory to explain the failure of NMDA antagonists to ameliorate global ischaemic injury builds upon the concept of spontaneous depolarisation. Similar electrophysiologically to the phenomenon of terminal depolarisation discussed above, spontaneous depolarisation is observed as an episodic and transient of loss of direct current potential within the marginally perfused penumbra of a focal ischaemic lesion.[11] As some blood flow persists, the tissue may be able to re-establish a polarised state, but this state remains precarious leading to episodic depolarisation and repolarisation of the tissue. Most troublesome is the large increase in metabolic demand caused by the repolarisation process. In normal tissue, CBF can be increased to meet this demand. In contrast, in ischaemic tissue the collateral vessels are already maximally dilated and thus are incapable of providing an appropriate response. Consequently, tissue oxygen content falls episodically below critical levels, causing secondary insults to penumbral tissue.[112] The frequency of such insults presumably defines the eventual fate of that tissue. This theory is supported by observations that NMDA and AMPA receptor antagonists effectively block spontaneous depolarisation, correlating with the known ameliorative effect of such compounds on size of infarct.[113 114] In contrast, during global ischaemia, spontaneous depolarisations have not been observed, and hence under such conditions this mechanism of action may not be available to NMDA receptor antagonists.

More recently, however, compounds that antagonise glutamate at the AMPA receptor have been found to be protective against both focal and global ischaemic injury.[110][115-118] Besides having the distinction that both types of ischaemia are amenable to therapy by AMPA receptor antagonism, these compounds do not apparently possess the psychomimetic side effects observed for the NMDA antagonists.[119] The mechanism by which AMPA receptor antagonists ameliorate global injury is not clear. It is speculated that because fast excitation is inhibited by AMPA receptor antagonism neither the NMDA nor the L type calcium channels become activated.

Several AMPA receptor antagonists are currently in development which may have clinical use.[110][120][121] An additional advantage for this approach to therapy is the absence of psychomimetic side effects for this class of drug. Such problems have plagued the clinical development of NMDA receptor antagonists which produce a mental state similar to that caused by ketamine. Similarly, psychomimetic effects seem to be absent for compounds which antagonise glutamatergic neurotransmission indirectly by competing with glycine at the NMDA recognition site. Glycine receptor antagonists have been found to be efficacious in animal models of focal (but not global) ischaemia and have even been demonstrated to have substantive anaesthetic potential as has also been found for NMDA and AMPA receptor antagonists (fig 11.6).[122-124]

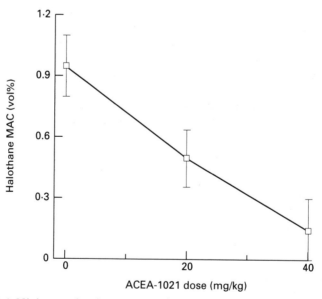

Fig 11.6 Minimum alveolar concentration (MAC) for halothane as a function of intravenous dose of the competitive glycine receptor antagonist ACEA-1021. Values = mean ± SD: (Recreated from McFarlane et al[124])

Brain death

Coexistent with advances made in the field of brain protection and resuscitation, equally important advances have occurred with respect to maintaining viability of other organ systems. Unfortunately, this may result in a patient with irreversible and total loss of cerebral function but persistent viability of remaining organ systems. A diagnosis of brain death has important medical, legal, ethical, and human implications because it may be the basis for termination of treatment or discontinuation of life support. Further, increasingly successful transplantation techniques have caused great demand for organs from beating heart donors. Consequently, it is necessary to have well defined and reliable criteria permitting the diagnosis of brain death with absolute certainty.

Although the concept of whole brain death had long been recognised and accepted by the medical community, clear diagnostic criteria were not developed until the late 1970s. In the United States of America, the President's Commission for the Study of Ethical Problems in Medicine and Biomedical and Behavioral Research proposed a model statute:[125] "Uniform determination of death act." In the statute, brain death is defined as the irreversible cessation of all functions of the entire brain, including the brain stem, determined in accordance with accepted medical standards. British criteria for brain stem death were established following a statement from the Conference of the Medical Royal Colleges and their Faculties.[126]

At present, many nations and institutions have adopted their own set of clinical criteria and technical investigations to determine irreversible loss of all brain functions (table 11.1).[127 128] As outcome from brain injury is less predictable in the very young, criteria for the diagnosis of brain death in adults are generally considered inadequate for infants and children.[125] Others, however, argue that standards used in adults apply also to children.[129] In any case, a diagnosis of brain death in infants and young children should be made by an experienced paediatrician.

Table 11.1 Diagnostic criteria for brain death

1 Establish aetiology of deep coma; exclude reversible causes of deep coma
2 Clinical neurological examination:
  Absence of cortical function:
    no spontaneous movement
    no response to external stimuli
  Absence of brain stem function:
    absent cephalic reflexes
    apnoea
3 Technical investigations:
  Electrical brain activity
  CBF: four vessel intracranial angiography is the most reliable test to demonstrate absence of
  intracerebral blood flow
4 Establish irreversibility

Clinical diagnosis of brain death

Brain death refers to the absence of neuronal function in the whole brain, including both cerebral hemispheres, the brain stem, and the cerebellum. In most countries, the diagnosis of brain death requires demonstration of loss of both cerebral cortical and brain stem function. In Britain, absence of brain stem function is considered to be indicative of absence of cortical function.[126]

A thorough neurological examination is the basis for a diagnosis of brain death, but a clinical diagnosis is valid only if reversible causes of deep coma can be excluded with absolute certainty. For example, hypothermia, endocrine and metabolic disorders, or residual effects of sedatives or neuromuscular blocking drugs make it impossible clinically to diagnose brain death from neurological examination alone. Hence, it is essential to establish the aetiology of the loss of consciousness. Analysis of blood and urine samples for drugs that depress brain function may be necessary.

Absence of cerebral cortical function
The following clinical criteria indicate loss of cerebral cortical function:

- Absence of spontaneous movement
- Absence of motor response to intensely painful external stimuli
- Movements resulting from spinal cord reflexes may persist after brain death and should not preclude the diagnosis of brain death[130]
- Decerebrate or decorticate posturing activity must be absent.[125]

Absence of brain stem function
Clinical criteria indicating brain stem death include failure to maintain respiration and absence of cephalic reflexes:

- Absence of spontaneous ventilation in the presence of a physiological stimulus for ventilation (apnoea) is a fundamental part of the diagnosis of brain stem death. Hypercapnia (documented $Pa_{CO_2} > 7 \cdot 32 – 7 \cdot 99$ kPa or $> 55 – 60$ mm Hg) is the stimulus most frequently used; passive oxygenation is usually provided by O_2 administration through a cannula placed in the endotracheal tube. In patients with a pre-existing reduced respiratory drive (for example, patients with severe chronic pulmonary disease), hypercapnia may not be a sufficient stimulus and some authors suggest use of hypoxaemia as a respiratory stimulus in those patients.[127]
- Absence of pupillary response to direct light stimulation (pupils are not necessarily dilated or equal). The pupillary light reflex may be absent for reasons unrelated to brain death (for example, dilating eye drops, atropine, hyoscine (scopolamine), glutethimide, opioids, neuromuscular blocking agents, eye disease, or eye trauma).
- Absence of blinking when lightly touching the cornea. The corneal reflex may be absent as a result of pre-existing facial weakness.

- Absence of oculocephalic reflex ("doll's eye phenomenon"): no eye movement when the head is turned from side to side.
- Absence of oculovestibular reflex (caloric test): no eye movement after irrigation of the external auditory canal with 30 ml of ice cold water (bilateral testing is necessary). The caloric test may be abolished by drugs (for example, sedatives, anticonvulsants, anticholinergics, tricyclic antidepressants, ototoxic antibiotics) or by disease of the labyrinth.
- No reaction to oropharyngeal or tracheal stimulation (for example, suctioning).
- Inactivity of the vagus nerve nuclei (atropine resistance): no increase of heart rate following the intravenous administration of atropine.

Vital organ function

Generally, vital organ functions are disturbed after brain death.[131] The following pathophysiological changes are frequently encountered, but have no diagnostic value:

- Haemodynamic instability (for example, dysrhythmias, ECG abnormalities, hypertension, hypotension)
- Hypothermia
- Diabetes insipidus
- Coagulopathy (disseminated intravascular coagulation).

In most institutions, a clinical diagnosis of brain death must be corroborated by a second physician. To establish irreversibility, many institutions request re-testing after a prescribed observation period, but there is no consensus about the optimal duration of the time interval. An interval of 24 hours is generally considered adequate,[125 127] but the increasing demand for transplant organs initiated a tendency towards accepting shorter intervals.[127 128] If the aetiology of the coma is known and irreversible, or if a four vessel angiography showed cessation of cerebral circulation, re-testing may not be necessary.

Technical investigations in the diagnosis of brain death

Several technical tests can be performed to support a clinical diagnosis of brain death and many institutions require or recommend such supplementary tests. Generally, these tests assess neuronal function or CBF.

Electroencephalogram

Although many countries recommend or require an isoelectric EEG trace to demonstrate absence of cortical function, EEG has some limitations as a diagnostic tool to confirm brain death.[127] Reversible causes of absence of EEG activity (for example, hypothermia or barbiturates) should be ruled out. Technical artefacts may complicate interpretation of the EEG trace and make it necessary to follow technical recommendations strictly for its recording in a potentially brain dead patient.[132 133] Analysis by an experienced observer is absolutely indicated to avoid errors of human interpretation. When these conditions are met, an isoelectric EEG trace indicates irreversible cessation of cortical function.[132 134]

Evoked potentials

Many consider brain stem death the critical criterion of brain death. In Britain, it is explicitly stated that loss of brain stem function implies loss of cortical function.[126] Most technical investigations, including EEG trace and CBF, do not examine brain stem function. Brain stem auditory evoked potentials and somatosensory evoked potentials respectively assess ascending auditory and sensory pathways of the brain stem and may be indicators of brain stem death.[135] The presence of brain stem auditory or somatosensory evoked potentials negates a diagnosis of brain death. The absence of auditory or somatosensory evoked responses may be caused by loss of brain stem function, but the possibility of false positive results reduces its reliability in the diagnosis of brain death. Damage to the peripheral auditory system or peripheral nerve damage, which cannot always be ruled out in comatose patients, may obliterate evoked responses. Therefore, when using evoked potentials to confirm brain death, sequential monitoring showing progressive disappearance of responses is more reliable than a single absent response.[136] As auditory evoked potentials test only part of the brain stem, their disappearance may occur before cessation of other brain stem functions.[136]

Cerebral blood flow measurement

Carotid and vertebral angiography showing cessation of blood flow to the brain is generally considered the ultimate criterion of brain death.[127] Although many nations and institutions consider clinical and EEG criteria sufficient for the diagnosis of brain death, angiographic demonstration of the cessation of intracerebral blood flow confirms the diagnosis with absolute certainty and is mandatory in a few countries. Four vessel angiography may be particularly indicated when the presence of drugs precludes a clinical diagnosis of brain death. It should be kept in mind, however, that cerebral angiography is invasive and potentially harmful to viable neurons. Intravenous or intra-arterial digital subtraction angiography has been shown to be as effective as conventional four vessel angiography to demonstrate cessation of intracerebral circulation, although it is easier and less time consuming to perform.[137]

Doppler ultrasonography of the extracranial arteries supplying blood to the brain displays a typical pattern in the case of intracranial circulatory arrest.[136] This method is reliable only when systolic blood pressure is normal and requires interpretation by an experienced investigator. Transcranial Doppler examination of blood flow in the middle cerebral artery also shows characteristic patterns after brain death.[138] An absent signal should not, however, be interpreted as a sign of brain death, because this may occur in the absence of cerebrovascular disturbances.[139] Extracranial or transcranial Doppler ultrasonography is useful for the early detection of disturbances or cessation of the intracranial circulation, and thus may be helpful in the determination of the right time for more invasive tests (angiography).[136] It cannot replace cerebral angiography as an unequivocal method for demonstrating cessation of brain circulation.

Other techniques for CBF measurement have been proposed as alternatives to conventional angiography in the diagnosis of brain death. Such tests include intravenous or intra-arterial radioisotope techniques,[140] and sequential computed cranial tomography.[141 142] These methods have gained popularity because they are less invasive or easier to perform than traditional four vessel angiography, but their reliability to demonstrate cessation of blood flow to the entire brain must be evaluated further.

Other tests

Several other technical investigations have been proposed in support of a clinical diagnosis of brain death.[143] Examples include: biochemical tests assaying enzymes and lactic acid in cerebrospinal fluid, determination of cerebral oxygen consumption, measurement of retinal blood flow, and electroretinography. These tests are not widely used and not sufficient to diagnose brain death.

In summary a clinical diagnosis of whole brain death is reliable if reversible causes of deep coma have been excluded, and if the cause of coma is known and explains the irreversible loss of all brain function sufficiently. Technical tests examining neuronal function and intracranial blood flow can confirm a clinical diagnosis of brain death, but only vertebral and carotid angiography is absolutely reliable as a diagnostic tool.

1 Wells B, Keats A, Cooley D. Increased tolerance to cerebral ischemia produced by general anesthesia during temporary carotid occlusion. *Surgery* 1963; **54**: 216–23.

2 Goldstein A, Wells B, Keats A. Increased tolerance to cerebral anoxia by pentobarbital. *Arch Int Pharmacodyn* 1966; **161**: 138–43.

3 Michenfelder J. The interdependency of cerebral function and metabolic effects following massive doses of thiopental in the dog. *Anesthesiology* 1974; **41**: 231–6.

4 Michenfelder JD, Theye R. Cerebral protection by thiopental during hypoxia. *Anesthesiology* 1973; **39**: 510–7.

5 Hoff J, Smith A, Hankinson H, Nielsen S. Barbiturate protection from cerebral infarction in primates. *Stroke* 1975; **6**: 28–33.

6 Michenfelder J, Milde J, Sundt T. Cerebral protection by barbiturate anesthesia: Use after middle cerebral artery occlusion in Java monkeys. *Arch Neurol* 1976; **33**: 345–50.

7 Nussmeier N, Arlund C, Slogoff S. Neuropsychiatric complications after cardiopulmonary bypass: Cerebral protection by a barbiturate. *Anesthesiology* 1986; **64**: 165–70.

8 Gisvold S, Safar P, Hendrickx H, Rao G, Moossy J, Alexander H. Thiopental treatment after global brain ischemia in pigtailed monkeys. *Anesthesiology* 1984; **60**: 88–96.

9 Brain Resuscitation Clinical I Study Group. Randomized clinical study of thiopental loading in comatose survivors of cardiac arrest. *N Engl J Med* 1986; **314**: 397–441.

10 Zaidan J, Klochany A, Martin W, Ziegler J, Harless D, Andrews R. Effect of thiopental on neurologic outcome following coronary bypass grafting. *Anesthesiology* 1991; **74**: 406–11.

11 Warner D, Deshpande J, Wieloch T. The effect of isoflurane on neuronal necrosis following near-complete forebrain ischemia in the rat. *Anesthesiology* 1986; **64**: 19–23.

12 Nehls D, Todd M, Spetzler R, Drummond J, Thompson R, Johnson P. A comparison of the cerebral protective effects of isoflurane and barbiturates during temporary focal ischemia in primates. *Anesthesiology* 1987; **66**: 453–64.

13 Gelb A, Boisvert D, Tang C, *et al*. Primate brain tolerance to temporary focal cerebral ischemia during isoflurane- or sodium nitroprusside-induced hypotension. *Anesthesiology* 1989; **70**: 678–83.

14 Warner D, Zhou J, Ramani R, Todd M. Reversible focal ischemia in the rat: Effects of halothane, isoflurane and methohexital anesthesia. *J Cereb Blood Flow Metab* 1991; **11**: 794–802.

15 Warner D, Hansen T, Vust L, Todd M. Distribution of cerebral blood flow during deep isoflurane vs. pentobarbital anesthesia in rats with middle cerebral artery occlusion. *J Neurosurg Anesth* 1989; **1**: 219–26.

16 Batjer H, Frankfurt A, Purdy P, Smith S, Samson D. Use of etomidate, temporary arterial occlusion, and intraoperative angiography in surgical treatment of large and giant cerebral aneurysms. *J Neurosurg* 1988; **68**: 234–40.

17 Warner D, McFarlane C, Todd M. Ludwig P, McAllister A. Sevoflurane and halothane reduce focal ischemic brain damage in the rat: Possible influence on thermoregulation. *Anesthesiology* 1993; **79**: 985–92.

18 Ridenour T, Warner D, Todd M, Gionet T. Comparative effects of propofol and halothane on outcome from temporary middle cerebral artery occlusion in the rat. *Anesthesiology* 1992; **76**: 807–12.

19 Verhaegen M, Todd M, Warner D. A comparison of cerebral ischemic flow thresholds during halothane/N_2O and isoflurane/N_2O anesthesia in rats. *Anesthesiology* 1992; **76**: 743–54.

20 Smith M-L, Auer R, Siesjö B. The density and distribution of ischemic brain injury in the rat following 2–10 min of forebrain ischemia. *Acta Neuropathol* 1984; **64**: 319–32.

21 Gionet T, Thomas J, Warner D, Goodlett C, Wasserman E, West J. Forebrain ischemia induces selective behavioral impairments associated with hippocampal injury in rats. *Stroke* 1991; **22**: 1040–7.

22 Sano T, Drummond J, Patel P, Grafe M, Watson J, Cole D. A comparison of the cerebral protective effects of isoflurane and mild hypothermia in a model of incomplete forebrain ischemia in the rat. *Anesthesiology* 1992; **76**: 221–8.

23 Smith A, Hoff J, Nielsen S, Larson C. Barbiturate protection in acute focal cerebral ischemia. *Stroke* 1974; **5**: 1–7.

24 Cole D, Shapiro H, Drummond J, Zivin J. Halothane, fentanyl/nitrous oxide, and spinal lidocaine protect against spinal cord injury in the rat. *Anesthesiology* 1989; **70**: 967–72.

25 Baughman V, Hoffman W, Thomas C, Miletich D, Albrecht R. Comparison of methohexital and isoflurane on neurologic outcome and histopathology following incomplete ischemia in rats. *Anesthesiology* 1990; **72**: 85–94.

26 Baughman V, Hoffman W. Neurologic outcome in rats following incomplete cerebral ischemia during halothane, isoflurane, or N_2O. *Anesthesiology* 1988; **69**: 192–8.

27 Hoffman W, Pelligrino D, Werner C, Kochs E, Albrecht R, Shulte am Esch J. Ketamine decreases plasma catecholamines and improves outcome from incomplete cerebral ischemia in rats. *Anesthesiology* 1992; **76**: 755–62.

28 Kochs E, Hoffman W, Werner C, Thomas C, Albrecht R, Schulte am Esch J. The effects of propofol on brain electrical activity, neurologic outcome, and neuronal damage following incomplete ischemia in rats. *Anesthesiology* 1992; **76**: 245–52.

29 Werner C, Hoffman W, Thomas C, Miletich D, Albrecht R. Ganglionic blockade improves neurologic outcome from incomplete ischemia in rats – partial reversal by exogenous catecholamines. *Anesthesiology* 1990; **73**: 923–9.

30 Warner D, Ludwig P, Pearlstein R, Brinkhous A. Halothane reduces focal ischemic injury in the rat when brain temperature is controlled. *Anesthesiology* 1995; **82**: 1237–45.

31 Rosomoff H. Hypothermia and cerebral vascular lesions. *Arch Neurol Psychol* 1957; **78**: 454–64.

32 Michenfelder J, Milde J. The effect of profound levels of hypothermia (below 14°C) on canine cerebral metabolism. *J Cereb Blood Flow Metab* 1992; **12**: 877–80.

33 Michenfelder J, Theye R. Hypothermia: Effect on canine brain and whole-body metabolism. *Anesthesiology* 1968; **29**: 1107–12.

34 Silverberg G, Reitz B, Ream A. Hypothermia and cardiac arrest in the treatment of giant aneurysms of the cerebral circulation and hemangioblastoma of the medulla. *J Neurosurg* 1981; **55**: 337–46.

35 Michenfelder J, Milde J. Failure of prolonged hypocapnia, hypothermia, or hypertension to favorably alter acute stroke in primates. *Stroke* 1977; **8**: 87–91.

36 Steen P, Milde J, Michenfelder J. The detrimental effects of prolonged hypothermia and rewarming in the dog. *Anesthesiology* 1980; **52**: 224–30.

37 Illievich U, Spiss C. Hypothermia therapy for the injured brain. *Curr Opin Anaesth* 1994; **7**: 394–400.

38 Busto R, Dietrich W, Globus M, Valdés I, Scheinberg P, Ginsberg M. Small differences in intraischemic brain temperature critically determine the extent of neuronal injury. *J Cereb Blood Flow Metab* 1987; **7**: 729–38.

39 Busto R, Dietrich W, Globus M, Ginsberg M. Postischemic moderate hypothermia inhibits CA1 hippocampal ischemic neuronal injury. *Neurosci Lett* 1989; **101**: 299–304.

40 Coimbra C, Wieloch T. Moderate hypothermia mitigates neuronal damage in the rat brain when initiated several hours following transient cerebral ischemia. *Acta Neuropathol* 1994; **87**: 325–31.

41 Dietrich W, Alonso O, Busto R, Globus M, Ginsberg M. Post-traumatic brain hypothermia reduces histopathological damage following concussive brain injury in the rat. *Acta Neuropathol* 1994; **87**: 250–8.

42 Clifton G, Allen S, Barrodale P, *et al.* A phase II study of moderate hypothermia in severe brain injury. *J Neurotrauma* 1993; **10**: 263–73.

43 Shiozaki T, Sugimoto H, Taneda M, *et al.* Effect of mild hypothermia on uncontrollable intracranial hypertension after severe head injury. *J Neurosurg* 1993; **79**: 363–8.

44 Marion D, Obrist W, Carlier P, Penrod L, Darby J. The use of moderate therapeutic hypothermia for patients with severe head injuries: a preliminary report. *J Neurosurg* 1993; **79**: 354–62.

45 Katsura K, Minamisawa H, Ekholm A, Folbergrova J, Siesjö B. Changes of labile metabolites during anoxia in moderately hypo- and hyperthermic rats: correlation to membrane fluxes of K^+. *Brain Res* 1992; **590**: 6–12.

46 Widmann R, Miyazawa T, Hoffmann K. Protective effect of hypothermia on hippocampal injury after 30 minutes of forebrain ischemia in rats is mediated by postischemic recovery of protein synthesis. *J Neurochem* 1993; **61**: 200–9.

47 Lei B, Tan X, Cai H, Xu Q, Guo Q. Effect of moderate hypothermia on lipid peroxidation in canine brain tissue after cardiac arrest and resuscitation. *Stroke* 1994; **25**: 147–50.

48 Jiang J, Lyeth B, Kapasi M, Jenkins L, Povlishock J. Moderate hypothermia reduces blood–brain barrier disruption following traumatic brain injury in the rat. *Acta Neuropathol* 1992; **84**: 495–500.

49 Cardell M, Boris-Moller F, Wieloch T. Hypothermia prevents the ischemia-induced translocation and inhibition of protein kinase-c in the rat striatum. *J Neurochem* 1991; **57**: 1814–18.

50 Chen Q, Chopp M, Bodzin G, Chen H. Temperature modulation of cerebral depolarization during focal cerebral ischemia in rats: correlation with ischemic injury. *J Cereb Blood Flow Metab* 1993; **13**: 389–94.

51 Baker K, Young W, Stone J, Kader A, Baker C, Solomon R. Deliberate mild intraoperative hypothermia for craniotomy. *Anesthesiology* 1994; **81**: 361–7.

52 Mellergård P, Nordström C. Intracerebral temperature in neurosurgical patients. *Neurosurgery* 1991; **28**: 709–13.

53 Frank S, Beattie C, Christopherson R, *et al.* Unintentional hypothermia is associated with postoperative myocardial ischemia. *Anesthesiology* 1993; **78**: 468–76.

54 Cheney F, Posner K, Caplan R, Gild W. Burns from warming devices in anesthesia: A closed claims analysis. *Anesthesiology* 1994; **80**: 806–10.

289

55 Myers R, Yamaguchi S. Nervous system effects of cardiac arrest in monkeys. Preservation of vision. *Arch Neurol* 1977; **34**: 65–74.
56 Ginsberg M, Welsh F, Budd W. Deleterious effect of glucose pretreatment on recovery from diffuse cerebral ischemia in the cat: I. Local cerebral blood flow and glucose utilization. *Stroke* 1980; **11**: 347–54.
57 Siemkowicz E, Gjedde A. Post-ischemic coma in rat: Effect of different pre-ischemic blood glucose levels on cerebral metabolic recovery after ischemia. *Acta Physiol Scand* 1980; **110**: 225–32.
58 Warner D, Smith M, Siesjö B. Ischemia in normo- and hyperglycemic rats: Effects on brain water and electrolytes. *Stroke* 1987; **18**: 464–71.
59 Lanier W, Stangland K, Scheithauer B, Milde J, Michenfelder J. The effects of dextrose infusion and head position on neurologic outcome after complete cerebral ischemia in primates: Examination of a model. *Anesthesiology* 1987; **66**: 39–48.
60 Pulsinelli W, Waldman S, Rawlinson D, Plum F. Moderate hyperglycemia augments ischemic brain damage: A neuropathologic study in the rat. *Neurology* 1982; **32**: 1239–46.
61 Swanson P. Acidosis and some metabolic properties of isolated cerebral tissues. *Arch Neurol* 1969; **20**: 653–63.
62 Rehncrona S, Rosen I, Siesjö B. Excessive cellular acidosis: an important mechanism of neuronal damage in the brain? *Acta Physiol Scand* 1980; **110**: 435–7.
63 Siesjö B, Smith M, Warner D. Acidosis and ischemic brain damage. In: Raichle E, Powers WJ (Eds), *Cerebrovascular diseases*. New York: Raven, 1987: 83–95.
64 Zasslow M, Pearl R, Shuer L, Leiberson R, Steinberg G, Larson JC. Hyperglycemia decreases neuronal ischemic changes after middle cerebral artery occlusion in the cat. *Anesthesia* 1987; **67**: A581.
65 Nedergaard M, Diemer N. Influence of hyperglycemia on ischemic brain damage after middle cerebral artery (MCA) occlusion in the rat. *J Cereb Blood Flow Metab* 1985; **5**: S231–2.
66 de Courten-Myers G, Kleinholz M, Wagner K, Myers R. Fatal strokes in hyperglycemic cats. *Stroke* 1989; **20**: 1707–15.
67 de Courten-Myers G, Myers R, Wagner K. Effect of hyperglycemia on infarct size after cerebrovascular occlusion in cats. *Stroke* 1990; **21**: 357.
68 Prado R, Ginsberg M, Dietrich W, Watson B, Busto B. Hyperglycemia increases infarct size in collaterally perfused but not end-arterial vascular territories. *J Cereb Blood Flow Metab* 1988; **8**: 186–92.
69 Ginsberg M. Glycolytic metabolism in brain ischemia. In: Weinstein PR, Faden AI (Eds), *Protection of the brain from ischemia*. Baltimore: Williams & Wilkins, 1990: 37–48.
70 Adams H, Olinger C, Biller J, *et al.* Usefulness of admission blood glucose in predicting outcome after severe cerebral infarction. *Stroke* 1987; **18**: 297.
71 Berger L, Hakim A. The association of hyperglycemia with cerebral edema in stroke. *Stroke* 1986; **17**: 865–71.
72 Candelise L, Landi G, Orazio E, Boccardi E. Prognostic significance of hyperglycemia in acute stroke. *Arch Neurol* 1985; **42**: 661–3.
73 Pulsinelli W, Levy D, Sigsbee B, Scherer P, Plum F. Increased damage after ischemic stroke in patients with hyperglycemia with or without established diabetes mellitus. *Am J Med* 1983; **74**: 540–4.
74 Lam A, Winn H, Cullen B, Sundling N. Hyperglycemia and neurological outcome in patients with head injury. *J Neurosurg* 1991; **75**: 545–51.
75 Woo J, Lam C, Kay R, Wong A, Teoh R, Nicholls M. The influence of hyperglycemia and diabetes mellitus on immediate and 3-month morbidity and mortality after acute stroke. *Arch Neurol* 1990; **47**: 1174–7.
76 van Kooten F, Hoogerbrugge N, Naarding P, Koudstaal P. Hyperglycemia in the acute phase of stroke is not caused by stress. *Stroke* 1993; **24**: 1129–32.
77 Lundy E, Ball T, Mandell M, Zelenock G. Dextrose administration increases sensory/motor impairment and paraplegia after infrarenal aortic occlusion in the rabbit. *Surgery* 1987; **102**: 737–42.
78 LeMay D, Zelenock G, D'Alecy L. The role of glucose uptake and metabolism in hyperglycemic exacerbation of neurological deficit in the paraplegic rat. *J Neurosurg* 1989; **71**: 594–600.

79 Drummond J, Moore S. The influence of dextrose administration on neurologic outcome after temporary spinal cord ischemia in the rabbit. *Anesthesiology* 1989; **70**: 64–70.

80 Sieber F, Smith D, Kupferberg J, *et al*. Effects of intraoperative glucose on protein catabolism and plasma glucose levels in patients with supratentorial tumors. *Anesthesiology* 1986; **64**: 453–9.

81 Fukuoka S, Yeh H, Mandybur T, Tew J. Effect of insulin on acute experimental cerebral ischemia in gerbils. *Stroke* 1989; **20**: 396–9.

82 Robertson C, Grossman R. Protection against spinal cord ischemia with insulin-induced hypoglycemia. *J Neurosurg* 1987; **67**: 739–44.

83 Strong A, Fairfield J, Monteiro E, *et al*. Insulin protects cognitive function in experimental stroke. *J Neurol Neurosurg Psychiatry* 1990; **53**: 847–53.

84 Warner D, Gionet T, Todd M, McAllister A. Insulin-induced normoglycemia improves ischemic outcome in hyperglycemic rats. *Stroke* 1992; **23**: 1775–81.

85 de Courten-Myers G, Kleinholz M, Wagner K, Myers R. Normoglycemia (not hypoglycemia) optimizes outcome from middle cerebral artery occlusion. *J Cereb Blood Flow Metabol* 1994; **14**: 227–36.

86 Longstreth W, Copass M, Dennis L, Rauch-Matthews M, Stark M, Cobb L. Intravenous glucose after out-of-hospital cardiopulmonary arrest: A community-based randomized trial. *Neurology* 1993; **43**: 2534–41.

87 Barsan W, Brott T, Broderick J, Haley E, Levy D, Marler J. Urgent therapy for stroke: Effects of a stroke trial on untreated patients. *Stroke* 1994; **25**: 2132–7.

88 Kirino T, Sano K. Selective vulnerability in the gerbil hippocampus following transient ischemia. *Acta Neuropathol* 1984; **62**: 201–8.

88a Smith M, Kalimo H, Warner D, Siesjö B. Morphologic lesions in the brain preceding the development of post-ischemic seizures. *Acta Neuropathol* 1988; **76**: 253–64.

89 Petito C, Feldman E, Pulsinelli W, Plum F. Delayed hippocampal damage in humans following cardiorespiratory arrest. *Neurology* 1987; **37**: 1281–6.

90 Kirino T, Tamura A, Sano K. Delayed neuronal death in the rat hippocampus following transient forebrain ischemia. *Acta Neuropathol* 1984; **64**: 139–47.

91 Pulsinelli W, Brierley J, Plum F. Temporal profile of neuronal damage in model of transient forebrain ischemia. *Ann Neurol* 1982; **11**: 491–8.

92 Smith M, Bendek G, Dahlgren N, Rosen I, Wieloch T, Siesjö B. Models for studying long-term recovery following forebrain ischemia in the rat. 2: A 2-vessel occlusion model. *Acta Neurol Scand* 1984; **69**: 385–401.

93 Benveniste H, Drejer J, Schousboe A, Diemer N. Elevation of the extracellular concentrations of glutamate and aspartate in rat hippocampus during transient cerebral ischemia monitored by intracerebral microdialysis. *J Neurochem* 1984; **43**: 1369–74.

94 Benveniste H, Jorgensen M, Sandberg M, Christensen T, Hagberg H, Diemer N. Ischemic damage in hippocampal CA1 is dependent on glutamate release and intact innervation from CA3. *J Cereb Blood Flow Metab* 1989; **9**: 629–39.

95 Suzuki R, Yamaguchi T, Li C, Klatzo I. The effects of 5-minute ischemia in Mongolian gerbils: II. Changes of spontaneous neuronal activity in cerebral cortex and CA1 sector of hippocampus. *Acta Neuropathol* 1983; **60**: 217–22.

96 Choi D, Maulucci-Gedde M, Kriegstein A. Glutamate neurotoxicity in cortical cell culture. *J Neurosci* 1987; **7**: 357–68.

97 Choi D. Ionic dependence of glutamate neurotoxicity in cortical cell culture. *J Neurosci* 1987; **7**: 369–79.

98 Siesjö B. Cell damage in the brain: A speculative synthesis. *J Cereb Blood Flow Metab* 1981; **1**: 155–85.

99 Siesjö B. Pathophysiology and treatment of focal cerebral ischemia. *J Neurosurg* 1992; **77**: 169–84.

100 Haley E, Kassell N, Torner J. A randomized trial of nicardipine in subarachnoid hemorrhage: angiographic and transcranial Doppler ultrasound results. *J Neurosurg* 1993; **78**: 548–53.

101 Haley E, Kassell N, Torner J. A randomized controlled trial of high-dose intravenous nicardipine in aneurysmal subarachnoid hemorrhage. *J Neurosurg* 1993; **78**: 537–47.

102 Haley EC, Truskowski L, Germanson T. A randomized trial of two doses of nicardipine in aneurysmal subarachnoid hemorrhage. *J Neurosurg* 1994; **80**: 788–96.

15>r>

103 Mohr J, Orgogozo J, Harrison M, et al. Meta-analysis of oral nimodipine trials in acute ischemic stroke. Cerebrovasc Dis 1994; 4: 197–203.

104 Forsman M, Aarseth H, Nordby H, Skulberg A, Steen P. Effects of nimodipine on cerebral blood flow and cerebrospinal fluid pressure after cardiac arrest: correlation with neurologic outcome. Anesth Analg 1989; 68: 436–43.

105 Mayer M, Westbrook G, Guthrie P. Voltage-dependent block by Mg^{2+} of NMDA responses in spinal cord neurons. Nature 1984; 309: 261–3.

106 Nowak L, Bregestovski P, Ascher P, Herbert A, Prochiantz A. Magnesium gates glutamate-activated channels in mouse central neurons. Nature 1984; 307: 462–5.

107 Baskys A. Metabotropic receptors and 'slow' excitatory actions of glutamate agonists in the hippocampus. Trends Neurol Sci 1992; 15: 92–6.

108 Oyzuart E, Graham D, Woodruff G, McCulloch J. Protective effect of the glutamate antagonist, MK-801 in focal cerebral ischemia in the cat. J Cereb Blood Flow Metab 1988; 8: 138–43.

109 Lanier W, Perkins W, Karlsson B, et al. The effects of dizocilpine maleate [MK-801], an antagonist of the N-methyl-D-aspartate receptor, on neurologic recovery and histopathology following complete cerebral ischemia in primates. J Cereb Blood Flow Metab 1990; 10: 252–61.

110 Nellgård B, Wieloch T. Postischemic blockade of AMPA but not NMDA receptors mitigates neuronal damage in the rat brain following transient severe cerebral ischemia. J Cereb Blood Flow Metab 1992; 12: 2–11.

111 Nedergaard M, Hansen A. Characterization of cortical depolarizations evoked in focal cerebral ischemia. J Cereb Blood Flow Metab 1993; 13: 568–74.

112 Back T, Kohno K, Hossman K-A. Cortical negative DC deflections following middle cerebral artery occlusion and KCl-induced spreading depression: Effect on blood flow, tissue oxygenation, and electroencephalogram. J Cereb Blood Flow Metab 1994; 14: 12–19.

113 Iijima T, Mies G, Hossman K. Repeated negative DC deflections in rat cortex following middle cerebral artery occlusion are abolished by MK-801 – effect on volume of ischemic injury. J Cereb Blood Flow Metab 1992; 12: 727–33.

114 Mies G, Kohno K, Hossmann K. Prevention of perinfarct direct current shifts with glutamate antagonist NBQX following occlusion of the middle cerebral artery in the rat. J Cereb Blood Flow Metab 1994; 14: 802–7.

115 Buchan A, Xue D, Huang Z, Smith K, Lesiuk H. Delayed AMPA receptor blockade reduces cerebral infarction induced by focal ischemia. Neurol Report 1991; 2: 473–6.

116 Buchan A, Li H, Pulsinelli W. The N-methyl-D-aspartate antagonist, MK-801, fails to protect against neuronal damage caused by transient, severe forebrain ischemia in adult rats. J Neurosci 1991; 11: 1049–56.

117 Le Peille TE, Arvin B, Moncada C, Meldrum B. The non-NMDA antagonists, NBQX and GYKI 52466, protect against cortical and striatal cell loss following transient global ischaemia in the rat. Brain Res 1992; 571: 115–20.

118 Gill R, Nordholm L, Lodge D. The neuroprotective actions of 2,3-dihydroxy-6-nitro-7-sulfamoyl-benzo(F)quinoxaline (NBQX) in a rat focal ischaemia model. Brain Res 1992; 580: 35–43.

119 Willetts J, Balster R, Leander J. The behavioral pharmacology of NMDA receptor antagonists. Trends in Pharmacological Sciences 1990; 11: 423–8.

120 Sheardown M, Nielsen E, Hansen A, Jacobsen P, Honore T. 2,3-Dihydroxy-6-nitro-7-sulfamoyl-benzo(F)quinoxaline: A neuroprotectant for cerebral ischemia. Science 1990; 247: 571–4.

121 Diemer N, Jorgensen M, Johansen F, Sheardown M, Honoré T. Protection against ischemic hippocampal CA1 damage in the rat with a new non-NMDA antagonist, NBQX. Acta Neurol Scand 1992; 86: 45–9.

122 Scheller M, Zornow M, Fleischer J, Shearman G, Greber T. The noncompetitive N-methyl-D-aspartate receptor antagonist, MK-801 profoundly reduces volatile anesthetic requirements in rabbits. Neuropharmacology 1989; 28: 677–81.

123 McFarlane C, Warner D, Todd M, Nordholm L. AMPA receptor competitive antagonism reduces halothane MAC in rats. Anesthesiology 1992; 77: 1165–70.

124 McFarlane C, Warner D, Dexter F, Nader A, Todd M. Glycine receptor antagonism: anesthetic effects in the rat. Anesthesiology 1995; 82: 963–8.

125 Brain Death. Guidelines for the determination of death. Report of the medical consultants on the diagnosis of death to the president's commission for the study of ethical problems in medicine and biomedical and behavioral research. *JAMA* 1981; **246**: 2184–6.

126 Brain Death. Conference of Medical Royal Colleges and their Faculties in the United Kingdom: Diagnosis of brain death. *BMJ* 1976; **2**: 1187–8.

127 Powner D. The diagnosis of brain death in the adult patient. *J Intensive Care Med* 1987; **2**: 181–9.

128 Mori K, Nakao S-i. Brain death. *Anaesthesia* 1994: 2565–76.

129 Black P. Brain death in the intensive care unit. *J Intensive Care Med* 1987; **2**: 177–8.

130 Ivan L. Spinal reflexes in cerebral death. *Neurology* 1973; **23**: 650–2.

131 Bodenham A, Park G. Care of the multiple organ donor. *Intensive Care Med* 1989; **15**: 1–9.

132 Black P. Brain death. *N Engl J Med* 1978; **299**: 338–44.

133 Brain Death. A definition of irreversible coma. Report of the ad hoc committee of the Harvard Medical School to examine the definition of brain death. *JAMA* 1968; **205**: 337–40.

134 Buchner H, Schuchardt V. Reliability of electroencephalogram in the diagnosis of brain death. *Eur Neurol* 1990; **30**: 138–41.

135 Facco E, Casartelli Liviero M, Munari M, Toffoletto F, Baratto F, Giron G. Short latency evoked potentials: New criteria for brain death? *J Neurol Neurosurg Psychiatry* 1990; **53**: 351–3.

136 Nau R, Prange H, Klingelöfer J, Kukowski B, Sander D, Tchorsch Rea. Results of four technical investigations in fifty brain dead patients. *Intensive Care Med* 1992; **18**: 82–8.

137 Vatne K, Nakstad P, Lundar T. Digital subtraction angiography (DSA) in the evaluation of brain death. A comparison of conventional cerebral angiography with intravenous and intra-arterial DSA. *Neuroradiology* 1985; **27**: 155–7.

138 Hassler W, Steinmetz H, Pirschel J. Transcranial Doppler study of intracranial circulatory arrest. *J Neurosurg* 1989; **71**: 195–201.

139 Ropper A, Kehne S, Wechsler L. Transcranial Doppler in brain death. *Neurology* 1987; **37**: 1733–5.

140 Korein J, Braunstein P, Kricheff I, Lieberman A, Chase N. Radioisotope bolus technique as a test to detect circulatory deficit associated with cerebral death. *Circulation* 1975; **51**: 924–39.

141 Arnold H, Kuhne D, Rohr W, Heller M. Contrast bolus technique with rapid CT-scanning – a reliable diagnostic tool for determination of brain death. *Neuroradiology* 1981; **22**: 129–32.

142 Rappaport Z, Brinker R, Rovit R. Evaluation of brain death by contrast-enhanced computerized cranial tomography. *Neurosurgery* 1978; **2**: 230–2.

143 Powner D, Pinkus R, Grenvik A. Decision-making in brain death and vegetable states – multiple considerations. In: Grenvik A, Safar P (Eds), *Brain failure and resuscitation*. New York: Churchill Livingstone, 1981: 239–59.

Index

Other titles in the series

CARDIOVASCULAR PHYSIOLOGY

Edited by H-J Priebe and K Skarvan

The first volume in this series for the newly qualified anaesthetist and intensive care specialist, this comprehensive yet concise text is a thoroughly up to date review of cardiovascular physiology written by an international group of renowned authors.

Readership: anaesthetists and trainees, intensive care doctors, trainees and nurses

ISBN 0 7279 0781 6   200 pages   September 1995   UK £29.95

Forthcoming titles for 1996
NEUROMUSCULAR TRANSMISSION
PAEDIATRIC INTENSIVE CARE

For further details contact your local bookseller, or in case of difficulty, contact the Books Division, BMJ Publishing Group, BMA House, Tavistock Square, London WC1H 9JR, UK (Tel +44 (0) 171-6245; Fax +44 (0) 171-383 6662)